Bladder Cancer

THIS VOLUME
IS ONE OF A SERIES

International Perspectives In Urology
EDITED BY
John A. Libertino, M.D.

CURRENT AND FORTHCOMING TITLES

McDougal and Persky
TRAUMATIC INJURIES OF THE GENITOURINARY SYSTEM

Javadpour
RECENT ADVANCES IN UROLOGIC CANCER

Jacobi and Hohenfellner
PROSTATE CANCER

deVere White
ASPECTS OF MALE INFERTILITY

Bennett
MANAGEMENT OF MALE IMPOTENCE

Roth and Finlayson
STONES: CLINICAL MANAGEMENT OF UROLITHIASIS

Donohue
TESTIS TUMORS

Marberger and Dreikorn
RENAL PRESERVATION

Lang
CURRENT CONCEPTS OF URORADIOLOGY

Johnston
MANAGEMENT OF VESICOURETERIC REFLUX

McGuire
CLINICAL EVALUATION AND TREATMENT OF
NEUROGENIC VESICAL DYSFUNCTION

International Perspectives In Urology

Volume 12

John A. Libertino, M.D.
series editor

Bladder Cancer

Edited by

Nasser Javadpour, M.D., F.A.C.S.

Professor and Director of Urologic Oncology
University of Maryland School of Medicine
Baltimore, Maryland
Consultant, National Naval Hospital
Bethesda, Maryland

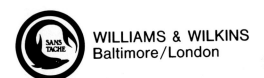

WILLIAMS & WILKINS
Baltimore/London

Editor: James L. Sangston
Associate Editor: Jonathan W. Pine, Jr.
Copy Editor: Caral Shields Nolley
Design: Bert Smith
Production: Anne G. Seitz

Accurate indications, adverse reactions, and dosage schedules for drugs are provided in this book, but it is possible that they may change. The reader is urged to review the package information data of the manufacturers of the medications mentioned.

Made in the United States of America

Library of Congress Cataloging in Publication Data

Main entry under title:

Bladder cancer.

   (International perspectives in urology ; v. 12)
   Includes index.
   1. Bladder—Cancer. I. Javadpour, N. 1937–
II. Series. [DNLM: 1. Bladder neoplasms.
W1 IN827K v. 12 /WJ 504 B6311]
RC280.B5B63 1984   616.99′462   84-2223
ISBN 0-683-04356-0

Composed and printed at the
Waverly Press, Inc.

Series Editor's Foreword

Cancer of the urinary bladder represents a formidable cause of cancer-related deaths annually. Although 75% of the 35,000 new tumors diagnosed annually in the United States are localized to the bladder, 10,000 people will succumb to this disease on an annual basis. Even though the majority of patients present with localized disease, the age-adjusted death rate has remained virtually the same since 1930. Clearly, advances have been made in the management of bladder cancer, it is reasonable for us from time to time to look at where we are and where we need to go with the management of any disease process.

With this in mind, Dr. Javadpour, Professor and Director of Urologic Oncology at the University of Maryland School of Medicine and consultant at the National Naval Hospital, has brought together the world's most outstanding international authorities on bladder cancer. Together they have provided us with a contemporary overview of bladder cancer, the epidemiologic considerations, pathology, natural history, and the clinical management of superficial and invasive bladder cancer.

This book represents the state of the art in terms of the diagnosis and treatment of bladder cancer. It is a reflection of Dr. Javadpour's commitment to uro-oncology and his dedication to the academic pursuit of our specialty. This textbook on bladder cancer represents the culmination of a great deal of effort on the part of Dr. Javadpour and the contributors, and we hope that it will stimulate others in our field to improve the longevity and quality of life of patients suffering from bladder cancer.

JOHN LIBERTINO

Preface

Cancer of the urinary bladder is a heterogenous disease involving several environmental factors and multistage processes. This disease has contributed to the understanding of carcinogenesis in human and laboratory animals. The first observation in gene-transferring technique was demonstrated in a line of bladder cancer. Also, the advent of cell surface isoantigens, T antigen, chromosomal banding, flow cytometry and utilization of cytology have improved the diagnosis and management of this cancer. In spite of some progress, a number of problems, including role of cystectomy, radiotherapy and finding effective chemotherapeutic regimen, remain unsolved. This book consists of two sections. The first section will review the progress in epidemiology, carcinogenesis, histopathology, cell markers, immunobiology, cytology, diagnosis and staging of bladder cancer. The second section will discuss surgery, radiotherapy, chemotherapy, combination therapy, management of superficial tumors, and clinical and experimental investigations in bladder cancer. A brief synopsis of an overview discusses the progress, problems and state of the art of the disease. This monograph is a part of a series, *International Perspective in Urology.* Its publication would have not been possible without the advice of John Libertino, M.D. of the Lahey Clinic and James Sangston, Senior Editor of Williams & Wilkins.

NASSER JAVADPOUR, M.D.

Contributors

Fernando Algaba, M.D.
Assistant Professor of Pathology
Autonomous University of
  Barcelona
Barcelona, Spain

Anwer Halim, Ph.D., F.R.C.S.
Senior Urologist
Tawam Hospital
Whittaker Corporation
Al Ain
United Arab Emirates

**R. Marian Hicks, Ph.D., D.S.c.,
  F.R.C.Path.**
School of Pathology
Middlesex Hospital Medical
  School
London, England

**Gerry B. Hill, M.B., Ch.B.,
  F.R.C.P.(C)**
Director, Department of
  Epidemiology
Alberta Cancer Board
Edmonton, Alberta, Canada

I. Hussain, M.B., F.R.C.S.
Senior Consultant and Head
Department of Urology
Central Hospital
Abu Dahbi
United Arab Emirates

Giovan Battista Ingargiola, M.D.
Institute of Urology
University of Palermo
Polyclinic Hospital
Palermo, Italy

**Nasser Javadpour, M.D.,
  F.A.C.S.**
Professor and Director of
  Urologic Oncology
University of Maryland School
  of Medicine
Baltimore, Maryland
Consultant, National Naval
  Hospital
Bethesda, Maryland

Alexander W. Miller, M.D.
Associate Director of Laboratory
  Services
Rush Presbyterian-St. Luke's
  Hospital
Chicago, Illinois

**Alvaro Morales, M.D.,
  F.R.C.S.(C), F.A.C.S.**
Professor and Chairman
Department of Urology
Queens University
Kingston, Ontario, Canada

William M. Murphy, M.D.
Pathologist, Baptist Memorial
  Hospital
Professor of Pathology and
  Urology
University of Tennessee
Center for the Health Sciences
Memphis, Tennessee

Kevin J. O'Connell, M.D.
Chairman, Department of
  Urology
National Naval Medical Center
Associate Professor of Surgery,
  Urology
Uniformed Services University
  of the Health Sciences
Bethesda, Maryland

Carlo Pavone, M.D.
Institute of Urology
University of Palermo
Polyclinic Hospital
Palermo, Italy

Michele Pavone-Macaluso, M.D.
Institute of Urology
University of Palermo
Polyclinic Hospital
Palermo, Italy

Howard M. Radwin, M.D.
Professor and Chairman
  Division of Urology
The University of Texas Health
  Science Center
San Antonio, Texas

Sameer Rafla, M.D., Ph.D.
Director and Chief of Radiation
  Therapy
The Methodist Hospital of
  Brooklyn
Lutheran Medical Center
Maimonides Medical Center
Clinical Professor of Radiation
  Oncology
State University of New York
College of Medicine
New York, New York

Jerome P. Richie, M.D.
Chief of Urologic Oncology
Departments of Surgery/Urology
  and Radiation Therapy
Brigham and Women's Hospital
  and Joint Center for Radiation
  Therapy
Harvard Medical School
Boston, Massachusetts

Francisco Solé-Balcells, M.D.
Associate Professor of Urology
Autonomous University of
  Barcelona
Barcelona, Spain

**Myron Tannenbaum, M.D.,
  Ph.D.**
Chief of Surgical Pathology and
  Cytopathology
Bronx Veterans Administration
  Medical Center
Bronx, New York
Professor of Pathology
Mt. Sinai School of Medicine
New York, New York

Maria Tripi, M.D.
Institute of Urology
University of Palermo
Polyclinic Hospital
Palermo, Italy

José Vicente, M.D.
Institute of Urology, Nephrology
  and Andrology
Fundacion Puigvert
Barcelona, Spain

Ralph R. Weichselbaum, M.D.
Departments of Surgery/Urology
  and Radiation Therapy
Brigham and Women's Hospital
  and Joint Center for Radiation
  Therapy
Harvard Medical School
Boston, Massachusetts

Ezzat Youssef, M.D.
Attending Radiotherapist
The Methodist Hospital of
  Brooklyn
Lutheran Medical Center
Maimonides Medical Center
Instructor, Downstate Medical
  Center
New York, New York

Eduardo Zungri, M.D.
Institute of Urology, Nephrology
  and Andrology
Fundacion Puigvert
Barcelona, Spain

Contents

1

Overview of Bladder Cancer

Nasser Javadpour, M.D., F.A.C.S.

Cancer of the bladder is a heterogeneous disease with a strong environmental and geographic propensity. The epidemiologic studies have pointed to several environmental factors including occupation, diet, coffee drinking, cigarette smoking, certain medications and chronic bladder infections (Table 1.1). Bladder cancer is considered as an environmental model of carcinogenesis with multistage processes including initiating and promoting factors. A number of carcinogens have been shown to possess synergism in induction of bladder cancer such as saccharin and nitrosamines in rats. The most remarkable progress in the understanding of bladder cancer has been in the recognition of the role of carcinogens, initiators, and promoters in a complex setting producing a hetergenous cancer, causing 3000–7000 deaths/year in the United States (Fig. 1.1). The potentiality of the urothelium is shown in Figure 1.2.

Recent investigations utilizing gene transfer technique and hybridizations with normal cell DNA has demonstrated the capability of oncogenes causing uncontrolled cell divisions when transferred to normal cell DNA (Fig. 1.3). As a matter of fact, the initial attempts to demonstrate transforming activity in human tumor DNA resulted in the recognition of an activated cellular oncogene from a cell line of bladder cancer. This development has opened a new avenue for possible detection, diagnosis, and preparation of therapeutic strategies against these targets.[1,2]

PREDICTORS OF RISK

Over the past several years, the advent of cell surface isoantigens, T-antigen, chromosomal analysis, flow cytometry and cytology have improved the detection of high risk and low risk bladder cancer (Table 1.2). Utilizing these markers, we have recognized a high risk, superficial low grade bladder cancer with loss of cell surface isoantigens, chromosomal abnormalities, abnormal cytology and flow cytometry that invariably invade and metastasize, and the patient succumbs. Recognition of this group that does not lend itself to identification by the conventional histopathologic examination allows appropriate initial therapy.

Table 1.1.
Environmental and Occupational Hazards in Bladder Cancer

Carcinogens	Exposure
Nicotine and caffeine	Smoking and ? coffee drinking
Nitrosamines, bracken ferm	Diets
Sweetner, tryptophane	Foods
Phenacetin, chlornaphazine	Medications
Bilharzial cystitis	Egypt and certain other countries
Chronic bladder irritation	Bladder exstrophy, chronic infection
Benzidine, β-naphthylamine	Aniline dye workers
Aromatic residues	Petroleum workers
Benzidine	Laboratory workers
Dye	Leather, textile workers, hairdressers, and spray painters.

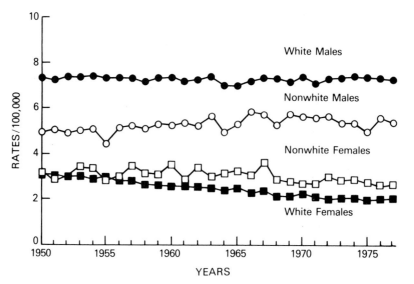

Figure 1.1. Age-adjusted mortality rates of bladder cancer.

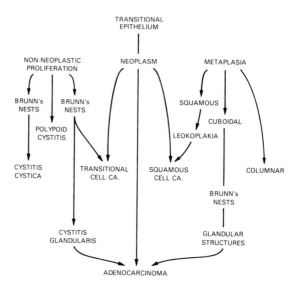

Figure 1.2. Potentialities of bladder epithelium. (From N. Javadpour, *Obstetrics and Gynecology* 35:600, 1970.)

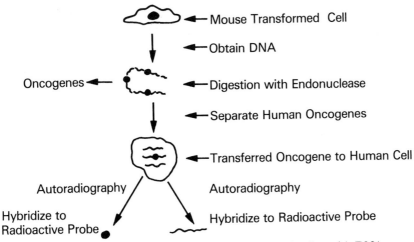

Figure 1.3. Transfer of oncogene and hybridization with DNA.

Table 1.2.
Factors Separating Low Risk and High Risk Groups of Bladder Cancer

Parameters	Low Risk	High Risk
Grades	I	III
Stages	0-A	B-D
ABO	Present	Absent
Chromosomes	Normal	Abnormal
Carcinoma *in situ*	Absent	Present
Recurrence	Less frequent	Frequent
Multiplicity	Less	More

tional histopathologic examination allows appropriate initial therapy. The improvements in immunocytochemical techniques, chromosomal banding technique and flow cytometry have made these procedures attractive and more reliable for clinical utilization.

DIAGNOSIS

Application of cytology, recognition of the natural history of carcinoma *in situ* and application of newer radioimaging techniques have improved the diagnosis and staging of these tumors. The use of fine needle aspirations of suspicious lymph nodes and utilization of computed tomograms have also been helpful. However, the clinical staging of the bladder cancer still needs improvement in reducing staging error. The pathology of carcinoma *in situ* has been better clarified. Mostofi has suggested designating carcinoma *in situ* as intraepithelial carcinoma, and grading them into three grades. Grade I represents less anaplastic (atypia), grade III represents more anaplastic (carcinoma *in situ*) and grade II will be an intermediate tumor (dysplasia). This classification is useful because it represents the degree of anaplasia, therefore, the natural history of the tumor. One may add cell surface antigen detection for grades I and II and predict the natural history and propensity for invasion; grade III already has an invasive natural history.

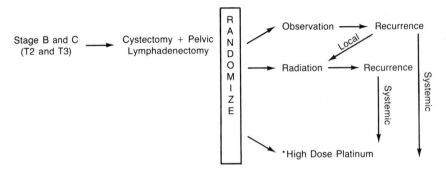

*200 mg/m^2 in 250 ml of 3% saline.

Figure 1.4. Randomized clinical trial with surgery, radiation and high dose platinum in invasive bladder cancer.

ADVANCES IN THERAPY

In treating bladder cancer, one should divide them into the high risk and low risk group based on grade, stage, multiplicity in time and space, cell markers, chromosome and other parameters. Although the low risk patient responds well with conservative endoscopic resection, the high risk group needs more intensive therapy such as radiation and/or cystectomy. Utilization of intravesical chemotherapy including doxorubicin, thiotepa and mitomycin have been shown effective in several controlled studies. The experience of European Organizations for Research and Treatment of Cancer (EORTC) have been reviewed in Chapter 14 on chemotherapy of the bladder cancer. However, doxorubicin, *cis*-platinum, and cytoxan appear to be effective in treatment of disseminated bladder cancer. The role of radiation and its timing is not clear. Randomized clinical trials are necessary to resolve these problems. The role of yttrium-aluminum-garnet (YAG) or Argon laser beam and hematoporphyrin-derivative phototherapy are currently under investigation. The role of immunotherapy, particularly utilization of BCG, has been discussed in a separate chapter. We are embarking on a protocol that randomized the infiltrative bladder cancer into cystectomy, cystectomy with radiation, and cystectomy with radiation and high dose *cis*-platinum. The completion of this protocol will establish the value of radiotherapy and high dose *cis*-platinum as adjuvant therapy in this disease (Fig. 1.4).

The role of clonogenic assay in bladder cancer, as in other cancers, is still experimental and the current technical problems and lack of controlled clinical trials precludes its clinical utilization. The future developments in radioimmunotherapy and chemoimmunotherapy may have potential in diagnosis and management of bladder cancer.

REFERENCES

1. Krontiris, T. G. The emerging genetics of human cancer. *N. Engl. J. Med. 307:*404, 1983.
2. Shih, C., Paddly L. C., Murray M., and Weinberg R. A. Transforming genes of carcinomas and neuroblastomas introduced into mouse fibroblasts. *Nature 290:*261, 1981.

2

Epidemiologic Considerations

Gerry B. Hill, M.B., Ch.B., F.R.C.P.(C)

Traditionally epidemiology has been defined as the study of the distribution of disease, and the determinants of disease, at the population level. The primary orientation of the discipline was always etiological, but it remained separate from other disciplines with similar aims, such as experimental pathology and toxicology. As knowledge concerning a particular group of diseases expands, and in particular when specific causal agents are identified, the relevant disciplines tend to merge.[1] Within this interdisciplinary activity the epidemiologist, although still concerned primarily with disease phenomena in humans, focuses his/her attention more often on small groups of special interest, and increasingly on the biochemical characteristics of such individuals. In addition the contribution of the epidemiologist is more often as a methodologist specializing in the design and interpretation of studies of disease in humans.

The group of diseases encompassed by the term "cancer" is an example of this interdisciplinary convergence. Although the precise mechanisms are not fully understood, a conceptual model in which malignant transformation is seen as a multistage process initiated by specific agents and promoted by others is generally accepted. The majority of tumors arise in the epithelial cells exposed to external carcinogens or to those present in excretions and secretions. The evidence for this hypothesis in relation to bladder cancer has been reviewed recently.[2]

Multidisciplinary research would look beyond etiology and include also the reaction of the host and the response to treatment. In the content of bladder cancer a coordinated multidisciplinary program of research has been described,[3] aimed at reducing the morbidity and mortality associated with the disease.

As part of the research effort underlying a rational program of cancer control, three separate but related roles for the epidemiologist emerge:

1. Quantifying the impact of the disease in terms of incidence, mobidity and mortality.
2. Quantifying the importance of known causal agents and identifying others.

3. Quantifying the effects of programs aimed at reducing exposure to causal agents or the early diagnosis of tumors in exposed individuals.

As the discipline has matured, epidemiologists have developed a corresponding typology of research methods which has now become fairly standard within the discipline[4] and increasingly recognized by others.

1. *Descriptive studies* using disease and death registration provide estimates of incidence and mortality rates. The variations of these over time, and between geographically and demographically defined groups, provides some validation for etiological hypotheses and suggests others. In addition, correlations of disease frequency with the prevalence of a particular agent provides somewhat stronger, but still very weak, evidence of association.
2. *Analytical studies* entail the study of such associations at the level of the individual, and are of two types. In *case-control studies* individuals with and without the disease are selected and previous exposure to various possible factors is determined. In *cohort studies* people exposed and not exposed to a particular factor are selected and their subsequent incidence of disease determined. Both approaches are fraught with many methodological pitfalls.[5] In general, case-control studies are easier to do but more susceptible to bias. Cohort studies are less so, but are usually difficult to mount, except in relation to occupational factors where exposed groups are more easily identified and followed up.

    Many possible factors can be studied in a simple case control study, and the incidence of many diseases can be measured in a cohort study. In both situations formal statistical tests of association are relevant only for a relationship stipulated *a priori*. Other associations should be regarded as chance findings until verified by other studies. An established association between exposure and disease does not imply causality, since it may be due to confounding with some other agent. A strict interpretation of causality would require evidence, from intervention studies, that manipulation of exposure produces corresponding changes in incidence. The characteristics of an association which would favour a causal interpretation in the absence of intervention studies have been generally accepted.[6]
3. Randomized controlled trials of the exposure of humans to carcinogenic agents are not feasible and controlled trials of reducing exposure are difficult. Observational studies of the effects of self-imposed reduction of exposure are susceptible to bias. Randomized studies of protective factors on incidence and of early detection programs on mortality are feasible and the need for such studies has been emphasized.[7]

Epidemiologists use precise terms to measure the impact of a disease and its association with etiological factors. Confusion arises when such terms are used loosely or incorrectly. The incidence of (number of new cases of) or mortality from (number of deaths due to) a disease are related to the appropriate person-years at risk and, in the case of cancer, expressed as rates/100,000. The latter are usually calculated for each sex separately and, if not specific for age also, are age-standardized, using a standard population, frequently the standard world population introduced by Segi *et al.*[7]

The measure of association of an etiological agent, or risk factor, with a disease is the *relative risk*, or risk ratio, defined as the ratio of the incidence rate of the disease among those exposed to the factor to that among those not exposed. The relative risk is measured directly in cohort studies and indirectly in case-control studies. The relative risk quantifies the importance of the risk factor for those exposed to it. A measure of the importance of the factor in relation to the incidence of the disease in the general population is the *attributable fraction*,[8] which is related to the relative risk (R) and the proportion of the population exposed to the factor (P) by the formula $P(R-1)/[P(R-1) + 1]$.

Other things being equal, mortality is the product of incidence and case-fatality, the latter being defined as the proportion of cases who succumb to the disease. Cancer mortality rates are often used as a proxy for incidence rates, but it is clear that changes in mortality reflect changes in incidence only if case-fatality is unchanged.

In one sense, the control of cancer in a population can be viewed as either reducing incidence, or case-fatality, or both. The importance of factors which influence case-fatality can be quantified in a manner similar to those affecting incidence.[9]

In the following sections the epidemiologic aspects of bladder cancer will be discussed under three headings: patterns of incidence and mortality, role of known etiological factors, and potential for prevention and early detection.

The epidemiology of bladder cancer has been the subject of several recent reviews.[10-14] These have been used extensively in writing this chapter, together with other more specialized reviews referenced separately.

PATTERNS OF INCIDENCE AND MORTALITY

Age and Sex

Both incidence and mortality rates for bladder cancer increase with age and are greater for males than females at all ages. Typical patterns of incidence and mortality by sex and age are shown in Figure 2.1, in which the logarithms of the rates are plotted against the logarithm of the mean age for each age group.

The graphs show that, with minor deviations, linear log-log relationships hold for both incidence and mortality. This relationship has been found for many epithelial tumors in different parts of the world, and its theoretical implications have aroused great interest.[15,16]

The lines for male and female incidence are virtually parallel, indicating that the male/female ratio for incidence does not vary with age. This is true for mortality also, but the vertical distance between the lines is smaller since the male/female ratio for mortality is less than that for incidence.

In both sexes, mortality increases with age more steeply than incidence, so that the mortality/incidence ratio increases with age. As indicated, the mortality/incidence ratio is a measure of case-fatality, and it is reasonable to conclude that this would increase with age, although it is possible that there could be an under reporting of incidence or over reporting of mortality at older ages.

International Variation

Table 2.1 shows the age-adjusted incidence and mortality rates by sex in the 10 countries for which national rates are available from recent

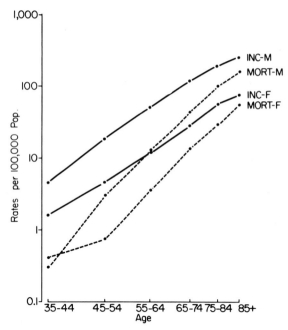

Figure 2.1. Cancer of the bladder incidence and mortality in Canada, 1971.

Table 2.1
Recent Estimates of Incidence[a] and Mortality[b] of Bladder Cancer in Selected Countries[c]

Country	Incidence			Mortality			Mortality/ Incidence	
	Males	Females	Ratio	Males	Females	Ratio	Males	Females
Denmark	22.0	5.6	3.9	7.5	2.0	3.8	0.37	0.37
Israel	19.0	4.0	4.8	6.0	1.2	5.0	0.32	0.30
Canada	17.5	4.8	3.6	5.2	1.5	3.5	0.30	0.33
Hong Kong	17.1	5.9	2.9	3.7	1.7	2.2	0.22	0.29
Scotland	16.5	4.8	3.4	8.2	2.6	3.2	0.50	0.54
Norway	14.6	4.0	3.7	4.9	1.9	2.6	0.34	0.48
Sweden	13.7	4.2	3.2	4.7	1.7	2.7	0.34	0.48
New Zealand	12.1	3.4	3.6	4.7	1.1	4.3	0.39	0.32
Finland	9.9	2.3	4.3	5.5	1.2	4.6	0.56	0.52
Singapore	6.1	1.7	3.6	2.3	0.8	2.9	0.38	0.47
Median	15.6	4.1	3.7	5.2	1.6	3.4	0.36	0.39

[a] Around 1975.[17]
[b] Around 1970.[18]
[c] Age-adjusted rates/100,000 world population.

World Health Organization publications.[17, 18] The countries are arranged in decreasing order of the incidence rates in males, with median 15.6/ 100,000. The median incidence rate for females among this group of countries is 4.1/100,000, and the ordering is similar to that in males, so that the male/female incidence ratio varies little about the median of 3.7. Exceptions are Hong Kong where the incidence in females is relatively high, and Israel and Finland where the female rates are comparatively low.

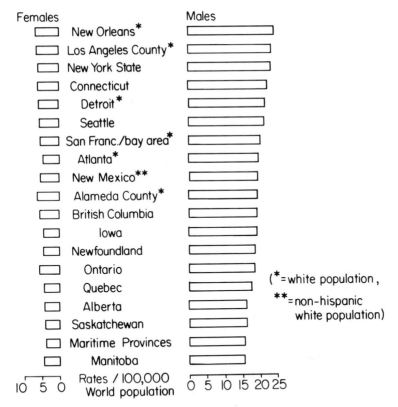

Figure 2.2. Cancer of the bladder. Age standardized incidence rates around 1975.

The median mortality rates are 5.2/100,000 for males and 1.6/100,000 for females, with the same consistency of the male/female ratio as seen for incidence, and with similar exceptions. On average, the male/female ratio is slightly smaller for mortality than for incidence.

The mortality/incidence ratio, which is a rough index of case fatality, is on average slightly higher in females (median 0.39) than in males (median 0.36). With the exception of Scotland and Finland, where the ratios exceed 0.5, and Hong Kong, where the ratios are under 0.3, the mortality/incidence ratios vary very little between countries.

Regional Variation

Figure 2.2 shows the most recent incidence estimates from cancer registries in North America.[17] Where possible the rates for white populations are shown, and the registries are listed in decreasing order of incidence in males, the order for females being similar.

In general the registries with high incidence are those based on urban or predominantly urban populations. Approximately 2-fold urban/rural ratios have been found in cancer registries in Norway[19,20] and the United Kingdom.[21]

Maps of cancer mortality by county have been published for the United States in 1950–1969[22] and Canada in 1966–1976.[23] In both countries the counties with high bladder cancer mortality were situated

Table 2.2
Incidence of Bladder Cancer by Ethnic Group and Sex in Selected Areas Around 1975[a]

Area	Amerindian		Black		Chinese		Japanese		Spanish		(Other) White	
	M	F	M	F	M	F	M	F	M	F	M	F
Alameda county, CA			12.0	4.5							19.6	6.1
Atlanta			9.1	3.8							19.8	4.8
Detroit			10.1	4.3							21.4	5.6
Los Angeles County			11.5	5.5	7.3	2.4	9.2	2.4	14.2	3.8	23.6	6.2
New Mexico	2.9	0.0							6.2	2.5	19.7	5.4
New Orleans			8.9	4.0							24.5	6.5
San Francisco bay area			10.7	4.1	10.6	2.0	6.5	3.2			20.0	5.5
Elsewhere												
Hawaii					8.4	1.2	9.9	3.4			23.5	3.9
Shanghai[b]					7.5	1.4						
Singapore					7.0	2.0						
Hong Kong[b]					17.1	5.9						
Japan[b]:Fukuoka							6.2	1.9				
Miyako							5.3	1.6				
Nagasaki							7.9	2.1				
Osaka							5.1	1.5				

[a] Age-standardized rates/100,000 world population.[17]
[b] Ethnic group not specified.

predominantly in the regions bordering on the Great Lakes and the Atlantic seaboard. Detailed analysis of the mortality by county in the United States[24,25] showed that the mortality rates in males were higher in countries where the chemical industry is concentrated.

Ethnic Group and Migration

The most recent age-standardized incidence rates by ethnic group in seven registration areas in the United States are shown in Table 2.2. In each area the rates are higher in whites than in any other ethnic group in both sexes.

On average the incidence in ethnic groups other than white is less than half that of whites of the same sex, with the exception of black females for whom the incidence is, on average, three-quarters of that of white females. These results are in keeping with those of an earlier review of cancer incidence and mortality in whites and nonwhites in the United States.[26]

Table 2.2 also allows a comparison of the incidence of bladder cancer among Chinese and Japanese who have migrated to Hawaii and California with the incidence of the same groups in Asia. The rates for Chinese in Hawaii and California resemble more closely those for Shanghai and for Chinese in Singapore than those for whites in Hawaii and California, which are similar. However, the rates in Hong Kong are considerably higher than those for Chinese elsewhere. A similar pattern of low rates among Japanese in Japan, Hawaii and California is also evident.

Table 2.3
Incidence of Cancer of the Bladder in Israel in 1960–1966[26] and 1972–1976[17]

Jews Born In	1960–1966[b]		1972–1976	
	Males	Females	Males	Females
Israel	13.5	2.8	15.4	3.7
Europe or America	14.2	3.4	18.3	4.4
Asia	9.0	2.4	17.0	2.7
Africa	23.3	3.1		
All Jews	15.8	3.4	20.9	4.5
Non Jews			8.6	1.2

[a] Age-standardized rates/100,000 world population.
[b] Includes cancer of urinary organs other than kidneys.

Table 2.3 gives the incidence of cancer of the bladder in Israel among Jews from different parts of the world and among non-Jews. The rates for Jews born in Israel, Europe or America are higher than for Jews born in Asia or non-Jews, while the rates for Jews born in Africa are high especially in males.

The mortality from bladder cancer among migrants from Europe to the United States[27] and to Canada[28] are compared with those of the donor and host countries in Table 2.4. Although the pattern of change is not uniform, among males in the majority of cases where the mortality in the donor country is less than that of the host, the mortality among migrants is greater than that in the donor country and *vice versa*. This tendency is less evident among females.

Social Class and Occupation

Cancer registries do not, in general, provide estimates of incidence by occupation and social class, but mortality rates based on statement of occupation on death registration and census enumeration in England and Wales are published periodically. Table 2.5 is taken from a recent review of cancer mortality from these reports.[29] In both men and married women the age-standardized mortality ratio at ages 15–64 is lowest in the professional class (I) and highest in unskilled workers (V). The progression from I to V is irregular, with high ratios for manual workers in Class III. Among the men the occupations with above average mortality were chemical workers, plumbers, bricklayers, painters and decorators, general laborers, postmen, bus-conductors, dock laborers, publicans and hairdressers.

Marital Status

Recent age-specific rates of mortality from cancer of the bladder by marital status in Canada are given in Table 2.6. In both sexes the married have the lowest rates at all ages, except for males in the oldest age group where the single have the lowest rate. On average, the mortality for single females and for the widowed and divorced of both sexes is 50% higher than for the married. These findings are qualitatively similar to those found in England and Wales in 1965–1967,[30] but the ratios are larger in the Canadian data.

Table 2.4
Age-adjusted Mortality Rate for Bladder Cancer Among Males

Country of Birth		Country of Origin, 1960	United States 1959–1961	Country of Origin, 1971	Canada, 1969–1973
United States	M		5.1	4.9	6.1
	F		1.8	1.6	1.8
Canada	M	5.7	6.8		5.4
	F	1.9	1.8		1.6
Austria	M		6.4	7.4	3.7
	F		1.6	1.5	1.3
Czechoslovakia	M		4.4	5.7	6.1
	F		0.9	1.1	1.6
Denmark	M			8.6	5.2
	F			2.2	1.9
Finland	M	5.1	4.1	4.0	7.0
	F	1.1	1.2	1.2	0.8
Germany	M		6.6	7.0	4.1
	F		1.9	1.5	0.8
Hungary	M		8.5	5.7	3.6
	F		1.4	1.1	1.3
Ireland	M	3.4	5.5		
	F	1.5	2.2		
Italy	M	5.0	5.8	6.8	4.2
	F	1.1	1.5	1.2	1.0
Lithuania	M		10.1		
	F				
Mexico	M		2.6		
	F		1.2		
Netherlands	M			6.6	4.0
	F			1.6	0.9
Norway	M	3.8	3.9	4.9	5.7
	F	1.8	2.8	1.5	1.7
Poland	M		5.5	5.4	4.6
	F		1.1	0.8	0.7
Romania	M			4.1	6.2
	F			0.9	2.9
Sweden	M	3.2	4.2	4.2	5.1
	F	1.4	1.7	1.4	1.8
United Kingdom	M	6.9	6.3	7.8	6.7
	F	2.1	2.1	2.2	1.7
U.S.S.R.	M		5.9		5.4
	F		1.3		1.1
Yugoslavia	M		4.5	3.3	4.9
	F		1.4	0.9	0.4

Trends in Incidence and Mortality

The changes in incidence reported by cancer registries with data available for periods around 1961 and 1975[17,19] are shown in Table 2.7. Over this period of approximately 14 years, incidence in males has increased in all areas, and the incidence in females has increased in all

Table 2.5
Bladder Cancer in England and Wales 1970–1972[27] Ages 15–64 (Standardized Mortality Ratio)

Social Class	Men	Married Women[a]
	%	%
I Professional	79	54
II Managerial	83	89
III Skilled workers	113	118
Nonmanual	91	71
Manual	120	131
IV Semiskilled workers	105	116
V Unskilled workers	115	123

[a] Social class based upon occupation of husband.

Table 2.6
Mortality from Cancer of the Bladder by Sex, Age and Marital Status. Canada 1975–1977[a]

Marital Status	Males (age)					Females (age)				
	25–44	45–64	65–74	75+	All Ages	25–44	45–64	65–74	75+	All Ages
Married	0.2	6.1	31.7	97.3	4.74	0.1	1.5	8.8	26.7	1.29
Single	0.1	6.2	42.7	76.6	4.87	0.1	3.6	10.9	36.3	1.98
		(1.02)[b]	(1.35)	(0.79)	(1.03)		(2.40)	(1.24)	(1.36)	(1.53)
Widowed & Divorced		12.9	46.5	122.5	7.23		3.4	11.8	35.4	1.94
		(2.11)[b]	(1.47)	(1.26)	(1.53)		(2.27)	(1.34)	(1.33)	(1.50)

[a] Rates/100,000.
[b] Ratio to rate for married.

areas but one. In both sexes the median percentage increase was 48%, corresponding to an average annual increase of about 3%.

Table 2.8 shows the changes in mortality from cancer of the bladder between 1958–1962 and 1968–1972 for eight countries with comparable data.[18] The average annual increase in this group of countries was about 2% in males and 1% in females.

Data from the second and third National Cancer Incidence Surveys in the United States[31] indicate increasing incidence of bladder cancer in males, both white and nonwhite, and decreasing incidence in females, both white and nonwhite, over the interval 1947–1948 to 1969–1971. The same reference[31] shows stable mortality rates from cancer of the bladder and other urinary organs, excluding kidney, in males and falling rates in females over a similar time interval.

Figure 2.3 shows the trends in the cumulative mortality at ages 25–64 in England and Wales by sex and social class.[29] Over the 50 years 1921–1971, mortality increased by over 60% among men in social classes III, IV and V but only by 22% in men in social class I and II. However, among married women over 40-year period 1931–1971, mortality increased less markedly in social classes III, IV and V, and fell slightly in social classes I and II.

Trends in age-standardized rates can obscure differences in trends by age. In particular, it is important to attempt to distinguish cohort trends (identified by year of birth) from secular trends (identified by year of death). This distinction is especially important in the interpretation of trends in chronic diseases such as tuberculosis[32] and cancer.[33] As an

Table 2.7
Trends in Incidence[a] of Bladder Cancer 1961–1975[17, 19]

Area	Males			Females		
	1961	1975	increase	1961	1975	increase
			%			%
Connecticut	16.9	22.3	32	5.1	6.0	18
Newfoundland	13.8	18.4	33	3.4	4.4	29
New York State	13.4	23.1	72	3.6	6.0	67
Saskatchewan	13.3	16.1	21	2.4	4.1	71
Manitoba	12.8	15.2	19	2.4	4.7	96
Israel	12.4	19.0	53	2.9	4.0	38
Denmark	12.4	22.0	77	3.8	5.6	47
Liverpool	11.4	16.4	44	3.2	4.0	25
New Zealand	10.4	12.1	16	2.3	3.4	48
Birmingham (UK)	10.2	17.1	68	2.3	4.5	96
Alberta	9.5	16.1	69	2.5	4.2	68
Sweden	8.4	13.7	63	2.9	4.2	45
Puerto Rico	7.9	8.4	6	3.7	2.8	−24
Finland	6.7	9.9	48	1.4	2.3	64
Norway	4.9	14.6	198	2.0	4.0	200
Slovenia	4.8	7.1	48	1.0	1.4	40
Singapore (Chinese)	2.1	7.0	233	0.5	2.0	300
Median	10.2	15.2	48	2.4	4.0	48

[a] Age-adjusted rates/100,000 world population.

Table 2.8
Trends in Mortality[a] from Cancer of the Bladder 1960–1970[18,]

Country	Males			Females		
	1958–1962	1968–1972	increase	1958–1962	1968–1970	increase
			%			%
Scotland	6.8	8.0	18	2.2	2.4	9
Italy	4.8	6.4	33	1.1	1.2	9
Israel	4.4	5.8	32	1.3	1.2	−8
Finland	4.2	4.9	17	0.9	1.0	11
France	4.1	5.6	37	1.2	1.3	8
N. Ireland	4.0	4.6	15	1.7	1.5	−12
Sweden	3.1	4.5	45	1.3	1.5	15
Japan	2.0	2.3	15	0.9	1.0	11
Median	4.2	4.3	25	1.3	1.3	9

[a] Age-adjusted rates/100,000 world populations.

example, Figure 2.4 shows, for each sex, age specific mortality rates in Canada displayed by year of death (*A, B*) and by year of birth (*C, D*). In each case an average mortality ratio is also shown. In both sexes there is a downward trend in the mortality ratio by year of death since 1946, more marked in females than in males. In males the mortality ratio by year of birth rises to a peak for men born about 1894 and then falls. In females there is no clear cohort trend. These patterns are similar to those found in mortality from bladder cancer in England and Wales,[34] though the downward secular trend was less evident.

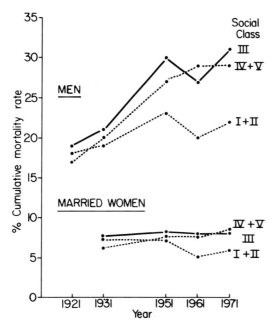

Figure 2.3. Cancer of the bladder cumulative mortality rate (percent) at ages 25–64 in England and Wales.

Histological Type

For statistical purposes neoplasms are classified primarily by site, but recently efforts have been made to classify incidence cases by histology in a uniform manner. Table 2.9 summarizes the information published in connection with reports on cancer incidence.[35, 36]

The completeness of reporting is not yet sufficient to enable estimates of the absolute incidence of different histological types to be made. Interest has focused on the ratio of squamous to transitional carcinomas.[35] It is clear from the table that, in relation to transitional carcinoma, squamous carcinoma is much more common in Africa and is least common in North America. Where the ratio is low it is lower in males than in females, and the data from registries with a high proportion of cases classified indicate that the difference is due chiefly to a relative excess of transitional carcinoma among males rather than to an excess of squamous carcinoma among females.

The overall ratios for Northern Europe and Eastern Europe are weighted by large series from two registries with above-average ratios in males.

ROLE OF KNOWN ETIOLOGIC FACTORS

The main groups of agents which are known or suspected to initiate or modify carcinogenesis are listed in Table 2.10, together with an indication of the evidence for their role in the etiology of human bladder cancer. There is no doubt that organic chemicals are the most important

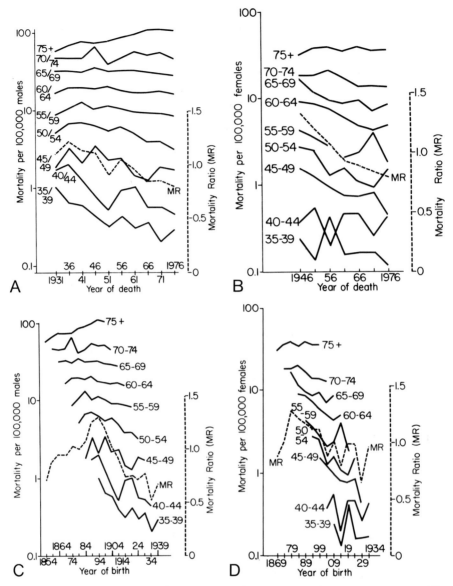

Figure 2.4. Mortality from cancer of the bladder in Canada. Age-specific mortality rates and mortality ratios by: year of death for *A*, males and *B*, females; and by: year of birth for *C*, males and *D*, females.

Table 2.9
Registrations of Bladder Cancer by Sex and Histology in Different Regions[35, 36]

Area	Squamous/Transitional Ratio	
	Male	Female
	%	%
Africa	196	193
South and Central America	7.1	17.1
North America	2.8	5.9
Asia	4.0	5.1
Northern Europe	8.1	11.9
(Excluding S. Thames)	5.8	10.1
Eastern Europe	20.5	30.2
(Excluding German D.R.)	4.5	35.3
Southern and Western Europe	8.2	8.6

Table 2.10
Agents Incriminated in the Etiology of Bladder Cancer

Agent	Evidence for Role in Bladder Cancer in Humans[a]
Biological	
Genetic and chromosomal abnormalities	D
Blood groups	C
Allergy and immunity	C
Viral infection	C
Bacterial infection	D
Schistosomal infection	B
Vitamin deficiency	C
Tryptophan metabolites	D
Balkan nephropathy	C
Physical	
Ionizing radiation	A
Chemical	
Aromatic amines	A
Others	See Table 2.8

[a] A, association consistently positive in analytical studies, including at least one cohort study, with evidence of dose response or experimental validation; B, association consistently positive in two or more analytical studies but no definite dose response or experimental validation; C, association positive in only one analytical study or inconsistent finding in multiple analytical studies; and D, association suggested by descriptive studies, case reports, or laboratory findings but not confirmed by analytical studies.

and these are discussed in more detail below, but first the evidence implicating other types of agent is reviewed briefly.

Genetic and Chromosomal Abnormalities

Bladder cancer is not one of the many types of cancer associated with single-gene abnormalities.[37] Chromosome studies of bladder tumors have found some numerical and morphologic changes but have not revealed any specific karyotypic change.[38] However some kindreds with a predisposition to urothelial cancer have been described.[39–41]

Blood Groups

An excess of blood group A in bladder cancer patients has been found in several studies, and, in the most recent, associations were found with HLA-B5 and HLA-CW4 but these findings need to be corroborated.[42]

Allergy and Immunity

An association between bladder cancer and a personal or family history of allergy has been reported in one case-control study.[43] Although prior administration of BCG vaccine inhibits the induction of experimental murine bladder cancer,[44] bladder cancer is not one of the malignancies which have been found in excess among patients with genetic or acquired immunodeficiency.[45,46]

Viral Infection

An RNA virus resembling known oncornaviruses was isolated from human bladder tumors.[47] Antibodies to DNA-containing viruses related to an oncogenic simian papovavirus have been found in bladder cancer patients[48,49] and in the general population,[50] but definite evidence of a causal relationship is lacking.

Bacterial Infection

Bladder cancer patients have reported previous urinary tract infection or obstruction more often than controls in several studies,[51-53] but such a history might be the effect rather than the cause of the cancer, or explained by recall bias. Uncontrolled studies have suggested an excess incidence of bladder cancer among patients with neurogenic bladder conditions,[54,55] and nitrosamines have been found in the urine of patients with chronic urinary tract infections.[56,57]

Schistosomal Infection

Recent reviews[10,14,15,58] cite clinical and descriptive epidemiological studies beginning in 1905 suggesting an association between bladder cancer and infection with *Schistosoma haematobium* in Egypt and East Africa. More recently informal case-control studies[59-61] have confirmed this association particularly in relation to squamous cell cancers. The tumors associated with *Bilharzia* are not concentrated in the trigonal region as are most bladder cancers.[62] Despite the lack of formal analytical studies the weight of the descriptive evidence, together with some positive experimental results,[63] make a causal relationship plausible. Bacteriuria is common among patients with schistosomiasis,[64] and nitrosamines have been found in *S. haematobium*-infected individuals also infected with nitrate-reducing bacteria.[65] This has led to the suggestion that the *S. haematobium* acts as a cocarcinogen for tumors initiated by nitrosamines.[66]

Vitamin Deficiency

Studies *in vitro* and in experimental animals indicate that vitamin A inhibits carcinogenesis and epidemiological studies of lung cancer suggest that this may be true in humans.[67] In a large case-control study of bladder cancer[68] an increased risk was found for lower levels of an index of Vitamin A intake.

Tryptophan Metabolites

Dietary tryptophan promotes the development of bladder tumors initiated by organic fluorine compounds in rats,[69,70] and patients with nonoccupational bladder cancer were found to excrete more of certain tryptophan metabolites than patients with occupational bladder cancer.[71,72] However this pattern of tryptophan metabolism is more frequent in females than males and is not specific to patients with bladder cancer, so that the role of tryptophan metabolites in bladder cancer needs further clarification.[10]

Balkan Nephropathy

A progressive form of kidney disease of unknown etiology is endemic in rural areas of Bulgaria, Rumania and Yugoslavia, and in these areas a high incidence of kidney and bladder tumors has also been noted. The incidence of nephropathy is higher in females than males.

In one of the affected areas, the Vrasta district of Bulgaria, the age-adjusted incidence rates for bladder tumors in villages where nephropathy is hyperendemic were 38.7/100,000 in males and 24.6 in females, compared with 8.9 in males and 2.1 in females in nonaffected villages.[73] The excess of tumors of the renal pelvis and ureter was even greater for females in affected villages. From the information on the two diseases in individuals it can be determined that the relative risk of urinary tract tumors for those with nephropathy is approximately 79. Both nephropathy and urinary cancer exhibit familial clustering but the cause is not known.

Ionizing Radiation

Epidemiological studies of the carcinogenic effects of radiation have been thoroughly reviewed recently.[74] Japanese atomic bomb survivors have been found to have an excess mortality from urinary cancer.[75] Excess risk of bladder cancer has also been reported in follow-up studies of women given radiotherapy for cervical cancer[76] and ovarian cancer,[77] but similar studies of women receiving radiation for benign pelvic conditions are equivocal.[78,79]

Chemical Carcinogens

Table 2.11 lists the situations in which exposure to chemical carcinogens is believed to produce bladder cancer in humans. The dominant model, based on clinical, epidemiological and experimental studies of industrial aromatic amines, involves uptake of a carcinogen by ingestion, inhalation or absorption through skin or mucous membrane, which produces cancer by direct contact of the excreted substances or a metabolite with the bladder epithelium.[80] This model is consistent with what is currently known about bladder cancer. In particular it has been shown that 2-acetylaminofluorene, a known dietary bladder carcinogen, also produces bladder cancer following intratracheal installation.[81] However studies of the urine of tobacco smokers has not, so far, established the presence of carcinogens derived from tobacco smoke,[82] and it has been suggested that inhaled carcinogens may produce cancer internally *via* the blood.[83]

Air Pollution

Apart from the general observation that the incidence of bladder cancer is higher in urban than rural areas, there is no evidence that pollution of the ambient air is implicated. Attention is usually focused on polycyclic aromatic hydrocarbons derived from incomplete combustion of fossil fuel, but such substances have been identified also in the soot produced by roasting coffee[84] and it has been suggested that this

Table 2.11
Exposure to Chemicals Incriminated in the Etiology of Human Bladder Cancer

Method of Exposure	Evidence for role in bladder cancer in humans[a]	Known or postulated chemical carcinogens[b]
Air pollution	D	PAH
Water treatment	C	Trihalomethanes
Occupation		
Agriculture and gardening	C	
Manufacturing and processing		
Aluminum	C	PAH
Chemicals and dyes	A	AA
Coal gas and tar	A	AA PAH
Food	C	
Glass	C	
Leather	B	
Machinery	B	PAH
Paint and pigment	B	AA
Petroleum	C	
Rubber and cable	A	AA
Textiles	B	AA
Wood	C	
Professions and services		
Cooking	C	
Hairdressing	B	AA
Medicine	B	AA
Photography	C	AA
Plumbing	B	
Seafairing	B	
Truck driving	B	
Diet		
Bracken fern	D	Shikimic acid
Fat and protein	D	
Artificial sweeteners	C	Saccharin, cyclamate
Lifestyle		
Coffee	B	Caffeine PAH
Tobacco	A	AA PAH
Hair dye	D	AA, lead
Opium	D	
Pharmaceutical		
Chlornaphazine	B	Specific compounds
Cyclophosphamide	D	Specific compounds
Azathioprine	D	Specific compounds
Isoniazid	D	Specific compounds
Phenacetin		

[a] See footnote to Table 2.10.
[b] PAH, polycyclic aromatic hydrocarbons; and AA, aromatic amines.

might contribute to the high incidence of bladder cancer in New Orleans.[85]

Water Treatment

In a thorough review of epidemiological studies of cancer and drinking water,[86] nine are listed in which an association between trihalomethanes and urinary cancer has been found, either directly, in terms of levels of trihalomethanes, or using the surrogate index of ratio of surface to ground water. Most of the studies were descriptive (ecological) and not all such studies were positive. The list included one case-control mortality study. In a case-control incidence study not included in the list,[53] the use of nonpublic rather than public water was a risk factor for bladder cancer in males, contrary to what one would expect if chlorination were the causal agent.

Occupation

Occupational bladder cancer has been extensively and repeatedly reviewed.[10-14, 80, 87-89] In the period immediately following the second world war epidemiologists began detailed cohort studies[90] which clarified the carcinogenicity of aromatic amines in the dyestuff industry established earlier by clinical[91] and experimental[92] studies. Later cohort studies established the increased risk of bladder cancer in other industries in which workers are exposed to aromatic amines, such as rubber and cable manufacture[93-97] and coal gas distillation.[98, 99]

Beginning in the late 1950s the case-control approach began to be used.[43, 51, 52, 100-109] These studies have, for the most part, confirmed the importance of industrial contact with aromatic amines, though two case-control studies[110, 111] failed to find any occupational risk. In addition the case-control studies have, with varying degrees of confirmation, indicated other industrial and occupational factors. Some of the latter, *e.g.* painters, textile workers, hairdressers, medical workers and photographers, were suspected *a priori* because of possible contact with aromatic amines. In others, such as leather workers, machinists, plumbers, sailors and truck drivers, elevated risks have been found in more than one study, but there is no evidence of involvement with aromatic amines. In some cases exposure to polycyclic aromatic hydrocarbons may be responsible. The increased risk in leather workers has been confirmed by a cohort study.[112]

Diet

Bladder cancer in cattle in northern Turkey was linked to their consumption of a species of bracken fern, *Pteris aquilina*,[113] and this was also found experimentally to produce bladder tumors in rats.[114] Japanese species of bracken, which are eaten by humans, were also found to contain carcinogens[115] one of which is shikimic acid.[116] There is no direct evidence incriminating bracken in relation to human cancer and no association with consumption of fiddlehead greens, a related species to bracken fern, was found in a case-control study of bladder cancer in Eastern Canada.[105]

International comparisons suggest an association between bladder cancer mortality and per capita consumption of fat and protein[117] but this has not been examined in analytic studies.

One of the most controversial issues in relation to bladder cancer is the role of artificial sweeteners. Saccharin has been available for a century.[118] Although an early study in rats showed saccharin to have some carcinogenic potential this was not pursued until 1970, following a ban on the use of cyclamate, an alternative to saccharin, which had been introduced in 1950. Cyclamate was banned following a 1969 study in rats in which bladder cancers were an incidental finding. Subsequent studies have shown that neither cyclamate nor its metabolites are carcinogenic.[119] Saccharin was submitted to intensive experimental study during the 1970s. Bladder tumors were found in rats, especially the male offspring of rats treated prior to mating, although a later study found bladder tumors in males of both generations.[119] Studies in rats have also shown that both saccharin and cyclamate can promote bladder cancer induced by N-methyl-N-nitrosourea.[120]

Reports of epidemiological studies of a possible association between use of artificial sweeteners and bladder cancer began in 1970. Descriptive studies of the trends in mortality in the United States, incidence in Connecticut, and cohort mortality in England and Wales showed no evidence of a trend consistent with that of consumption of artificial sweeteners.[121, 122] Cohort mortality studies of diabetics in the United States[123] and England and Wales[124] revealed no excess of bladder cancer despite the fact that 23% of the diabetics in one of the studies reported taking saccharin for at least 10 years.[124] The lack of association between diabetes and bladder cancer death was also indicated by an analysis of the frequency with which diabetes was mentioned on the certificates of people dying from cancer in England and Wales.[125]

A review in 1981[118] summarized the results of 11 case-control studies of bladder cancer and artificial sweeteners,[43, 88, 110, 126–132] all based in the United States or Canada. Since then three further case-control studies have been reported,[107, 133, 134] including results from England and Japan. In general the studies have shown no increased risk of bladder cancer in relation to intake of artificial sweeteners in the form of tablets or drops, or as an ingredient of soft drinks. One of the earlier studies[128] showed a small but statistically significant relative risk of 1.6 for males, but a reduced, though not statistically significant relative risk of 0.6 for females. Since this report appeared at a time when the results of experimental studies showing excess cancer in male rats were leading to governmental regulation, the study became extremely controversial. The generally negative results of subsequent reports, including a major study involving 3010 cases and 5783 controls in the United States,[132] have calmed the debate. There seems to be a consensus that if a risk does exist then it can only be small in magnitude, although widespread use would make even a small increase important. An interesting feature of the results of the case-control studies is that the majority of them showed a protective effect for use of artificial sweeteners by females. This was not found in the large study in the United States,[132] but the overall relative risk for females from the other studies, using the method of Mantel and Haenszel[135] is 0.7. The meaning of this is not clear. The use of artificial sweeteners among control subjects is correlated with many characteristics other than those usually adjusted for in case-control studies[136] and it is possible that these correlations differ between the sexes. It is not unreasonable to imagine that women are more prone than men to use artificial sweeteners for weight control, and this might be associated with a greater intake of vitamin A or cruciferous vegetables which may be protective.[68]

Life-style

Of the three culturally acceptable drug addictions—alcohol, caffeine and nicotine—only the first has not been implicated in the etiology of bladder cancer. Where an association with alcohol has been sought it has not been found.[52, 137]

The carcinogenicity of caffeine has not been adequately tested in animals,[138] but it has been shown to be a potentiator for several carcinogens in animal experiments.[139] Coffee drinking has been found to be associated with several cancer sites in epidemiological studies and the coffee which is drunk may contain polycyclic hydrocarbons.[84] Interest in coffee drinking as a risk factor for bladder cancer was aroused by the 1971 report of a case-control study in eastern Massachusetts,[140] in which relative risk of 1.24 in men and 2.58 in women were found. This was an unanticipated finding since a previous mortality study had shown no correlation of bladder cancer mortality with national coffee consumption.[141] A subsequent correlation of bladder cancer incidence and imports of coffee in 10 countries, and of trends in incidence and trends in coffee imports in 2 countries also provided little support for the association.[142]

The publication of the Massachusetts study stimulated a further analysis[143] of data from an earlier case-control study in New Orleans,[52] and increased risks for coffee drinking were found which persisted after adjustment for age and cigarette smoking, the risk being greatest, 5.65 for black females. The results of a retrospective analysis of another earlier set of data also provided partial confirmation of the association.[144] Since then the relationship has been addressed in several case-control studies, some of which[43, 88, 104, 110, 126] have been reviewed in detail[13] and others published subsequently.[107, 145, 146] In general these case-control studies show weak overall associations in both sexes, the median of the reported relative risks being 1.5 for males and 1.1 for females. A major problem in the interpretation of these studies is the possible confounding effect of cigarette smoking. However, as has been pointed out,[147] in some studies[88, 144, 146] there is a clear dose-response for coffee consumption after adjustment for cigarette smoking, at least in males. Where the type of coffee has been distinguished the association has been found for ground, instant and decaffeinated coffee although in the most recent study[146] the dose relationship was strongest for regular coffee.

The association between tobacco smoking and bladder cancer has been thoroughly investigated, and the studies up to 1980 have been reviewed thoroughly.[13, 14] A positive relationship has been found consistently in descriptive, case-control and cohort studies. Geographic studies have found positive correlations of mortality[148] and incidence[142] with cigarette consumption, and mortality from bladder cancer is correlated with that from lung cancer.[149] Cohort analyses of incidence in the United States and Denmark[150] and mortality in England and Wales[122, 150, 151] showed an associated with consumption of tobacco in those countries.

Since 1956 smoking has also been studied in many case-control studies[43, 51, 52, 88, 100, 104, 110, 111, 152–156] in the United States, Canada, France,

Italy, Japan, and Poland. In the majority of studies the risk is elevated only for cigarette smokers and the relative risk is higher in males (median 2.2) than in females (1.8). In most studies, too, a dose-response has been demonstrated, at least for cigarette smoking in males, though not as consistent as for lung cancer.[136] In one study a dose-response was found for male pipe smokers.[53] In general, ex-smokers have elevated risks compared with nonsmokers, but less than those of current smokers. The conclusion from analysis of duration of smoking suggests that the latent interval for bladder cancer with respect to cigarette smoking is as long as 20 years.[13] A difference between the risk for smokers of filtered rather than nonfiltered cigarettes is not as marked as for lung cancer. It has been suggested that this could be due to the comparatively smaller relative risk involved, or to the failure of mechanical filtration to remove the agent responsible for bladder cancer.[136]

The association between tobacco smoking and bladder cancer in males has been confirmed in several cohort studies.[157-160] This, together with the dose-relationship and the indirect evidence in animal experiments makes a causal relationship between tobacco smoking and bladder cancer very plausible.

Hair dyes contain aromatic amines which have been found to be carcinogenic in rodents and have been shown to penetrate the skin.[161] Lead acetate, which is used to darken gray hair, has also been shown to produce tumors in rats and can also be absorbed when used by humans.[161] Elevated risks of bladder cancer have been demonstrated in barbers and hairdressers.[51, 52, 101] However, where an association between personal use of hair dyes and bladder cancer has been sought in case-control studies no elevated risk has been found.[162-164]

It has been suggested that opium addiction might account for the extremely high male/female ratio of bladder cancer observed in southern Iran.[165]

Pharmaceuticals

Chlornaphazine is a naphthylamine mustard first introduced for use in leukemia and lymphoma, but later used to treat polycythemia vera. An association between polycythemia and bladder cancer was subsequently noticed,[166] and chlornaphazine identified as the responsible agent.[167] Bladder cancer has also been reported in patients treated with other alkylating agents—cyclophosphamide[168-171] and azathioprine.[172]

Isoniazid, like many other hydrazine derivatives, has been shown to produce tumors in animals.[138] Two case-control studies[43, 173] have failed to show any significant association between bladder cancer and exposure to isoniazid but the numbers involved were too small to draw definite conclusions. A cohort study of patients treated for tuberculosis with isoniazid also failed to show any excess of bladder cancer.[174]

Phenacetin is an aromatic amine and both the compound itself and one of its metabolites have been shown to be carcinogenic in rodents.[138] Phenacetin is, therefore, the prime suspect in relation to the excess risk of urinary tract tumors found in those abusing analgesic compounds.[175-178] The tumors in such patients are transitional cell carcinomas but are more frequently in the renal pelvis then in the bladder, the reverse of the situation with tumors produced by occupational exposure to aromatic amines. The reason for this is not clear.[13]

In a recent case-control study of bladder cancer in women less than 50 years old, the relative risk of reported heavy use of phenacetin-containing drugs prior to diagnosis was 6.5.[179]

A slight elevation of risk in males for use of aspirin-containing analgesics has also been reported.[53]

Incidence and Mortality in Relation to Etiology

Perusal of Tables 2.10 and 2.11 shows that the agents for which a causal relationship with human bladder cancer can be deemed established are radiation, occupational exposure to aromatic amines, and exposure to one or more of the chemical agents in tobacco smoke. Other agents for which the evidence of a causal relationship is strong, but not yet established, are schistosomal infection, coffee drinking and occupational or medical exposures not necessarily involving aromatic amines.

It is of some interest to consider how far the observed variation in incidence and mortality could be explained by these etiological factors. It must be emphasized, of course, that differences in incidence or mortality between regions or between time periods are affected by many statistical artifacts due to lack of comparability in reporting, access to medical care, diagnostic practice and coding. Overlooking these artifacts we can ask how far the differentials by sex, age, social class, ethnic group, urban/rural residence, marital status, as well as geographic differences and time trends, might be congruent with the findings of etiological studies.

Unfortunately information on the differences in the prevalence of the etiological agents with respect to these demographic and temporal factors is not, in general, precisely known. In some cases proxy indexes can be used, for example the proportion of the work force employed in different industries, or the per capita consumption of tobacco or coffee. Where these have been correlated with geographic differences in incidences or mortality, the results have been in relation to employment in the chemical industry[24, 25] and tobacco consumption[142, 148] but equivocal in relation to coffee consumption.[141, 142]

Changes in incidence and mortality over time have also been shown to be consistent with cohort changes in tobacco consumption.[122, 150, 151] If smoking is the dominant etiological factor, then the male/female ratio in incidence should eventually diminish. Smoking could also explain, at least in part, the observed differences by social class, marital status and ethnic group.

POTENTIAL FOR PREVENTION AND EARLY DETECTION

Although reduction in mortality is not the only goal of a cancer control program it is indubitably the most important. Since mortality is the product of incidence and case-fatality, it follows that these are the two main targets. It is helpful conceptually to express this algebraically, writing M for mortality, I for incidence and F for case fatality: $M = I \times F$.

If we assume for simplicity that the cancer is produced by a causal agent to which each individual is either exposed or not, that the incidence of cancer with or without the factor is I_1 or I_0, and that the proportion of individuals exposed to the agent is P, then $I = PI_1 + (1-P)I_0$.

In similar fashion assume for simplicity that those who develop the cancer fall into two classes, those who present "late" and those who present "early," with corresponding case-fatalities F_1 and F_0, and that the proportion of individuals presenting late is Q, then $F = QF_1 + (1-Q)F_0$. Substituting in the first equation we get: $M = I \times F = [PI_1 + (1-P)I_0] \times [QF_1 + (1-O)F_0] = [PD + I_0] \times [QT + F_0]$ where $D = I_1 - I_0$ = the "risk difference," and, correspondingly, $T = F_1 - F_0$ = the "treatment difference."

It is now apparent that there are four subgoals for cancer control:

1a. Reduce I by reducing P the proportion of the population exposed to risk.
1b. Reduce I by reducing D, the risk difference, by reducing the susceptibility of those exposed.
2a. Reduce F by reducing Q, the proportion of cases treated late.
2b. Reduce F by reducing T, the treatment difference, by improving the prognosis for late cases.

It is not difficult to show that the marginal effects on mortality of these strategies are DF, PF, IT and IQ, respectively. The elasticity for changes in P or D, which equals the proportional reduction in M obtained by reducing P or D, to zero is PDF/M and it is easy to show that this reduces to the formula for the "attributable fraction" given above. In like manner the elasticity for changes in Q or T is IQT/M which might be called the "therapeutic fraction" by analogy.

The attributable fraction (sometimes called the population attributable risk percent, Levin's attributable risk, or the etiologic fraction) is, therefore, the basic measure of the importance of a particular risk factor in a given population. It is not unreasonable to assume that the risk difference is constant between different populations, though this is less likely to be true if there is some other risk factor which may "interact" with the factor in question. If we also assume that risk factor does not influence case-fatality, but only incidence, then the attributable fraction will be directly proportional to P, the prevalence of the risk factor.

The fractions of the incidence of bladder cancer attributable to various factors have been estimated from several case-control studies and these are shown in Table 2.12. These are not completely comparable since some are unweighted estimates based on the prevalence of the factor among the controls, which are usually matched for age with the cases and hence not representative of the population as a whole. However there are some consistencies apparent across the six studies in four developed countries. In particular it is clear that cigarette smoking accounts for more male bladder cancer (39–61%) than any other factor, and smoking is also important in females (26–31%). Analyses of cohort trends in bladder cancer mortality in England and Wales have also indicated that cigarette smoking is the most important factor.[122, 151] In

Table 2.12
Fraction of Bladder Cancer Incidence Attributable to Various Etiological Factors as Estimated from Case-Control Studies

Area	Sex	Percentage attributable to:				
		Cigarette Smoking	Pipe Smoking	Coffee Drinking	High Risk Occupation	Artificial Sweetener Consumption
Eastern Massachusetts[102, 142, 153]	M	39		24	18	
	F	29		49	6	
Canada, 3 Provinces[105]	M	61	12	21	8	7
	F	26		12	1	
Six U.S. Cities[88]	M	48		32[a]	1[a]	
	F	31		6[a]		
Connecticut[146]	M	40[a]		24		
	F	26[a]		25		
Manchester, England[145]	M	43[a]				
Nagoya, Japan[146]	M	40[a]				

[a]Unweighted estimates calculated using the prevalence of the factor among the controls.

one study[151] the estimate of the attributable fraction was 78% for males and 30% for females.

The next most important factor, assuming it is causal, is coffee drinking with attributable fractions ranging from 21–32% in males and 6–49% in females. However, it should be noted that these estimates for coffee drinking are restricted to studies from the United States and Canada.

The fraction of all bladder cancer attributed to high risk occupation is small in these areas. The results of reviews of case histories or death certificates in England and Wales[101, 180, 181] produced estimates of occupational exposure in males ranging from 10–34%.

If two etiological factors are eliminated, it does not follow that the fraction of the disease thus eliminated will equal the sum of the attributable fractions for the two factors. A sufficient condition for this to be true is that the two factors are distributed independently in the population and the risk difference for one factor is the same whether or not the other factor is present. The prevalence of smoking is not independent of coffee drinking or occupation. Recent case-control studies suggest that the risks of smoking and occupation are not additive in men[156] and the risks of smoking and coffee drinking are not additive in women.[88, 146]

Some empirical confirmation of these theoretical results is obtained from a comparison of the incidence of cancer among Mormons and non-Mormon populations in Utah.[182] The incidence of bladder cancer among non-Mormons differed very little from that observed among U.S. whites in the Third National Cancer Survey, but the incidence among Mormons was 26% lower in males and 23% lower in females. Since the Mormon religion proscribes the use of tobacco and coffee, insofar as this proscription is followed these results provide an estimate of the reductions which might be obtained in practice by life-style modification.

The potential reduction in bladder cancer mortality that could be obtained by early detection in the United States can be estimated from published data on survival following treatment.[183] Estimating case fatality as 1—the 5-year survival rate, and taking "early" to be "localized" cases as defined in Reference 183, the values of Q, F_1 and F_0 (see p. 26) for white patients are estimated as 0.18, 0.84 and 0.45, respectively. Hence the theoretical potential reduction in mortality, estimated by the formula $Q(F_1-F_0)/[Q(F_1-F_0) + F_0]$, is 0.13. In other words, 13% of the mortality could be avoided if all patients had the same prognosis as those presenting with localized disease.

Just as the potential reduction in incidence due to eliminating a risk factor is meaningful only if (1) the factor is truly causal, and (2) elimination of exposure is practicable, so the potential reduction in mortality due to detecting all cases in an early stage is meaningful only if (1) diagnosis in the presymptomatic stage improves prognosis, and (2) a safe, acceptable and efficient method of early detection exists. The only conclusive evidence for the effectiveness of early detection in reducing mortality is obtained from a randomized controlled trial. Although a noninvasive screening test for bladder cancer is provided by urinary cytology, no controlled trials of its effectiveness have been reported. Even if the value of early detection is taken for granted, the efficiency of screening the general population for bladder cancer is doubtful.[184] On the initial screening of a population with a perfectly sensitive test, the number of cases detected will be, on average, the yearly incidence multiplied by the mean duration of detectable disease. The utility of this must be weighed against the disutility of screening the population and the unnecessary investigation of false-positive results. No accurate estimates of the mean duration of the detectable presymptomatic stage of bladder cancer have been made, but from the experience of screening an industrial population[185] it would appear that the mean duration is less than 1 year. Thus the prevalence of the disease in the general population in the age group being screened is likely to be of the order of 10–30/100,000. With a false negative rate of about 12%[185] the detection rate in a single screening will be approximately 1/4,000 to 1/11,000. These estimates are consistent with the results of screening hospital patients without urinary symptoms in which 6500 patients were screened without detecting any cancer.[184]

Screening of workers in high risk industries has been used for several decades[184-186] and there has been some evidence of increased survival compared with other patients, but no formal controlled study of mortality in screened and unscreened groups has been reported.

SUMMARY AND CONCLUSIONS

The incidence of bladder cancer, primarily transitional cell carcinoma, varies considerably both between and within countries, increases with age, is about 4 times higher in males than females, and is generally increasing with time at an average annual rate of 3%. Mortality rates from cancer of the bladder vary between one-third and one-half of incidence rates and are increasing at a smaller rate than incidence, 2%/year in males and 1% in females. Incidence and mortality rates among migrant groups show some change towards the rates of the host country.

The results of epidemiological studies have established that radiation, occupational exposure to aromatic amines, and exposure to one or more of the chemical agents in tobacco smoke are causally related to cancer of the bladder. There is strong evidence, also, that associations with schistosomal infection, coffee drinking and other occupational or medical exposures may be causal. Differences in occupation or tobacco smoking can explain, at least in part, the observed demographic, geographic and temporal differentials in incidence and mortality. The quantitative results of epidemiological studies, primarily in North America, indicate that about one-half of the incidence of bladder cancer in males, and about one-quarter of that in females is attributable to cigarette smoking, the proportion attributable to occupation is much less and is more variable. If the association of bladder cancer with coffee-drinking is causal then this could account for about one-quarter of the incidence of the disease.

Based on the difference in survival between patients treated for localized disease and patients treated for more advanced disease, and on the proportions of patients so treated, it can be estimated that a reduction of 13% in mortality could be achieved by early detection. However, no controlled trials of the effectiveness of screening have been undertaken. Nonexperimental studies of cytological screening of industrial populations at high risk suggest an increase in survival but no formal trials have been reported.

From the epidemiological perspective, further research is required in the following areas:

1. Determination of the agents in tobacco smoke which cause bladder cancer.
2. Clarification of the role of schistosomiasis, coffee-drinking and some industrial exposures, and isolation of the agents involved.
3. Information on the interaction between different etiological agents and their prevalence in different regions and population subgroups.
4. Controlled trials of the effectiveness of cytological screening in high risk groups.

Acknowledgements. I thank Brenda Sykes, Diane Harding and Ladislav Ferenczi for their help in preparing this review, and the Alberta Cancer Board for granting me study leave to write it.

REFERENCES

1. Lower, G. M. Concepts in causality: chemically induced human urinary bladder cancer. *Cancer 49*:1056–1066, 1982.
2. Hicks, R. M. Multistage carcinogenesis in the urinary bladder. *Br. Med. Bull. 36*:39–46, 1980.
3. Friedell, G. H., Greenfield, R. E., Hilgar, A. G., and Ellwein, L. B. Overview of the national bladder cancer project and conference objectives. *Cancer Res. 37*:2745–2751, 1977.
4. Last, J. M. (ed) *A Dictionary of Epidemiology.* Oxford University Press, New York, 1983.
5. Sackett, D. L. Bias in analytic research. *J. Chron. Dis. 32*:51–63, 1979.
6. Hill, A. B. The environment and disease: association or causation. *Proc. R. Soc. Med. 58*:295–300, 1965.
7. Segi, M., Hattori, H., and Segi, R. *Age-Adjusted Death Rates for Selected Sites (A-Classification) in 46 Countries in 1975.* Segi Institute of Cancer Epidemiology, Nagoya, 1980.

8. Walters, S. D. The estimation and interpretation of attributable risk in health research. *Biometrics 32:*829–849, 1976.
9. Hill, G. B., Romeder, J. M. Calcul en prévention: un modéle pour la planification de programmes de santé communautaire. In *Systems Science in Health Care*, edited by C. Tilquin. Pergamon, Oxford, 1981.
10. Oyasu, Y., and Hopp, M. L. The etiology of cancer of the bladder. *Surg. Gynecol. Obstet. 138:*97–108, 1974.
11. Morrison, A. S., and Cole, P. Epidemiology of bladder cancer. *Urol. Clin. North. Am. 3:*13–29, 1976.
12. Parkes, H. G. The epidemiology of the aromatic amine cancers. In *Chemical Carcinogens*, edited by C. E. Searle. American Chemical Society, Washington D.C., 1976.
13. Matanoski, G. M., and Elliott, E. A. Bladder cancer epidemiology. *Epidemiol. Rev. 3:*203–229, 1981.
14. Morrison, A. S., and Cole, P. Urinary Tract. In *Cancer Epidemiology and Prevention*, edited by D. Schottenfeld and J. F. Fraumeni, Jr. Saunders, Philadelphia, 1982.
15. Cook, P., Doll, R., and Fellingham, S. A. A mathematical model for the age distribution of cancer in man. *Int. J. Cancer 4:*93–112, 1969.
16. Doll, R. Age. In *Host Environment Interactions in the Etiology of Cancer in Man*, edited by R. Doll, and I. Vodopija. International Agency for Research on Cancer, Lyon, 1973.
17. Waterhouse, J., Muir, C., Shanmugaratnam, K., and Powell, J. *Cancer Incidence in Five Continents*, Vol. 4. International Agency for Research on Cancer, Lyon, 1982.
18. Staszewski, J. Cancer of the urinary bladder: international mortality patterns and trends. *World Health Stat. Quart. 33:*27–41, 1980.
19. Doll, R., Muir, C., and Waterhouse, J. *Cancer Incidence in Five Continents*, Vol. 2. Springer-Verlag, Berlin, 1970.
20. Waterhouse, J., Muir, C., Correa, P., and Powell, J. *Cancer Incidence in Five Continents*, Vol. 3. International Agency for Research on Cancer, Lyon, 1976.
21. Registrar General. Statistical review of England and Wales for the two years 1966–1967, supplement on cancer. Her Majesty's Stationery Office, London, 1972.
22. Mason, T. J., McKay, F. W., Hoover, R., Blot, W. J., and Fraumeni, J. F. *Atlas of Cancer Mortality for U.S. Counties 1950–1969*. U.S. Department of Health, Education and Welfare, Washington D.C., 1975.
23. Health and Welfare Canada, Statistics Canada. *Mortality Atlas of Canada*, Vol. 1, *Cancer*. Minister of Supply and Services Canada, Hull, Quebec, 1980.
24. Hoover, R., and Fraumeni, J. F. Cancer mortality in U.S. Counties with chemical industries. *Environ. Res. 9:*196–207, 1975.
25. Blot, W. J., and Fraumeni, J. F., Jr. Geographic patterns of bladder cancer in the United States. *J. Natl. Cancer Inst. 61:*1017–1023, 1978.
26. Steinitz, R., and Costin, C. Cancer in Jewish immigrants. *Israel J. Med. Sci. 7:*1413–1436, 1971.
27. Lilienfeld, A. M., Levin, M. L., and Kessler, I. I. *Cancer in the United States.* Harvard University Press, Cambridge, Mass., 1972.
28. Billette, A., Dewar, R., Hill, G., Nagnur, D., Silins, J., and Smith, M. Cancer mortality in Canada by place of birth. (To be published).
29. Logan, W. P. D. Cancer mortality by occupation and social class 1851–1971. Her Majesty's Stationery Office, London, and International Agency for Research on Cancer, Lyon, 1982.
30. Registrar General. Statistical Review of England and Wales for the Year 1967. Part III. Commentary. Her Majesty's Stationery Office, London, 1971.
31. Devesa, S. S., and Silverman, D. T. Cancer incidence and mortality trends in the United States: 1935–74. *J. Natl. Cancer Inst. 60:*545–571, 1978.
32. Frost, W. H. Age selection of mortality from tuberculosis in successive decades. *Am. J. Hyg. 30:*91–96, 1939.
33. Case, R. A. M. Cohort analysis of mortality rates as a historical or narrative technique. *Br. J. Prev. Soc. Med. 10:*151–171, 1956.
34. Osmond, C., Gardner, M. J., and Acheson, E. D. Analysis of trends in cancer mortality in England and Wales during 1951–1980 separating changes associated with period of birth and period of death. *Br. Med. J. 284:*1005–1008, 1982.
35. Tulinius, H. Frequency of some morphological types of neoplasm of five sites. In

Cancer Incidence in Five Continents, Vol. 2, edited by R. Doll, C. Muir, and J. Waterhouse. Springer-Verlag, Berlin, 1970.

36. Shanmuguratnam, K., and Powell, J. Special study on histomorphological types of cancer. In *Cancer Incidence in Five Continents*, Vol. 4, edited by J. Waterhouse, C. Muir, K. Shanmuguratnam, and J. Powell. International Agency for Research on Cancer, Lyon, 1982.

37. Mulvihill, J. J. Congenital and genetic diseases. In *Persons at High Risk of Cancer. An Approach to Cancer Etiology and Control*, edited by J. F. Fraumeni, Jr. Academic Press, New York, 1975.

38. Sandberg, A. A. Chromosome studies in bladder cancer. In *Carcinoma of the Bladder*, edited by J. G. Connolly. Raven Press, New York, 1981.

39. Fraumeni, J. F., and Thomas, L. B. Malignant bladder tumors in a man and his three sons. *JAMA 201:*507–509, 1967.

40. McCullough, D. L., Lamon, D. L., McLaughlin, A. P., and Gittes, R. F. Familial transitional cell carcinoma of the bladder. *J. Urol. 113:*629–635, 1975.

41. Lynch, H. T., and Walzak, M. P. Genetics in urogenital cancer. *Urol. Clin. N. Am. 7:*815–829, 1980.

42. Herring, D. W., Cartwright, R. A., and Williams, D. D. R. Genetic associations of transitional cell carcinoma. *Br. J. Urol. 51:*73–77, 1979.

43. Miller, C. T., Neutel, C. I., Nair, R. C., *et al.* Relative importance of risk factors in bladder carcinogenesis. *J. Chron. Dis. 31:*51–56, 1978.

44. Pang, A. S. D., and Morales, A. Immunoprophylaxis of a murine bladder cancer with high dose BCG immunizations. *J. Urol. 127:*1006–1009, 1982.

45. Kersey, J. H., and Spector, B. D. Immune deficiency diseases. In *Persons at High Risk of Cancer. An Approach to Cancer Etiology and Control*, edited by J. F. Fraumeni, Jr. Academic Press, New York, 1975.

46. Kinlen, L. J. Immunologic factors. In *Persons at High Risk of Cancer. An Approach to Cancer Etiology and Control*, edited by J. F. Fraumeni, Jr. Academic Press, New York, 1975.

47. Elliott, A. Y., Frayley, E. E., Castro, A. E., *et al.* Isolation of an RNA virus from transitional cell tumors of the human urinary bladder. *Surgery 74:*46–50, 1973.

48. Shah, K. V. Investigation of human malignant tumors in India for simian virus 40 etiology. *J. Natl. Cancer Inst. 42:*139–145, 1969.

49. Shah, K. V., Palma, L. D., and Murphy, G. P. The occurrrence of SV 40-neutralizing antibodies in sera of patients with genitourinary carcinoma. *J. Surg. Oncol. 3:*443–450, 1971.

50. Gardner, S. D. Prevalence in England of antibody to human polyomavirus (BK). *Br. Med. J. 1:*77–78, 1973.

51. Wynder, E. L., Onderdonk, J., and Mantel, N. An epidemiological investigation of cancer of the bladder. *Cancer 16:*1388–1407, 1963.

52. Dunham, L. J., Rabson, A. S., Stewart, H. L., Frank, A. S., and Young, J. L., Jr. Rates, interview and pathology study of cancer of the urinary bladder in New Orleans, Louisiana. *J. Natl. Cancer Inst. 41:*683–709, 1968.

53. Howe, G. R. An epidemiologic study of bladder cancer. In *Carcinoma of the Bladder*, edited by J. G. Connolly. Raven Press, New York, 1981.

54. Melzack, J. The incidence of bladder cancer in paraplegia. *Paraplegia 4:*85–96, 1966.

55. Davies, J. M. Two aspects of the epidemiology of bladder cancer in England and Wales. *Proc. R. Soc. Med. 70:*411–413, 1977.

56. Hicks, R. M., Walters, C. L., Elsebai, I., *et al.* Demonstration of nitrosamines in human urine: preliminary observations on a possible etiology for bladder cancer in association with chronic urinary tract infections. *Proc. R. Soc. Med. 70:*413–417, 1977.

57. Radomski, J. L., Greenwald, D., Hearn, W. L., Block, N. L., and Woods, F. M. Nitrosamine formation in bladder infections and its role in the etiology of bladder cancer. *J. Urol. 120:*48–50, 1982.

58. Burton, G. J. Parasites. In *Cancer Epidemiology and Prevention*, edited by D. Schottenfeld, and J. F. Fraumeni, Jr. Saunders, Philadelphia, 1982.

59. Mustacchi, P., and Shimkin, M. B. Cancer of the bladder and infestation with Schistosoma haematobium. *J. Natl. Cancer Inst. 20:*825–842, 1958.

60. Gelfand, M. Weinberg, R. W., and Castle, W. M. Relation between carcinoma of the bladder and infestation with *Schistosoma haematobium. Lancet 1:*1249–1251,

1967.

61. Hinder, R. A., and Schmaman, A. Bilharziasis and squamous carcinoma of the bladder. *S. Afr. Med. J. 43:*617–618, 1969.

62. El-Boulkany, M. N., Ghoneim, M. A., and Mansour, M. A. Carcinoma of the bilharzial bladder in Egypt: clinical and pathological features. *Br. J. Urol. 44:*561–570, 1972.

63. Kuntz, R. E., Cheever, A. W., and Myers, B. J. Proliferative epithelial lesions of the urinary bladder of nonhuman primates infected with *Schistosoma haematobium. J. Natl. Cancer Inst. 48:*223–245, 1972.

64. Laughlin, L. W., Farid, Z., Mansour, N., *et al.* Bacteriuria in urinary schistosomiasis in Egypt. A prevalence survey. *Am. J. Trop. Med. Hyg. 27:*916–918, 1978.

65. Hicks, R. M., Ismail, M. M., Walters, C. L., *et al.* Association of bacteriuria and urinary nitrosamine formation with *Schistosoma haematobium* infection in the Qalyub area of Egypt. *Trans. R. Soc. Trop. Med. Hyg. 76:*519, 1982.

66. Hicks, R. M. The canopic worm: role of bilharziasis in the aetiology of human bladder cancer. *J. R. Soc. Med. 76:*16–22, 1983.

67. Armstrong, B. K., McMichael, A. J., and MacLennan, R. Diet. In *Cancer Epidemiology and Prevention*, edited by D. Schottenfeld, and J. F. Fraumeni, Jr. Saunders, Philadelphia, 1982.

68. Mettlin, C., and Graham, S. Dietary risk factors in human bladder cancer. *Am. J. Epidemiol. 110:*255–263, 1979.

69. Dunning, W. F., Curtis, M. R., and Maun, M. E. The effect of added dietary tryptophan on the occurrence of 2-acetylaminofluorene-induced liver and bladder cancer in rats. *Cancer Res. 10:*454–459, 1950.

70. Cohen, S. M., Arai, M., Jacobs, J. B., and Friedell, G. H. Promoting effect of saccharin and DL-tryptophan in urinary bladder carcinogenesis. *Cancer Res. 39:*1207–1217, 1979.

71. Brown, R. R., Price, J. M., Satter, E. J., and Wear, J. B. The metabolism of tryptophan in patients with bladder cancer. *Acta Univ. Int. Cancer 16:*299–303, 1960.

72. Boyland, E., and Williams, D. C. The metabolism of tryptophan-II the metabolism of tryptophan in patients suffering from cancer of the bladder. *Biochem. J. 64:*578–582, 1956.

73. Nicolor, I. G., Chernozemsky, I. N., Petkova-Bocharova, T., *et al.* Epidemiologic characteristics of urinary system tumors and Balkan nephropathy in an endemic region of Bulgaria. *Eur. J. Cancer 14:*1237–1242, 1978.

74. Boice, J. D., Land, C. E. Ionizing radiation. In *Cancer Epidemiology and Prevention*, edited by D. Schottenfeld and J. F. Fraumeni, Jr. Saunders, Philadelphia, 1982.

75. Beebe, G. W., Land, C. E., and Kato, H. Studies of the mortality of A-bomb survivors. 6. Mortality and radiation dose, 1950–1974. *Radiat. Res. 75:*138–201, 1978.

76. Dickson, R. J. Late results of radium treatment of carcinoma of the cervix. *Clin. Radiol. 23:*528–535, 1972.

77. Reimer, R. R., Hoover, R., Fraumeni, J. F., Jr., and Young, R. C. Second neoplasms following ovarian cancer. *J. Natl. Cancer Inst. 61:*1195–1197, 1978.

78. Palmer, J. P., and Spratt, D. W. Pelvic carcinoma following irradiation of benign gynecologic diseases. *Am. J. Obstet. Gynecol. 72:*497–505, 1956.

79. Smith, P., and Doll, R. Late effects of X-irradiation in patients treated for metropathia hemorrhagica. *Br. J. Radiol. 49:*224–232, 1976.

80. Hueper, W. C. *Occupational and Environmental Cancer of the Urinary System.* Yale University Press, New Haven, 1969.

81. Oyasu, R., Kitajima, T., Hopp, M. L., and Sumie, H. Induction of bladder cancer in hamsters by repeated intratracheal administration of 2-acetylaminofluorene. *J. Natl. Cancer Inst. 50:*503–506, 1973.

82. Wynder, E. L., and Hoffman, D. Tobacco. In *Cancer Epidemiology and Prevention*, edited by D. Schottenfeld, and J. F. Fraumeni, Jr. Saunders, Philadelphia, 1982.

83. Winkelstein, W., Jr. Smoking and cancer of the cervix. *Br. J. Cancer 43:*736–737, 1981.

84. Kuratsumie, M., and Hueper, W. C. Polycyclic aromatic hydrocarbons in coffee soots. *J. Natl. Cancer Inst. 20:*37–51, 1958.

85. Hueper, W. C., and Payne, W. W. Carcinogenic studies on soot of coffee-roasting

plants. *Arch. Pathol. 69*:716–727, 1960.

86. Shy, C. M., and Struba, R. J. Air and water pollution. In *Cancer Epidemiology and Prevention*, edited by D. Schottenfeld, and J. F. Fraumeni, Jr. Saunders, Philadelphia, 1982.

87. Tola, S. Occupational cancer of the urinary bladder. In *Occupational Cancer and Carcinogenesis*, edited by H. Vainio, M. Sorsa, and K. Hemminki. Hemisphere Publishing Corporation, Washington, 1981.

88. Wynder, E. L., and Goldsmith, R. The epidemiology of bladder cancer. A second look. *Cancer 40*:1246–1268, 1977.

89. Clayson, D. B. Recent research into occupational bladder cancer. In *Carcinoma of the Bladder*, edited by J. G. Connolly. Raven Press, New York, 1981.

90. Case, R. A. M., Hosker, M. E., McDonald, M. B., *et al.* Tumours of the urinary bladder in workmen engaged in the manufacture and use of certain dyestuff intermediates in the British chemical industry. *Br. J. Indust. Med. 11*:75–104, 213–216, 1954.

91. Rehn, L. Blasengeschwulste bei Fuchsin-Arbeitern. *Arch. Klin. Chir. 50*:588–600, 1895.

92. Heuper, W. C. "Aniline tumors" of the bladder. *Arch. Pathol. 25*:858–899, 1938.

93. Case, R. A. M., and Hosker, M. E. Tumour of the urinary bladder as an occupational disease in the rubber industry in England and Wales. *Br. J. Prev. Soc. Med. 8*:39–50, 1954.

94. Davies, J. M. Bladder tumours in the electric-cable industry. *Lancet 2*:143–146, 1965.

95. Fox, A. J., Lindars, D. C., and Owen, R. A survey of occupational cancer in the rubber and cablemaking industries: Results of five-year analysis, 1967–1971. *Br. J. Ind. Med. 31*:140–151, 1974.

96. McMichael, A. J., Spirtas, R., Gable, J. F., *et al.* Mortality among rubber workers; relationship to specific jobs. *J. Occup. Med. 18*:178–185, 1976.

97. Monson, R. R., and Nakano, K. K. Mortality among rubber workers. I. White male union employees in Akron, Ohio. *Am. J. Epidemiol. 103*:284–296, 1976.

98. Doll, R., Fisher, R. E. W., Gammon, E. J., *et al.* Mortality of gasworkers with special reference to cancers of the lung and bladder, chronic bronchitis, and pneumoconiosis. *Br. J. Ind. Med. 22*:1–12, 1965.

99. Doll, R., Vessey, M. P., Bearsley, R. W. R., *et al.* Mortality of gasworkers—final report of a prospective study. *Br. J. Ind. Med. 29*:394–406, 1972.

100. Lockwood, K. On the etiology of bladder tumors in Kobenhavn-Frederiksberg: an inquiry of 369 patients and 369 controls. *Acta. Pathol. Microbiol. Scand. 51*(Suppl. 145):1–166, 1961.

101. Anthony, H. M., and Thomas, G. M. Tumors of the urinary bladder: an analysis of the occupations of 1030 patients in Leeds, England. *J. Natl. Cancer Inst. 45*:879–895, 1970.

102. Cole, P., Hoover, R., and Friedell, G. H. Occupation and cancer of the lower urinary tract. *Cancer 29*:1250–1260, 1972.

103. Checkoway, H., Arp, E., Holbrook, R. H. *et al.* A case-control study of bladder cancer in the rubber industry (meeting abstract). *Am. J. Epidemiol. 106*:243, 1977.

104. Miller, A. B. The etiology of bladder cancer from the epidemiological viewpoint. *Cancer Res. 37*:2939–2942, 1977.

105. Howe, G. R., Burch, J. D., Miller, A. B., *et al.* Tobacco use, occupation, coffee, various nutrients and bladder cancer. *J. Natl. Cancer Inst. 64*:701–713, 1980.

106. Chapman, J. A., Connolly, J. G., and Rosenbaum, L. Occupational bladder cancer: a case-control study. In *Carcinoma of the Bladder*, edited by J. G. Connolly. Raven Press, New York, 1981.

107. Sullivan, J. W. Epidemiologic survey of bladder cancer in Greater New Orleans. *J. Urol. 128*:281–283, 1982.

108. Silverman, D. T., Hoover, R. N., Albert, S., and Graff, K. M. Occupation and cancer of the lower urinary tract in Detroit. *J. Natl. Cancer Inst. 70*:237–245, 1983.

109. Wigle, D. T. Bladder cancer: possible new high risk occupation. *Lancet 2*:83–84, 1977.

110. Morgan, R. W., and Jain, M. G. Bladder cancer: smoking, beverages and artificial sweeteners. *Can. Med. Assoc. J. 110*:1067–1070, 1974.

111. Tyrell, A. B., McCaughey, W. T. E., and MacAirt, J. G. Occupational and nonoc-

cupational factors associated with vesical neoplasm in Ireland. *J. Irish Med. Assoc. 64*:213–217, 1971.

112. DeCoufle, P. Cancer risks associated with employment in the leather and leather products industry. *Arch. Environ. Health 34*:33–37, 1979.

113. Pamukcu, A. M., Goksoy, S. K., and Price, J. M. Urinary bladder neoplasms induced by feeding bracken fern (*Pteris aquilina*) to cows. *Cancer Res. 27*:917–924, 1967.

114. Pamukcu, A. M., and Price, J. M. Induction of intestinal and urinary bladder cancer in rats by feeding bracken fern (*Pteris aquilina*). *J. Natl. Cancer Inst. 43*:275–281, 1969.

115. Hirono, I., Shilbuya, C., Fushimi, K., *et al.* Studies on carcinogenic properties of bracken *Pteridium aquilinum. J. Natl. Cancer Inst. 45*:179–188, 1970.

116. Evans, I. A., and Osman, M. A. Carcinogenicity of bracken and shikimic acid. *Nature 250*:348–349, 1974.

117. Armstrong, B., and Doll, R. Environmental factors and cancer incidence and mortality in different countries with special reference to dietary practices. *Intl. J. Cancer 15*:617–631, 1975.

118. Howe, G. R., and Chapman, J. A. W. Artificial sweeteners and human bladder cancer: a review of the epidemiologic evidence. In *Carcinoma of the Bladder*, edited by J. G. Connolly. Raven Press, New York, 1981.

119. Grice, H. C., Clegg, D. J., Coffin, D. E., *et al.* Carcinogens in foods. In *Carcinogens in Industry and the Environment*, edited by J. M. Sontag. Marcel Dekker, New York, 1981.

120. Hicks, R. M. Carcinogenesis in the urinary bladder: a multistage process. In *Carcinoma of the Bladder*, edited by J. G. Connolly. Raven Press, New York, 1981.

121. Burbank, F., Fraumeni, J. F., Jr. Synthetic sweetener consumption and bladder cancer trends in the United States. *Nature 227*:296–297, 1970.

122. Armstrong, B., and Doll, R. Bladder cancer mortality in England and Wales in relation to cigarette smoking and saccharin consumption. *Br. J. Prev. Soc. Med. 28*:233–240, 1974.

123. Kessler, I. I. Cancer mortality among diabetics. *J. Natl. Cancer Inst. 44*:673–686, 1970.

124. Armstrong, B., Lea, A. J., Adelstein, A. M., *et al.* Cancer mortality and saccharin consumption in diabetics. *Br. J. Prev. Soc. Med. 30*:151–157, 1976.

125. Armstrong, B., and Doll, R. Bladder cancer mortality in diabetics in relation to saccharin consumption and smoking habits. *Br. J. Prev. Soc. Med. 29*:73–81, 1975.

126. Simon, D., Yen, S., and Cole, P. Coffee drinking and cancer of the lower urinary tract. *J. Natl. Cancer Inst. 54*:587–591, 1975.

127. Kessler, I. I., and Clark, J. P. Saccharin, cyclamate and human bladder cancer. *J. Am. Med. Assoc. 240*:349–355, 1978.

128. Howe, G. R., Burch, J. D., Miller, A. B., *et al.* Artificial sweeteners and human bladder cancer. *Lancet 2*:578–581, 1977.

129. Wynder, E. L., and Stellman, S. D. Artificial sweetener use and bladder cancer: a case-control study. *Science 207*:1214–1216, 1980.

130. Morrison, A. S., and Buring, J. E. Artificial sweeteners and cancer of the lower urinary tract. *N. Engl. J. Med. 302*:537–541, 1980.

131. Connolly, J. G., Rider, W. D., Rosenbaum, L., and Chapman, J. A. W. Relation between the use of artificial sweeteners and bladder cancer. *Can. Med. Assoc. J. 119*:408, 1978.

132. Hoover, R. N., and Strasser, P. H. Artificial sweeteners and human bladder cancer. Preliminary results. *Lancet 1*:837–840, 1980.

133. Cartwright, R. A., Adib, R., Glashen, R., *et al.* The epidemiology of bladder cancer in West Yorkshire. A preliminary report on nonoccupational aetiologies. *Carcinogenesis 2*:343–347, 1981.

134. Morrison, A. S., Verhock, W. G., Leck, I., *et al.* Artificial sweeteners and bladder cancer in Manchester, U.K. and Nagoya, Japan. *Br. J. Cancer 45*:332–336, 1982.

135. Mantel, N., and Haenszel, W. Statistical aspects of the analysis of data from retrospective studies of disease. *J. Natl. Cancer Inst. 22*:719–748, 1959.

136. Wynder, E. L., and Stellman, S. D. Environmental factors in the causation of bladder cancer. In *Carcinoma of the Bladder*, edited by J. G. Connolly. Raven Press, New York, 1981.

137. Williams, R. R., and Horm, J. W. Association of cancer sites with tobacco and

alcohol consumption and socioeconomic status of patients: interview study from the third national cancer survey. *J. Natl. Cancer Inst. 58:*525–547, 1977.

138. Clayson, D. B. Therapeutic agents and procedures in cancer induction. In *Carcinogens in Industry and the Environment*, edited by J. M. Sontag. Marcel Dekker, New York, 1981.
139. Berg, J. W. Diet. In *Persons at High Risk of Cancer. An Approach to Cancer Etiology and Control*, edited by J. F. Fraumeni, Jr. Academic Press, New York, 1975.
140. Cole, P. Coffee-drinking and cancer of the lower urinary tract. *Lancet 1:*1335–1337, 1971.
141. Stocks, P. Cancer mortality in relation to national consumption of cigarettes, solid fuel, tea and coffee. *Br. J. Cancer 24:*215–225, 1970.
142. Morrison, A. S. Geographic and time trends of coffee imports and bladder cancer. *Eur. J. Cancer 14:*51–54, 1978.
143. Fraumeni, J. F., Jr., Scotto, J., and Dunham, L. F. Coffee-drinking and bladder cancer. *Lancet 2:*1204, 1971.
144. Bross, I. D. J., and Tidings, J. Another look at coffee-drinking and cancer of the urinary bladder. *Prev. Med. 2:*445–451, 1973.
145. Morrison, A. S., Buring, J. E., Verhock, W. G., *et al.* Coffee drinking and cancer of the lower urinary tract. *J. Natl. Cancer Inst. 68:*91–94, 1982.
146. Marrett, L. D., Walter, S. D., and Meigs, J. M. Coffee drinking and bladder cancer in Connecticut. *Am. J. Epidemiol. 117:*113–127, 1983.
147. Weinberg, D. M., Ross, R. K., Mack, T. M., *et al.* Bladder cancer etiology. A different perspective. *Cancer 51:*675–680, 1983.
148. Fraumeni, J. F., Jr. Cigarette smoking and cancers of the urinary tract: geographic variation in the United States. *J. Natl. Cancer Inst. 41:*1205–1211, 1968.
149. Lea, A. J. Cigarette smoking and cancer of the lungs and bladder. *Lancet 1:*590–591, 1966.
150. Hoover, R., and Cole, P. Population trends in cigarette smoking and bladder cancer. *Am. J. Epidemiol. 94:*409–418, 1971.
151. Stevens, R. G., and Moolgavkar, S. H. Estimation of relative risk from vital data: smoking and cancers of the lung and bladder. *J. Natl. Cancer Inst. 63:*1351–1357, 1979.
152. Lilienfeld, A. M., Levin, A. J., and Moore, G. E. The association of smoking with cancer of the urinary bladder in humans. *Arch. Intern. Med. 98:*129–135, 1956.
153. Cole, P., Monson, R. R., and Haning, H. Smoking and cancer of the lower urinary tract. *N. Engl. J. Med. 284:*129–134, 1971.
154. Schwartz, D., Flamant, R., Lellouch, J., *et al.* Results of a French survey on the role of tobacco, particularly inhalation, in different cancer sites. *J. Natl. Cancer Inst. 26:*1085–1108, 1961.
155. Staszewski, J. Smoking and cancer in Poland. *Br. J. Cancer 14:*419–436, 1960.
156. Vineis, P., Segman, N., Costa, G., and Terracini, B. Evidence of a multiplicative effect between cigarette smoking and occupational exposures in the aetiology of bladder cancer. *Cancer Lett. 14:*285–290, 1981.
157. Hammond, E. C. Smoking in relation to death rates of one million men and women. In *Epidemiological Approaches to the Study of Cancer and Other Chronic Diseases. National Cancer Institute Monograph No. 19*, edited by W. Haenszel. Department of Health, Education and Welfare, Washington, 1966.
158. Kahn, H. A. The Dorn study of smoking and mortality among U.S. Veterans: report on eight and one-half years of observation. In *Epidemiological Approaches to the Study of Cancer and Other Chronic Diseases. National Cancer Institute Monograph No. 19*, edited by W. Haenszel. Department of Health, Education and Welfare, Washington, 1966.
159. Weir, J. M., and Dunn, J. E., Jr. Smoking and mortality: a prospective study. *Cancer 25:*105–112, 1970.
160. Doll, R., and Peto, R. Mortality in relation to smoking: 20 years observation on male British doctors. *Br. Med. J. 2:*1525–1536, 1976.
161. Marzulli, F. N., and Weisburger, E. K. Cosmetics. In *Carcinogens in Industry and the Environment*, edited by J. M. Sontag. Marcel Dekker, New York, 1981.
162. Jain, M., Morgan, R. W., and Elinson, L. Hair dyes and bladder cancer. *Can. Med. Assoc. J. 117:*1131–1132, 1977.
163. Neutel, C. I., Nair, R. C., and Last, J. M. Are hair dyes associated with bladder

cancer? *Can. Med. Assoc. J. 119:*307–308, 1978.

164. Hennekens, Ch., Speizer, F. E., Rosner, B., *et al.* Use of permanent hair dyes and cancer among registered nurses. *Lancet 1:*1390–1393, 1979.
165. Sadeghi, A., and Behmard, S. Cancer of the bladder in southern Iran. *Cancer 42:*353–356, 1978.
166. Videback, A. Polycythaemia vera, course and prognosis. *Acta. Med. Scand. 138:*179–187, 1950.
167. Thiede, T., Chievitz, E., and Christensen, B. C. Chlornaphazine as a bladder carcinogen. *Acta. Med. Scand. 175:*721–725, 1964.
168. Pearson, R., and Solway, M. S. Does cyclophosphamide induce bladder cancer? *Urology 11:*437–447, 1978.
169. Seltzer, S. E., Benazzi, R. B., and Kearney, G. P. Cyclophosphamide and carcinoma of the bladder. *Urology 11:*352–356, 1978.
170. Plotz, P. H., Klippel, J. H., Decker, J. L., *et al.* Bladder complications in patients receiving cyclophosphamide for systemic lupus erythematosus or rheumatoid arthritis. *Ann. Intern. Med. 91:*221–223, 1979.
171. Fairchild, W. V., Spence, C. R., Solomon, H. D., *et al.* The incidence of bladder cancer after cyclophosphamide therapy. *J. Urol. 122:*163–164, 1979.
172. Scharf, J., Nahir, M., Eidelman, S., *et al.* Carcinoma of the bladder with azothiaprine therapy. *JAMA 237:*152, 1977.
173. Glassroth, J. L., Snider, D. E., and Conistock, G. W. Urinary tract cancer and isoniazid. *Am. Rev. Resp. Dis. 116:*331–333, 1977.
174. Howe, G. R., Lindsay, J., Coppock, E., and Miller, A. B. Isoniazid exposure in relation to cancer incidence and mortality in a cohort of tuberculosis patients. *Int. J. Epidemiol. 8:*305–312, 1979.
175. Angervall, L., Bengtsson, U., Zetterlund, C. G., and Zsigmond, M. Renal pelvic carcinoma in a Swedish district with abuse of phenacetin-containing drug. *Br. J. Urol. 41:*401–405, 1969.
176. Kung, L. G. Hypernephroides Karzinom und Karzinom der arbeitenden harnwege nach Phenacetin-abusus. *Schweiz Med. Wochenschr. 106:*47–51, 1976.
177. Johansson, S., and Wahlgvist, L. Tumours of urinary bladder and ureter associated with abuse of phenacetin-containing analgesics. *Acta. Pathol. Microbiol. Scand. 85:*768–774, 1977.
178. Mahoney, J. F., Storey, B. G., Ibanez, R. C., and Stewart, J. H. Analgesic abuse, renal parenchymal disease and carcinoma of the kidney or ureter. *Aust-NZ J. Med. 7:*463–469, 1977.
179. Piper, J., and Matanoski, G. Bladder cancer in young women (meeting abstract). *Am. J. Epidemiol. 118:*440, 1983.
180. Veys, C. A. Two epidemiological inquiries into the incidence of bladder tumors in industrial workers. *J. Natl. Cancer Inst. 43:*219–226, 1969.
181. Davies, J. M., Somerville, M., and Wallace, D. M. Occupational bladder tumour cases identified during ten years' interviewing of patients. *Br. J. Urol. 48:*561–566, 1976.
182. Lyon, J. L., Klauber, M. R., Gardner, J. W., and Smart, C. R. Cancer incidence in Mormons and non-Mormons in Utah 1966–70. *N. Engl. J. Med. 294:*129–133, 1976.
183. Axtell, L. M., Asire, A. J., and Myers, M. H. *Cancer Patient Survival.* Department of Health Education and Welfare, Washington, 1976.
184. Trott, P. A. Cytological screening for cancer of the bladder. *Proc. R. Soc. Med. 69:*496–498, 1976.
185. Parkes, H. G. Occupational bladder cancer. *Practitioner 214:*80–86, 1975.
186. Cartwright, R. A., Gadian, T., Garland, J. B., and Bernard, S. M. The influence of malignant cell cytology screening on the survival of industrial bladder cancer cases. *J. Epidemiol. Community Health 35:*35–38, 1981.

3

Carcinogenesis—
A Multistage Process

R. Marian Hicks, Ph.D., D.Sc., F.R.C.Path.

The possibility that carcinogenesis could involve a stepwise, multi-stage process in any tissue other than the mouse skin, has only very recently gained credence. There has been a natural reluctance to abandon the simple cause-and-effect explanation which was all that seemed to be required to account for the development of cancer following exposure of people or animals to massive doses of single chemical carcinogens such as 2-naphthylamine or benzidine. Epidemiological studies have shown, however, that less than 10% of human bladder cancer is attributable to exposure to such identified chemical carcinogens. The major risk factor for bladder cancer, as for lung cancer, is cigarette smoking rather than occupational exposure to industrial chemicals. Even after allowing for the major contribution of cigarette smoking, the causes of a substantial proportion of human bladder cancers are still not positively identified, although many diverse factors, varying from dietary habits to infections with *Schistosoma haematobium* have been shown to increase risk for bladder cancer. Some of these factors, even though they increase the age-related prevalence of bladder cancer, are not carcinogenic *per se* when tested in experimental animal models or *in vitro* model systems.

In order to accommodate the currently available epidemiological and experimental data, it is necessary to postulate that carcinogenesis in the bladder, as in the mouse skin, is able to proceed by a multistage process. If it is assumed that the process is analogous to that which takes place in the skin, then it can be assumed to involve a temporal sequence of events in which the different stages can be brought about by different factors, not all of which need be carcinogens in their own right.

At this point, it is important to stress that there is no theoretical reason why carcinogenesis should not follow more than one developmental pathway. The development of some tumors may involve a series of discrete step functions, but others may well develop by another biological pathway which does not require the intervention of any factor other than exposure to a powerful complete carcinogen.

RESPONSE OF THE BLADDER TO SINGLE CARCINOGENS

Several specific bladder carcinogens have been identified which on their own can cause bladder cancer to develop. These include aromatic amines such as 2-naphthylamine, benzidine, 4-aminobiphenyl and chlornaphazine in man and 2-acetylaminofluorene in rodents. Examples of effective solitary carcinogens for the rodent bladder include N-butyl-N-(4-hydroxybutyl)nitrosamine (BBN),[30] N-methyl-N-nitrosourea (MNU)[25] and N-(4-(5-nitro-2-furyl)-2-thiazolyl)formamide (FANFT).[15] With either MNU or BBN, it is possible to induce a low incidence of bladder cancer in rats with a single, relatively high dose,[25] (and Turton and Hicks, unpublished observations) but, in general, in order to produce a high yield of autonomously-growing neoplasms, these carcinogens have to be administered over a prolonged period of time, usually for a few weeks. Thus, 0.05% BBN in drinking water is not carcinogenic if withdrawn within 4 weeks, but will produce a 100% incidence of bladder cancer if maintained in the diet for 16 weeks or longer. Similarly, 0.2% FANFT in the diet is not usually carcinogenic after 6 weeks feeding, but after 10 weeks feeding all rats develop bladder cancer.

Tumor incidence is, as a rule, directly proportional to the total dose of carcinogen administered, whereas there is an inverse relationship between the dose and the latent period before tumors develop. These dose-relationships have been shown to hold for the induction of bladder cancer in rats when low dose levels of MNU, BBN and FANFT are used. However, the absolute dose-relationship is substantially modified by duration of dosing and the aliquot size used. For any given total dose of carcinogen, small aliquots administered over a long period of time produce a higher tumor incidence than will the same total dose given as fewer, larger aliquots, or as a single dose. We observed this first with MNU,[21,45] and subsequently when using BBN (Turton and Hicks, unpublished). The cancer incidence obtained in the rat bladder with three different dose levels of BBN is shown in Figure 3.1. At all time intervals, there is a clear dose-related response. The absolute response, however, is drastically modified by aliquot size as is shown in Figure 3.2. It can be seen, for example, that the tumor incidence produced by 600 mg BBN given as three equal aliquots of 200 mg each is actually lower than that produced by 300 mg BBN given as 6 aliquots of 50 mg each, or 150 mg given as 12 aliquots of 12.5 mg each. Similar results were reported by McCormick et al.[37] in a mouse bladder cancer model also using BBN as the carcinogen.

These observations can be explained partly by the genotoxicity of carcinogens. The higher the dose, the greater will be the ratio of lethal to mutagenic damage to the genome, and the fewer the number of cells which will survive which are potentially able to generate neoplasms. If, however, carcinogenesis is progressing by a series of step-functions, the greater efficacy of multiple doses may also reflect the ability of carcinogens to bring about more than one step in this multistage process.

A very important conclusion can be drawn from these observations, namely that the effect of prolonged exposure to very low doses of

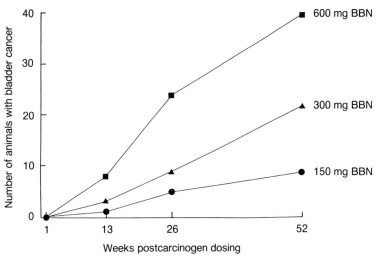

Figure 3.1. Dose-related incidence of bladder cancer in rats treated with *N*-butyl-*N*-(4-hydroxybutyl)nitrosamine (BBN).

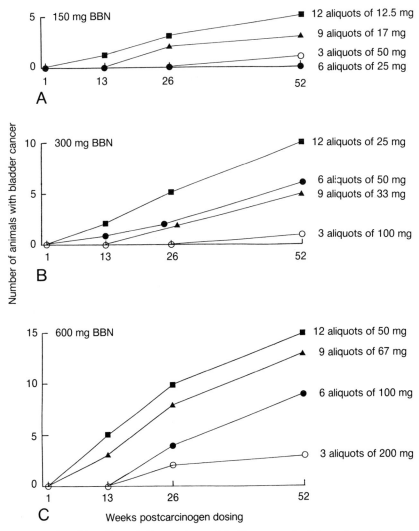

Figure 3.2. The effect of aliquot size on bladder cancer incidence in rats treated with *N*-butyl-*N*-(4-hydroxybutyl)nitrosamine (BBN).

carcinogens, such as may result from environmental or occupational exposure, is potentially far more hazardous than a single accidental exposure to a massive dose of even a quite potent solitary carcinogen.

RESPONSE OF THE BLADDER TO MULTIPLE FACTORS

The first unequivocal demonstration that carcinogenesis could involve a multistage process in the bladder, resulted from work with rats pretreated with a subcarcinogenic dose of MNU instilled directly into the bladder lumen.[26] When these MNU-treated animals were subsequently given sodium saccharin in the diet or drinking water, or sodium cyclamate in the diet, approximately 50% developed benign and/or invasive bladder tumors. In the 2-year duration of the trial, bladder tumors developed in only a low percentage (approximately 1%) of animals fed sweetener-containing diets but not pretreated with MNU, and none developed in MNU-treated rats fed a normal diet. Similar observations were subsequently made with rats fed low doses of FANFT followed by either sodium saccharin or DL-tryptophan,[11, 16] and also with rats exposed briefly either to BBN or to 2-acetylaminofluorene (2-AAF) and given sodium saccharin in the drinking water.[31] In these examples, a low yield of bladder tumors was produced by brief exposure of the animals to the carcinogens FANFT, BBN or 2-AAF, but the yield was greatly increased by subsequent oral administration of saccharin, cyclamate or tryptophan, none of which were significantly carcinogenic in their own right.

Dietary tryptophan increases the yield of bladder tumors in mice pretreated with FANFT and in dogs pretreated with 4-aminobiphenyl or 2-naphthylamine,[36, 42] and phenacetin enhances the carcinogenic effect of BBN in rats. Other factors which increase the time-related prevalence of bladder cancer in carcinogen-treated bladders include the male sex hormone, testosterone,[5, 40] deficiency of vitamin A,[7] nonspecific irritation of the urothelium either by a calculus[8] or by calcified and live ova of the parasite *Schistosoma haematobium*,[27] and a component of normal rat urine.[41] Similarly, methyl methanesulfonate increases the incidence of bladder cancer following a low dose of MNU,[49] and cyclophosphamide increases the yield after FANFT.[2] The experimental data underlying these and other examples have been reviewed recently in some detail[10, 22] and collectively they provide evidence that carcinogenesis in the urinary bladder can progress by a multistage developmental process.

The parallel between multistage carcinogenesis in the rat urinary bladder and initiation and promotion in the mouse skin is obvious, and it is important to determine whether the biological process involved is identical in the two tissues, or whether there are fundamental differences between these two models of animal cancer. If the biological events underlying the different stages of carcinogenesis are identical in bladder and skin, then the very extensive data obtained with the mouse skin model may also have implications for the understanding, etiology, prognosis and treatment of cancer of the urinary bladder in man.

EQUIVALENCE OF MULTISTAGE CARCINOGENESIS IN RODENT URINARY BLADDER AND MOUSE SKIN CANCER MODELS

Multistage Carcinogenesis in the Skin

Current understanding and terminology relating to multistage carcinogenesis are extensions from the original two-stage initiation and promotion model developed by Rous and Berenblum in the 1940s. This model was proposed in order to explain the observation that when mouse skin, previously exposed to a low, subcarcinogenic dose of benzo(*a*)pyrene (BP), is wounded or painted with croton oil there is a greatly increased yield of skin tumors. The subsequent studies of van Duuren, Boutwell and Hecker and more recently of Slaga,[46] Weinstein,[51] and others, have confirmed the existence of several discrete operational stages in tumor development in mouse skin and elucidated some of the biochemical events underlying these stages.

INITIATION

In the mouse skin model, carcinogenesis can be considered as an operational process during which a normal cell and its progeny are converted over a period of time into cancer cells which fail to respond to normal growth control factors in their environment. The first step in this process, initiation, is the result of a covalent reaction of an initiating carcinogen with the DNA of the target cell thus producing a heritable modification of the genome. If a relatively high dose of carcinogen is used, cancer may develop directly without the cooperation of any other factor providing the dose used was not cytotoxic. By contrast, a low dose of carcinogen may introduce into a few cells only, random permanent damage in normally supressed areas of the genome which, therefore, will not be expressed as a new phenotype unless the cell is also exposed to additional factors which modulate gene expression. Characteristically, initiation is a rapid event, will occur during a single exposure to the carcinogen, is directly dose-related to the carcinogen, and involves only a small proportion of the possible target cells. If the initiating event has taken place in one of the basal stem cells, which are immortal in the lifetime of the host, unless the damage is rapidly repaired before the cell divides, the initiating change in the genome will be permanent. Because it is not expressed, however, there will no change of phenotype and no recognizable biochemical or behavioral difference between the initiated and normal epithelium. Initiating carcinogens, since they react chemically with the genome, may produce lethal, mutagenic, or initiating lesions depending on the dose used.

PROMOTION

The next stage in multistage carcinogenesis in the skin, promotion, involves an altered pattern of gene expression thus permitting the damage introduced by the initiating agent to be expressed as a new phenotype. The definitions of promotion and the terminology in current use have been reviewed recently.[23] In mouse skin, two stages of promotion have been identified. Stage 1 promotion involves a rapidly induced change in cell differentiation thus permitting the cells to acquire an altered proliferative capacity, i.e. the initiated cell is converted into a preneoplastic cell. Stage 2 promotion, by contrast, involves the selective proliferation of preneoplastic cells with the consequent formation of a benign tumour, i.e. clonal expansion of the population of premalignant cells.

In the mouse skin, stage 1 promoters act primarily at the cell membrane where, in the presence of calcium and a phospholipid, they bind to and activate protein kinase C. Within minutes, alterations occur in membrane phospholipid metabolism, membrane structure and membrane function.[51] Protein kinase C controls the degree of phosphorylation of serine and threonine residues in certain regulatory cell proteins which, in turn, control many cell functions including gene expression. By activating protein kinase C, stage 1 promoters can thus modulate the activity of various hormones and growth factors. A promoter, in its reaction with the cell membrane, is thus analogous to insulin, epidermal growth factor or platelet-derived growth factor, all of which bind to another protein kinase, namely tyrosine kinase. Prolonged exposure to the promoting agent is not necessary for stage 1 promotion; these effects can be observed within seconds or minutes of a single exposure of skin to the promoter 12-O-tetradecanoylphorbol-13-acetate (TPA). Not all stage 1 promoters by themselves, however, can cause tumors to develop in initiated skin and, operationally, they are incomplete promoters unless they can also bring about stage 2 events.

For stage 2 promotion to occur, there must be selective proliferation of the preneoplatic (stage 1-promoted) cells, in order to permit expansion of this preneoplastic cell population at the expense of neighboring normal tissue to form a benign, noninvasive tumor. Stage 2 promotion is dependent on a sustained proliferative stimulus which enables the altered growth potential of the preneoplastic cells to be expressed. Stage 2 promoters therefore induce enzymes such as ornithine decarboxylase (ODC) whose products accelerate the rate of cell division. ODC is the rate-limiting enzyme for synthesis of the polyamines putrescine, spermidine and spermine which in turn modulate the rate of synthesis of DNA, RNA and proteins; it thus plays a decisive role in the control of cell division.[17] Most growth-promoting stimuli, including growth-promoting hormones and epidermal growth factor, will act as stage 2 promoters, but unless they are also stage 1 promoters, they will not on their own promote tumor growth in initiated skin.

MALIGNANT CONVERSION

The final step in this process of multistage carcinogenesis in the skin is malignant conversion of one or more of the preneoplastic cells in the benign tumor to a fully committed cancer cell which, because it fails to respond normally to its immediate environment, can give rise to an autonomously growing invasive cancer. For such malignant conversion of a cell to occur, an additional genetic event is required, akin to, but not necessarily identical with, initiation. This second genetic event probably involves transposition of genetic material, as for example from an oncogenic virus or by sister chromatid exchange, rather than covalent reaction of the carcinogen with the genome.[38] This final stage of malignant transformation has been less well investigated than the preceding stages of initiation and promotion in multistage carcinogenesis in the skin.

Thus the process of multistage carcinogenesis in the mouse skin model can be described with some accuracy. The question now is whether the multistage process of carcinogenesis in the bladder involves the same or different stages as those of initiation, promotion and malignant conversion in the mouse skin.

Multistage Carcinogenesis in the Urinary Bladder

INITIATION

It is generally accepted that the process of initiation of a urothelial cell in the bladder is analogous to initiation of an epidermal cell in the skin and involves covalent binding of the carcinogen with the urothelial cell DNA. The exact nature of the DNA adducts formed by various carcinogens may well differ; there is some evidence that damage to the genome produced by FANFT is more readily repaired than damage produced by N-nitroso compounds such as MNU or BBN. The breakdown products of MNU or BBN alkylate various residues of DNA, most of which are rapidly repaired with the exception of O-6-alkylguanine which persists for many weeks. FANFT gives rise to a deformylated product ANFT, which is metabolised *via* prostaglandin endoperoxide synthetase to another intermediate capable of binding to DNA. The adducts formed between urothelial cell DNA and the metabolites of 2-acetylaminofluorene or 2-naphthylamine are different again, but in all instances the operational effect is the same; covalent reaction of the carcinogenic metabolite with DNA causes a permanent modification of the genome and results in the formation of an initiated cell. What is not yet fully understood is the basis of the quite remarkable specificity exhibited by some initiating carcinogens for their particular target tissue.

PROMOTION

There is considerably more disagreement as to whether promotion in the bladder involves the same biological phenomena as it does in the skin. The essential definition of a promoter, as it is generally understood and as it was originally used by Berenblum, is a compound that will increase the time-related yield of visible tumors in initiated epidermis. He defined promoters as factors which were not carcinogenic on their own, but which would increase tumor yield if applied after, but not before, treatment of the skin with a subcarcinogenic dose of an initiating carcinogen; he emphasized that prolonged exposure to a promoter was required for it to be effective, and that the early stages of promotion appeared to be reversible. A wider definition of promotion is now needed to encompass both this operational definition and the more recent biochemical division of promotion into stage 1 and stage 2 events. Various agents including saccharin, cyclamate and tryptophan as described above, appear to fit Berenblum's operational definition of a promoter, in that they increase the yield of bladder cancers in animals pretreated with a low dose of an initiating carcinogen.

It must be emphasized, however, that promotion in the bladder has not been studied as extensively as it has been in the skin. So far, none of the promoters of carcinogenesis in the bladder strictly fulfills all the criteria developed to define a promoter in skin. But nor do most skin promoters. For example, it is generally stated that promoters are not carcinogenic *per se*, and yet TPA on its own will produce a few tumors in uninitiated mouse skin.[6,43] Similarly, 7-bromomethyl-benz(*a*)anthracene is an effective promoter of carcinogenesis in mouse skin previously initiated with 7,12,-dimethylbenz(*a*)anthracene, but it is also a complete carcinogen on its own.[44] Indeed, there is no *a priori* reason why any one compound should not be able to effect more than one process in multistage carcinogenesis, for the underlying biochemical events differ at the different stages.

Saccharin, which is perhaps the most extensively investigated of the bladder promoters, as well as increasing the yield of tumors in preinitiated rat bladders, on its own can increase bladder cancer incidence in male offspring when tested in two-generation studies. Furthermore, in numerous studies, it has been observed that more bladder cancers are consistently found in rats fed saccharin than in those which are not,[26,47,48] although the number of animals used in any single study was too few to permit a statistically significant conclusion to be reached. The mechanism by which saccharin can act as a very weak solitary bladder carcinogen is not yet understood. Unlike classical initiating carcinogens, it is not capable of reacting covalently with DNA, and must be used at high dose levels to be effective. It is possible that at high concentrations most of the factors identified as promoters of bladder carcinogenesis (see above) have more in common with stage 2 than with stage 1 promoters in the skin. Stage 2 promoters are all hyperplastic agents and cause some degree of basal cell hyperplasia in their target tissue following the induction of ODC activity. Physical or chemical damage to the urothelium, such as is caused by a calculus, *S. haematobium* ova or administration of cyclophosphamide, is known to significantly increase the time-related incidence of cancer in initiated bladders, and they may act simply by supplying the proliferative stimulus required to permit clonal expansion of preneoplastic cells already present in the urothelium. However, wounding has been identified as a stage 1 promoter in mouse skin[46] so it is not impossible that these factors also can act as complete promoters.

Vitamin A deficiency also increases mitotic activity in the basal cells of the urothelium leading first to hyperplasia and later to epidermalisation.[19,20] Similarly, there is a component in rat urine which not only increases tumor incidence, but also causes urothelial hyperplasia in the urothelium of preinitiated, heterotopically transplanted rat bladders.[29] Saccharin also, is a hyperplastic agent for the rat bladder *in vivo*[9,39] and for both rat and human bladder maintained as organ cultures *in vitro*.[24,34] This effect is not attributable to crystalluria but is a direct effect of saccharin on the urothelium.[9,13]

Some of these promoting agents in the bladder, including saccharin, a metabolite of tryptophan namely 3-hydroxyanthranilic acid, and the heat-stable promoting factor from rat urine, are capable of inducing ODC activity in their target tissue, as also is the skin promoter TPA.[32,41] Epidermal growth factor and insulin, which act as stage 2 promoters in skin, also induced ODC activity in the urothelial cells but TPA was by far the most effective. Recently, it was reported that when directly instilled into the bladder (3H)TPA binds to the urothelium with a comparable specificity to its binding in skin.[50]

These observations are consistent with the hypothesis that the various agents shown to have tumor-promoting activity in the urinary bladder are analogous to stage 2 skin promoters in their biological effect on the bladder urothelium. Whether or not they can also act as stage 1 promoters is not known as yet. The fact that there is high affinity binding of TPA to the urothelium, in itself indicates that the appropriate phosphokinase C receptor sites are present in bladder cell membranes as well as in skin. Whether saccharin, or other bladder cancer promoters are capable of similar high affinity binding to specific receptor sites in the urothelium has not yet been investigated. Indirect evidence for interaction of saccharin and tryptophan with the cell membrane has been produced by Kakizoe and his co-workers,[33] who have studied the concanavalin A-agglutinability of rat urothelial cells. They found that urothelial cells from rats treated with an initiating dose of a bladder carcinogen developed a transient increased agglutinability which is not maintained by 5% sodium chloride in the diet but is maintained either by 5% sodium saccharin or 2% DL-tryptophan in the diet. This certainly indicates that saccharin and tryptophan modify the cell membrane, but not necessarily by the same mechanism as does TPA.

The morphological effects in the urothelium produced by saccharin and other bladder cancer promoters have been reviewed elsewhere and related to the effect of skin promoters on the epidermis.[10,22,24]

MALIGNANT CONVERSION

Even less is known about the final stage of multistage carcinogenesis in the urinary bladder than is known about malignant conversion in the skin. Undoubtedly, invasive bladder cancer in man and rodents is frequently preceded by papillary and/or nodular hyperplasia.[31,35] There is considerable evidence that these benign proliferative lesions represent an expanded population of preneoplastic cells, within which the occasional cell may develop malignant potential in response to an as yet unidentified stimulus. This may involve activation of a latent oncogene following transposition of genetic material either from an infective agent such as the papilloma virus, or alternatively as a result of induced rearrangement of genetic material within in the urothelial cell DNA. In this context, it is notable that saccharin at high concentrations, although not consistently mutagenic, does cause some sister chromatid exchange in both human and hamster cells *in vitro*.[1,52] Such transposition of genetic material is known to be capable of activating normally suppressed gene sequences and could well permit expression of a late-stage oncogene. At high concentrations saccharin may also interfere with the tertiary structure of DNA and thereby trigger clastogenic changes.[3]

CONCLUSIONS

There is sufficient and diverse experimental evidence to support the thesis that carcinogenesis in the urinary bladder can develop by a multistage process. Evidence is incomplete but circumstantially convincing, that the stages are analogous to those described as initiation, promotion and malignant conversion in multistage carcinogenesis in the skin. There has been some opposition to accepting the possibility that these processes in the two tissues are indeed analogous, largely because of the recent widespread abuse of the term promoter. It is becoming increasingly common to find this term incorrectly applied to any factor enhancing tumor incidence in response to a carcinogenic stimulus, irrespective of whether or not it fulfils any of the basic criteria proposed by Berenblum for promotion. For example, gross dietary factors such as increased total lipid or total caloric intake have been referred to as promoters, as have factors which increase the susceptibility of the animal to initiating carcinogens by inducing those enzymes which metabolize the carcinogen to its ultimate reactive species. Such factors may correctly be referred to as cocarcinogens, but they do not participate directly in the temporal sequence of events described by the terms initiation, promotion and malignant conversion.

There are important theoretical and practical reasons for accepting that carcinogenesis in the urinary bladder can proceed by a multistage process. It provides a unifying theory which satisfactorily accommodates most of the experimental and epidemiological evidence for a multifactorial etiology for bladder cancer. Because even brief exposure to a low dose of a first-stage carcinogen can produce permanently initiated cells, it is important to realize that there is no such thing as a safe dose of a known bladder carcinogen below which there is no effect. Because physical damage to the urothelium can act as a promoting stimulus to a bladder exposed to an initiating carcinogen some time previously, irritation of the bladder by an indwelling catheter, or repeat biopsies of the tissue, or the presence of urinary calculi, or the use of drugs such as cyclophosphamide which are cytotoxic for the urothelium, may well lead to unexpected complications and increase the risk for bladder cancer for the patient.

On the other hand, recognition that the promotion phase of tumor development occupies a considerable period of time, probably many years in man, offers the opportunity to develop new therapeutic modalities designed to delay the progression of initiated urothelial cells to invasive bladder cancers. Recent work on antipromoters, particularly on retinoids which in skin specifically antagonize stage 2 promotion,[46] has demonstrated that the onset of symptomatic bladder cancer in carcinogen-treated experimental animals can be delayed by including retinoids in the diet.[4, 18, 28] The development of specific inhibitors for the various postinitiation stages in multistage carcinogenesis offers great potential for the control of bladder cancer in patients who have been successfully treated for their first neoplasm but who, nevertheless, are still at high risk for developing further cancers.

There is considerable public concern about the possible danger arising from exposure to carcinogens in the environment and/or workplace, which is based on the widespread assumption that all carcinogens have a direct and inevitable causal role. A wider acceptance of the multistage nature of carcinogenesis, and a concomitant realization that late-stage carcinogens, *i.e.* promoting factors, are equally important in the etiology of the disease would be a useful advance in public health education. As emphasized by Doll and Peto[14], if cells must be exposed to more than one factor in the right temporal sequence before they can develop into an autonomous cancer, then avoidance of exposure to either the early (initiating) or the late-stage (promoting) factors, will reduce the risk of developing cancer. The only determinant of which is the most important risk factor is that which is more easily avoided, and indeed in terms of human cancer prevalence, removal of exposure to late-stage factors has a more immediate effect on the subsequent relative risk of developing cancer than does removal of exposure to initiating carcinogens.[12, 14] This has already been demonstrated by the reduced risk for lung cancer seen after cessation of cigarette smoking which is known to contain factors active at the penultimate stage in lung carcinogenesis. Similar advances in the understanding, avoidance and treatment of carcinoma of the bladder may be expected to follow from further exploration of the biology and modulation of multistage carcinogenesis in the urothelium.

Acknowledgments. Most of this work has been made possible by generous support over many years by the British Cancer Research Campaign. I am also indebted to all my colleagues who have worked with me on problems of multistage carcinogenesis including J. St. J. Wakefield, J. Chowaniec, N. Severs, R. J. Tudor, and J. A. Turton.

REFERENCES

1. Abe, S., and Sasaki, M. Chromosome aberrations and sister chromatid exchanges in Chinese hamster cells exposed to various chemicals. *J. Natl. Cancer Inst. 58:*1635, 1977.
2. Arai, M., Cohen, F. M., and Friedell, G. H. Promoting effect of cyclophosphamide (CP) on rat urinary bladder carcinogenesis following initiation by *N*-(4-(5-nitro-2-furyl)-2-thiazolyl) formamide (FANFT). In Proceedings of the Japanese Cancer Association: 36th Annual Meeting, October 1977, Tokyo, p. 39. Japanese Cancer Association, Tokyo. 1977.
3. Ashby, J. Short-term tests—saccharin and cyclamates. European Toxicology Forum, Geneva, October 1983, *2:*317, The Toxicology Forum, Washington, 1983.
4. Becci, P. J., Thompson, H. J., Grubbs, C. J., Brown, C. C., and Moon, R. C. Effect of delay in administration of 13-*cis*-retinoic acid on the inhibition of urinary bladder carcinogenesis in the rat. *Cancer Res. 39:*3141, 1979.
5. Bertram, J. F., and Craig, A. W. Specific induction of bladder cancer in mice by butyl-(4-hydroxybutyl)nitrosamine and effects of hormonal modification on the sex difference in response. *Eur. J. Cancer 8:*587, 1972.
6. Boutwell, R. K., Bosch, B. K., and Rusch, M. P. On the role of croton oil in tumor formation. *Cancer Res. 17:*71, 1957.
7. Capurro, P., Angrist, A., Black, J., and Moumgis, B. Studies in squamous metaplasia in rat bladder. I. Effects of hypovitaminosis A, foreign bodies and methylcholanthrene. *Cancer Res. 20:*563, 1960.
8. Chapman, W. H., Kirchheim, D., and McRoberts, J. W. Effect of urine and calculus formation on the incidence of bladder tumors in rats implanted with paraffin wax pellets. *Cancer Res. 33:*1225, 1973.
9. Chowaniec, J., and Hicks, R. M. Response of the rat to saccharin with particular reference to the urinary bladder. *Br. J. Cancer 39:*355, 1979.
10. Cohen, F. M. Promotion in urinary bladder carcinogenesis. *Environ. Health Perspect. 50:*51, 1983.

11. Cohen, F. M., Arai, M., Jacobs, J. B., and Friedell, G. H. Promoting effect of saccharin and D,L-tryptophan in urinary bladder carcinogenesis. *Cancer Res. 39:*1207, 1979.
12. Day, N. E., and Brown, C. C. Multistage models and primary prevention of cancer. *J. Natl. Cancer Inst. 64:*977, 1980.
13. Demers, D. M., Fukushima, F., and Cohen, F. M. Effect of sodium saccharin and L-tryptophan on rat urine during bladder carcinogenesis. *Cancer Res. 41:*108, 1981.
14. Doll, R., and Peto, R. The causes of cancer: quantitative estimates of avoidable risks of cancer in the United States today. *J. Natl. Cancer Inst. 66:*1193, 1981.
15. Erturk, E., Cohen, S. M., Price, J. M., and Bryan, D. T. Pathogenesis, histogenesis, histology and transplantability of urinary bladder carcinoma induced in albino rats by oral administration of *N*-(4-(5-nitro-2-furyl)-2-thiazolyl)formamide. *Cancer Res. 29:*2219, 1969.
16. Fukushima, S., Friedell, S.H., Jacobs, J. B., and Cohen, F. M. Effect of L-tryptophan and sodium saccharin on urinary bladder carcinogenesis initiated by *N*-(4-(5-nitro-2-furyl)-2-thiazolyl)formamide. *Cancer Res. 41:*3100, 1981.
17. Gaugas, J. M. (ed) Polyamines in biomedical research. John Wiley, New York, 1980.
18. Grubbs, C. J., Moon R. C., Squire, R. A. Farrow, G. M., Stinson, S. F. Goodman, D. G., Brown, C. C., and Sporn, M. B. 13-*cis*-retinoic acid: inhbition of bladder carcinogenesis induced in rats by *N*-butyl-*N*-(4-hydroxybutyl)nitrosamine. *Science 198:*743, 1977.
19. Hicks, R. M. Hyperplasia and cornification of the transitional epithelium in the vitamin A-deficient rat. *J. Ultrastruct. Res. 22:*206, 1968.
20. Hicks, R. M. Nature of the keratohyalin-like granules in hyperplastic and cornified areas of transitional epithelium in the vitamin A-deficient rat. *J. Anat. 104:*327, 1969.
21. Hicks, R. M. Multistage carcinogenesis in the urinary bladder. *Br. Med. Bull. 36:*39, 1980.
22. Hicks, R. M. Effect of promoters on incidence of bladder cancer in experimental animal models. *Environ. Health Perspect. 50:*37, 1983.
23. Hicks, R. M. Commentary. Pathological and biochemical aspects of tumor promotion. *Carcinogenesis 4:*1209, 1983.
24. Hicks, R. M. Promotion: Is saccharin a promoter in the urinary bladder? European Toxicology Forum, Geneva, October 1983, *1:*232, The Toxicology Forum, Washington, 1983.
25. Hicks, R. M., and Wakefield, J. St. J. Rapid induction of bladder cancer in rats with *N*-methyl-*N*-nitrosourea. 1. Histology. *Chem.-Biol. Interact. 5:*139, 1972.
26. Hicks, R. M., Wakefield, J. St. J., and Chowaniec, J. Evaluation of a new model to detect carcinogens or co-carcinogens: results obtained with saccharin, cyclamate and cyclophosphamide. *Chem.-Biol. Interact. 11:*225, 1975.
27. Hicks, R. M., James, C., and Webbe, G. Effect of *Schistosoma haematobium* and *N*-butyl-*N*-(4-hydroxybutyl)nitrosamine on the development of urothelial neoplasia in the baboon. *Br. J. Cancer. 42:*730, 1980.
28. Hicks, R. M., Chowaniec, J., Turton, J. A., Massey, E. D., and Harvey, A. The effects of dietary retinoids on experimentally induced carcinogenesis in the rat bladder. In *Molecular Interrelations of Nutrition and Cancer, 34th Annual Symposium on Fundamental Cancer Research*, University of Texas System Cancer Center and M. D. Anderson Hospital and Tumor Institute, pp. 419–447, edited by M. S. Arnot, J. van Eys and Y.-M. Wang. Raven Press, New York, 1982.
29. Hirao, Y., Izumi, K., and Oyasu, R. The effect of normal rat urine on mucosal regeneration in heterotopic urinary bladder. *Lab. Invest. 42:*76, 1980.
30. Ito, N., Hyasa, Y., Tamai, A. Okajima, E., and Kitamura, H. Histogenesis of urinary bladder tumours induced by *N*-butyl-*N*-(4-hydroxybutyl)nitrosamine in rats. *Gann 60:*401, 1969.
31. Ito, N., Fukushima, S., Shirai, T., and Nakanishi, K. Effects of promoters on *N*-butyl-*N*-(4-hydroxybutyl)nitrosamine-induced urinary bladder carcinogenesis in the rat. *Environ. Health Perspect. 50:*61, 1983.
32. Izumi, K., Hirao, Y., Hopp, L., and Oyasu, R. *In vitro* induction of ornithine decarboxylase in urinary bladder carcinoma cells. *Cancer Res. 41:*450, 1981.
33. Kakizoe, T., Komatso, H., Niijima, T., Kawachi, T., and Sugimura, T. Maintenance by saccharin of membrane alterations of rat bladder cells induced by subcarcinogenic treatment with bladder carcinogens. *Cancer Res. 41:*4702, 1981.
34. Knowles, M. A., Summerhayes, I. C., and Hicks, R. M. Carcinogenesis studies using

cultured and rat mouse bladder. In *In Vitro Models for Cancer Research*, edited by M. E. Webbe. CRC Press, Boca Raton, Florida, (In press) 1984.

35. Koss, L. G. Mapping of the urinary bladder: its impact on the concepts of bladder cancer. *Hum. Pathol. 10:*533, 1979.

36. Matsushima, M. The role of the promoter *N*-tryptophan on tumorigenesis in the urinary bladder. 2. Urinary bladder carcinogenicity of FANFT (initiating factor) and L-tryptophan (promoting factor) in mice. *Japan. J. Urol. 68:*731, 1979.

37. McCormick, D. L., Ronan, S. S., Becci, P. J., and Moon, R. C. Influence of total dose and dose schedule on induction of urinary bladder cancer in the mouse by *N*-butyl-*N*-(4-hydroxybutyl)nitrosamine. *Carcinogenesis 2:*251, 1981.

38. Moolgavkar, S. H., and Knudson, A. G. Mutation and cancer: a model for human carcinogenesis. *J. Natl. Cancer Inst. 66:*1037, 1981.

39. Nakanishi, K., Hagiwara, A., Shibata, M., Imalda, K., Tatematsu, M., and Ito, N. Dose response of saccharin in induction of urinary bladder hyperplasia in Fischer 344 rats pretreated with *N*-butyl-*N*-(4-hydroxybutyl)nitrosamine. *J. Natl. Cancer Inst. 65:*1005, 1980.

40. Okajima, E., Hiramatsu, T., Iriya, K., Ijuin, F., Matsushima, S., and Yamada, K. Effects of sex hormones on development of urinary bladder tumors in rats induced by *N*-(4-hydroxybutyl)nitrosamine. *Urol. Res. 3:*73, 1975.

41. Oyasu, R., Babaya, K., Ozono, S., Morikawi, A., and Chmiel, J. S. Urinary components capable of enhancing ornithine decarboxylase (ODC) activity promote bladder tumorigenicity. *Proc. Am. Assoc. Cancer Res. 24:*419, 1983.

42. Radomski, J. L., Radomski, T., and MacDonald, W. E. Carcinogenic interacton between D,L-tryptophan and 4-aminobiphenyl or 2-naphthylamine in dogs. *J. Natl. Cancer Inst. 58:*1831, 1977.

43. Roe, S. G. C. The development of malignant tumours of mouse skin after "initiating" and "promoting" stimuli. III. The carcinogenic action of croton oil. *Br. J. Cancer. 10:*72, 1956.

44. Scribner, N. K., and Scribner, J. D. Separation of initiating and promoting effects of the skin carcinogen 7-bromomethylbenz(*a*)anthracene. *Carcinogenesis 1:*97, 1980.

45. Severs, N. J., Barnes, S. H., Wright, R., and Hicks, R. M. Induction of bladder cancer in rats by fractionated intravesicular doses of *N*-methyl-*N*-nitrosourea. *Br. J. Cancer. 45:*337, 1982.

46. Slaga, T. J. Overview of tumor promotion in animals. *Environ. Health Perspect. 50:*3, 1983.

47. Taylor, J. M., and Friedman, L. Combined chronic feeding and 3-generation reproduction study of sodium saccharin in the rat. *Toxicol. Appl. Pharmacol. 29:*154, 1974.

48. Tisdell, M. O., Nees, P. O., Harris, D. L. *et al.* Long-term feeding of saccharin in rats. In *Cancer Testing Technology and Saccharin*, pp. 57–60. Office of Technology Assessment, U. S. Government Printing Office, Washington, 1977.

49. Tudor, R. J., Severs, N. J., and Hicks, R. M. The induction of urothelial hyperplasia by methyl methanesulphonate and ethyl methanesulphonate. *Br. J. Cancer. 48:*289, 1983.

50. Verma, A. K., Renzikoff, C. A., Erturk, E., and Bryan, G. T. Specific-binding, stimulation of urinary bladder epithelial ornithine decarboxylase (ODC), and induction of transitional cell hyperplasia by the tumor promoter 12-*O*-tetradecanoylphorbol-13-acetate (TPA). *Proc. Am. Assoc. Cancer Res. 24:*218, 1983.

51. Weinstein, I. B. Protein kinase, phospholipid and control of growth. *Nature, 302:*750, 1983.

52. Wolff, F., and Rodin, B. Saccharin-induced sister chromatid exchanges in Chinese hamster and human cells. *Science 200:*543, 1978.

4

Pathology of Urothelial Cancers

Myron Tannenbaum, M.D., Ph.D.

Transitional epithelium of the urinary bladder or urothelium presents histologically a large variety of patterns that can be easily demonstrated on conventional light histology. The classification of the histopathology of urinary bladder carcinomas has been well documented extensively by numerous authors.[1-3] Even though there is a large amount of information and atlases on the pathology of these neoplasms, there remains much that is an enigma to those people who are in a daily position of evaluating the pathology of these tumors. There is a need to communicate this information to the chemotherapist, the radiologist, and now the environmentalist but lastly, yet most importantly, the urologic surgeon. It is the purpose of this chapter to bring into focus from the point of view of the uropathologist what might be some of the points of confusion about the pathology and, consequently, the evaluation of the data needed by the various medical disciplines who deal with the urothelial cancer problem, *e.g.* carcinoma *in situ*, nonpapillary carcinomas and atypical urothelial hyperplasia.

Carcinoma *in situ*

Three decades ago the term, "carcinoma *in situ*," was applied to that neoplastic urothelium seen in histologic sections which was interposed (cystoscopically nonexophytic urothelium) between surrounding overt papillary tumors of the urinary bladder removed by cystectomy.[4,5]

Now more than 20 years later, employing urinary cytology, a group of patients was selected out of an even larger group of patients who had cancer of the urinary bladder.[6] The former patients showed evidence of positive cytology or cancer cells in the urine. When these patients were examined cystoscopically, they were found to be free of visible tumors with the only evidence of malignancy being detected by urinary cytological study. They were then followed for varying periods of time ranging from 3 months to 7 years before there were any cystoscopic visible lesions or recurrences within the urinary bladder.

At our medical center, a similar disease pattern has also been seen. It is now routine to obtain random biopsies of the bladder mucosa but especially from the lateral and posterior walls above the trigone where the incidence of carcinoma *in situ* is the highest. If multiple tissue levels are taken of the carcinoma *in situ*, in approximately 30% of the patients so examined there will be an early invasive or early stage A invading urothelial cancer. In some instances, the carcinoma *in situ* urothelium contains intraepithelial blood vessels that are not observed by the urologist on cystoscopic examination. The cytologic characteristics of the carcinoma *in situ* cells can be further shown to be pleomorphic when they are compared cytologically with normal cells that are present within the same microscopic field. In these early biopsy specimens, the carcinoma *in situ* process is readily demonstrated not only to be present beneath the normal urothelium and above the basement membrane, but also in Brunn's nests, cystitis cystica and, in many instances, in the periurethral prostatic ducts. The nuclei of many of these carcinoma *in situ* areas are usually 2–3 times the nuclear size of the normal urothelium. These urothelial lesions are usually found over a highly vascularized area of microcapillaries.

These urothelial cancers are believed to begin in the lower basal cell layer and then to extend outward to the lumen replacing the intermediary cell layer as well as the surface cell layer. Each one of these three cell layers has certain ultrastructural characteristics that readily identify it as originating from a particular layer of the urothelium. Transmission electron microscopy when used in conjunction with scanning electron microscopy, reveals even more incipient cellular characteristics that can label these cells as malignant even before conventional light histology and light cytologic techniques. The cell surface of the normal bladder cell has asymmetrical membranes whereas these structures disappear when the cell has been committed towards the malignant state.

By mapping, Koss *et al.*[7] has studied this type of lesion in 20 surgically removed bladders. He has demonstrated carcinoma *in situ* and related lesions, *i.e.* atypical hyperplasias in those areas adjacent to or distant from visible tumors. He has also found numerous areas of occult invasive carcinoma to be derived from such abnormal epithelium. These histological findings suggest that the areas of the bladder most frequently involved by these precancerous lesions are the left and right lateral walls and the posterior wall. The trigone and dome regions are less frequently involved.

In a retrospective light histology study of carcinoma *in situ* of the urinary bladder, Tannenbaum and Romas[8] were able to observe 140 cases of carcinoma *in situ* of the urinary bladder with a follow-up period of 14–21 years. The patient records in all of their cases indicated no previous history of urothelial or bladder cancer. Eighty percent of the cases presented with symptoms of dysuria or microscopic hematuria. There was an initial histological documentation of carcinoma *in situ* for each patient before they were included in the study. In a period of 4–6 years, 40% of the patients progressed from a stage A to B_1 lesion. Ten percent were stage B_2 to stage C. At the 10-year follow-up period, 60% of these patients were stage A to B_1, 20% were B_2 to C, whereas the remaining patients expired. When the same patients were examined 15–21 years after the initial documentation of their cystoscopically flat carcinoma *in situ*, 40% had died from their disease with the remaining majority being classified as stage B_2 to stage D. This initial retrospective

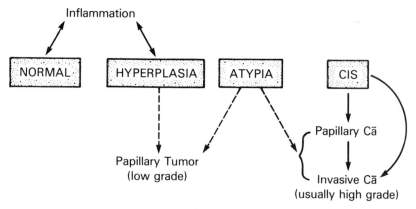

Figure 4.1. Evolution of carcinoma *in situ.*

study strongly suggests that urothelial carcinoma *in situ* is a biological aggressive and nonretrogressive disease. It is only through cytological studies and random biopsies of the cystoscopically normal urothelium under the most fastidious cystoscopic conditions and pathologic fixation that these early urothelial cancers can be documented.

Similar morphologic and clinical observations in lesions that were detected by positive urinary cytology in patients without any previous urothelial neoplasms have also been observed at the Mayo Clinic.[9] They noted that the evolution of these tumors was considerably longer than they had previously documented.[10]

The natural history of this lesion has yet to be resolved. On the basis of serial biopsies and mapping studies of cystectomy specimens,[11-13] it is readily recognized that there may be a progression of normal urothelium to flat carcinoma *in situ* (cystoscopically flat erythematous areas) through the possible stages of hyperplasia and atypia as illustrated in Figure 4.1.[14] The various histological features that exemplify carcinoma *in situ* also characterize cytologically those features found in higher grade papillary transitional cell tumors, i.e. grades II or III. This clearly represents a loss of the superficial umbrella cells. With the sole utilization of light histology, there are no specific histological features of the early phases of low grade carcinoma *in situ* (nonexophytic) that can be recognized. Perhaps it is the vascular pattern in the underlying lamina propria, a feature emphasized by Koss[12,13] that might provide valuable early histological as well as cystoscopic identification of the potentially dangerous hyperplastic or atypical urothelium that might progress into carcinoma *in situ.*

PATHOLOGY OF INVASIVE UROTHELIAL TUMORS

As soon as the tumor is detected cytologically and cystoscopically, a biopsy specimen is obtained and several variegated patterns of tumor spread are revealed. The possible life cycle of untreated tumors of the urinary bladder has been postulated at Columbia-Presbyterian Medical Center.[15] In order to invade, many of these tumors, both in the flat as well as in the exophytic papillary form, must have cell extension beyond the basement membrane. Once this occurs, there is invasion through the lamina propria and then, with the course of time which is ill-defined, invasion of both muscle and/or lymphatics. Frequently these tumors of the solid nonpapillary type can spread laterally. At the same time, they may perforate the submucosa and spread as finger-like projections into the muscularis of the bladder. At first, the papillary tumors are exophytic into the bladder lumen and consequently they are readily seen cystoscopically. Both forms, the flat *in situ* cancer and the papillary exophytic type tend to shower off cells into the lumen of the bladder. Depending on the grade of the tumor, they can be readily detected by urinary cytology. The higher the grade, the easier it is to detect the cancer by means of urinary cytology. Many of the papillary tumors will also bleed because the tumor has delicate fibrovascular stalks that contain blood vessels without smooth muscle. If these tumors twist, branches of the tumor break off into the urine and blood will also pulsate out from the vessels in the tumor branches. The papillary tumors also break through the basement membrane that envelops their base and they then invade the lamina propria or submucosa and perhaps, in some instances, the muscularis. All types eventually become ulcerated and infected. At this time, it becomes difficult to determine whether the tumors were originally of the solid or papillary form. If urinary cytology is used with increased frequency, many of these tumors can be detected at very early stages, *i.e.* before they reach stages B_1 or B_2. Consequently, they should be detected at an early stage as represented in the upper third of Figure 4.2. At all times it is extremely difficult for any pathologist to critically separate the advanced stage B_1 from the early B_2 lesions. This difficulty is compounded when the specimens are cauterized, and especially when there is no specific orientation of the specimens for histological sectioning.

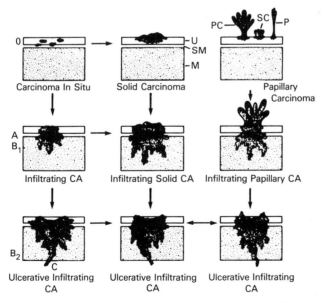

Figure 4.2. Schematic representation of the natural history of bladder tumors. (Reproduced by permission from M. M. Melicow. Tumors of the bladder: a multifaceted problem. *Journal of Urology 112*:467, 1974.)

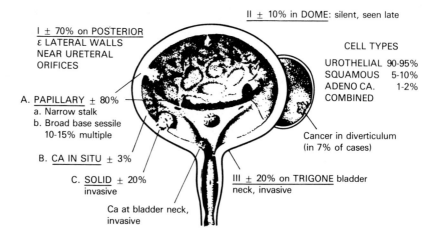

Figure 4.3. Usual sites and shapes of bladder neoplasms. (Reproduced by permission from M. M. Melicow. Tumors of the bladder: a multifaceted problem. *Journal of Urology 112:*467, 1974.)

The topographical distribution and cell types of bladder tumors are seen in Figure 4.3. The majority of bladder tumors (70%) are located on the posterior and lateral walls near the ureteral orifices. Most of the tumors in this category are papillary as they have fibrovascular stalks. The remaining 20% are in a solid invasive form and have no fibrovascular formation. They also commonly extend through the basement membrane that surrounds the nests of Brunn. There is also a varying amount of carcinoma *in situ* which is found associated with these bladder neoplasms about 3% of the time.[15] However, it is our impression that this percentage is a very variable one. It is greatly dependent upon whether the pathologist, in cooperation with the urologist, spends a considerable amount of time looking for this lesion in the associated biopsy specimens—that should be taken within 1 cm distance from these tumors. If this is done, the incidence of carcinoma *in situ* is considerably greater than 3%. These figures vary at each institution depending upon many factors, *i.e.* the fixatives, the methods of handling the specimen and whether the pathologists spend the time looking for these lesions.

As can be seen from Figure 4.3, a small proportion of the urothelial tumors are also noted in the dome of the bladder (10%). There is, however, a significant percentage of these urothelial tumors which occur in the region of the bladder neck (20%). The majority of these cell types are 90–95% urothelial. About 5% demonstrate a squamous cell component. Approximately 1% are adenocarcinoma in cell type. It is a common occurrence that there can be varying percentages of each of these cell types associated with the other. However, it is rare that all three types are found together.

When eight hundred and forty primary vesical tumors were studied over a period of 10 years, there was a varying distribution of the grades, incidence, age, group and sex. It was noted that 97% of the tumors developed after the patient was over 40 years old. The greatest incidence in the series studied by Melicow[15] occurred between the ages of 50 and

79. The male-to-female ratio was approximately 3:1. The extremely well differentiated grade I and grade II tumors reached a peak of incidence within the 6th–7th decade of life and then showed a relative decrease within the next decade. The grade III and IV tumors were fewer in number but continued to be relatively prominent from the 7th decade on.

GRADING OF UROTHELIAL TUMORS

Similar to the stage, the grade of the urothelial tumor has prognostic significance. On different occasions, how reproducible is the grading of the same urothelial tumor by the same pathologist and between different pathologists? Ooms et al.[16] performed an analysis of the performance of pathologists on the grading of bladder tumors. Fifty-seven transurethrally resected bladder tumors were analyzed to determine whether using the World Health Organization grading system, different pathologists graded the same bladder tumor differently (interindividual consistency) and whether the same pathologist graded a bladder tumor differently at different times (intraindividual consistency). Disturbingly high interindividual and intraindividual inconsistencies in the grading of bladder tumors were found. All pathologists showed essentially the same degree of intraindividual inconsistency. In almost 50% of the cases, the tumor was graded differently at different times by the same pathologist. In clinical decision making, the inconsistencies might invalidate the usefulness of bladder tumor grading. The same group has also subsequently performed morphometric grading of bladder tumors in comparison with histologic grading by various pathologists. They[17] have described the results of grading of bladder tumors using morphometry and then compared these with the results of histologic grading of the same tumor by different pathologists. The nuclear sizes of cells obtained from the superficial and deep cell layers of each carcinoma and from giant cells were measured in 27 cases in which the histologic grading by different pathologists was unequivocal. In cells from all three areas, the nuclear area increased with higher grades of tumor. However, tumors of grades I and II showed significant differences in the size only of the large cells. It can be seen from their study that morphometry is a valuable tool in the objective grading of bladder tumors with the exception of carcinoma *in situ* lining the bladder lumen.

UROTHELIAL DYSPLASIA

The clinical significance of urothelial dysplasia is beginning to be appreciated. There is good circumstantial evidence that as a pathological diagnosis it may precede overt urothelial cancer. In a retrospective study of resected flat urothelium adjacent to exophytic urothelial cancer, Althausen et al.[18] found that 9 of 25 patients with urothelial dysplasia developed invasive cancers within a 5-year follow-up period. Similarly, Murphy et al.[19] studied prospectively selected urothelial biopsies from patients followed for urothelial cancer. Eleven of twenty-nine patients (38%) had documented recurrences after the appearance of these "premalignant lesions" as compared to only five of thirty-two (16%) individuals with normal urothelium at the selected biopsy sites.

Urothelial dysplasia or *urothelial atypia* is a relatively recent pathologic term that will need further clinical definition as there is increasing pathological recognition of this lesion. The disease is multifocal and is frequently encountered in those patients who are being followed for bladder cancer. Their frequency in pathological specimens varies considerably.[18,20-22] It is present with great frequency in radical cystectomy specimens and can also be found in urothelial biopsies with no apparent clinical disease.[1,9,19] Many of the patients with urothelial atypia are middle-aged males without any history of urinary tract infections. They, however, complain of frequency and dysuria. The urothelial atypia or dysplastic lesions cannot be localized endoscopically. These lesions like carcinoma *in situ* commonly exfoliate cells into the urine. The recognition of these cells cannot be readily differentiated from the atypical cells that are commonly found with the urothelial atypia of regenerating urothelium seen in repair associated with trauma or infection.

Urothelial atypia or dysplasia describes a spectra of histologic abnormalities between normal urothelium and carcinoma *in situ*.[23] These lesions can be divided into three degrees of morphologic severity, i.e. mild, moderate and severe. Lesions of the lowest grade may not be readily distinguished from reactive, regenerating, and/or reparative urothelium. On occasion, the highest grade may be difficult to distinguish from unequivocal carcinoma.

REFERENCES

1. Koss, L. G. Tumors of the urinary bladder. In *Atlas of Tumor Pathology, Second Series, Part II, Fascicle 8.* Armed Forces Institute of Pathology, Washington, 1974.
2. Pugh, R. C. B. The pathology of bladder tumours. In *Tumours of the Bladder*, Vol. 2, edited by D. M. Wallace. Livingstone, Edinburgh, 1959.
3. Mostofi, F. K. Pathology of malignant tumours of urinary bladder. In *The Biology and Clinical Management of Bladder Cancer*, edited by E. H. Cooper and R. E. Williams. Blackwell Scientific Publishers, Oxford, 1975.
4. Melicow, M. M. Histological study of vesical urothelium intervening between gross neoplasms in total cystectomy. *J. Urol. 68:*261, 1952.
5. Melicow, M. M., and Hollowell, J. W. Intraurothelial cancer; carcinoma *in situ*, Bowen's disease of the urinary system: discussion of thirty cases. *J. Urol. 68:*763, 1952.
6. Melamed, M. D., Vousta, N. G., and Grabstald, H. Natural history and clinical behavior of *in situ* carcinoma of the human urinary bladder. *Cancer 17:*1533, 1964.
7. Koss, L. G., Nakanishi, I., and Freed, S. Z. Non-papillary carcinoma *in situ* and atypical hyperplasia in cancerous bladders. Further studies of surgically removed bladders by mapping. *Urology 9:*442, 1977.
8. Tannenbaum, M., and Romas, N. A. The pathobiology of early urothelial cancers. In *Genitourinary Cancer*, edited by D. G. Skinner and J. B. deKernion. Saunders, Philadelphia, 1978.
9. Farrow, G. M., Utz, D. C., and Rife, C. C. Morphological and clinical observations of patients with early bladder cancer treated with total cystectomy. *Cancer Res. 36:*2495, 1976.
10. Utz, D. C., Hanash, K. A., and Farrow, G. M. The plight of the patient with carcinoma *in situ* of the bladder. *J. Urol. 111:*491, 1974.
11. Cooper, P. H., Waisman, J., Johnston, W. H., and Skinner, D. G. Severe atypia of transitional epithelium and carcinoma of the urinary bladder. *Cancer 31:*1055, 1973.
12. Koss, L. G. Cytology in the diagnosis of bladder cancer. In *The Biology and Clinical Management of Bladder Cancer*, edited by E. H. Cooper and R. E. Williams. Blackwell

Scientific Publishers, Oxford, 1975.

13. Koss, L. G. Mapping of the urinary bladder: its impact on the concept of bladder cancer. *Hum. Pathol. 10:*533, 1979.

14. Pugh, R. C. B. Histological staging and grading of bladder tumours. In *Bladder Cancer: Principles of Combination Therapy*, edited by R. T. D. Oliver, H. J. G. Bloom, and W. F. Hendry. Butterworths, London, 1981.

15. Melicow, M. M. Tumors of the bladder: a multifaceted problem. *J. Urol. 112:*467, 1974.

16. Ooms, E. C. M., Anderson, W. A. D., Alons, C. L., Boon, M. E., and Veldhuizen, R. W. Analysis of the performance of pathologists in the grading of bladder tumors. *Hum. Pathol. 14:*140, 1983.

17. Ooms, E. C. M., Kurver, P. H. J., Veldhuizen, R. W., Alons, C. L., and Boon, M. E. Morphometric grading of bladder tumors in comparison with histologic grading by pathologists. *Hum. Pathol. 14:*144, 1983.

18. Althausen, A. F., Prout, G. R., Jr., and Daly, J. J.: Non-invasive papillary carcinoma *in situ. J. Urol. 166:*575, 1976.

19. Murphy, W. M., Nagy, G. K., Rao, M. K. *et al.* "Normal" urothelium in patients with bladder cancer. *Cancer 44:*1050, 1979.

20. Schade, R. O. K., and Swinney, J. Pre-cancerous changes in bladder epithelium. *Lancet 2:*943, 1968.

21. Eisenberg, R. B., Roth, R. R., and Schweinberg, M. H. Bladder tumors and associated proliferative mucosal lesions. *J. Urol. 84:*544, 1960.

22. Soloway, M. S., Murphy, W. M., Rao, M. K., *et al.* Serial multiple site biopsies in patients with bladder cancer. *J. Urol. 120:*57, 1978.

23. Murphy, W. M., and Soloway, M. S. Developing carcinoma (dysplasia) of the urinary bladder. In *Pathology Annual*, Vol. 17, edited by S. C. Sommers and P. P. Rosen, Appleton-Century-Crofts, New York, 1982.

5

Natural History, Etiology, Diagnosis and Staging of Bladder Cancer

Nasser Javadpour, M.D., F.A.C.S.

Accurate diagnosis and staging of the bladder tumors depends upon a meticulous history and physical examination, as well as radiologic, laboratory, endoscopic, operative and histopathologic findings. The clinical features of tumors of the bladder include pain, disturbances of urination, hematuria, pyuria, and mass. Although the recent advances in endoscopic and radiologic techniques may delineate the exact extent of tumors of the urinary bladder, these procedures should not replace a thorough history and physical examination.

A careful bimanual examination of the lower urinary tract including rectum should be part of any endoscopic examination and preferably should be performed under anesthesia.[17]

The objectives of this chapter are to review the natural history, etiology, pathology, diagnosis, tumor markers and staging of the bladder cancer.

NATURAL HISTORY

Over the past several years, important progress, including a better insight into environmental etiology, and recognition of the natural history and carcinogenesis has provided a better understanding of bladder cancer. Although some progress has been made in the basic understanding and diagnosis of bladder cancer, meaningful clinical progress in terms of management has been confined to tumor markers, cytology, ultrasonography and computed tomography. Many problems remain unsolved, including lack of controlled clinical trials and unavailability of highly effective chemotherapy as an adjuvant to surgery or as primary treatment in disseminated bladder cancer.

The incidence of bladder cancer varies in different countries, and it is a worldwide problem. The incidence of this disease in the United

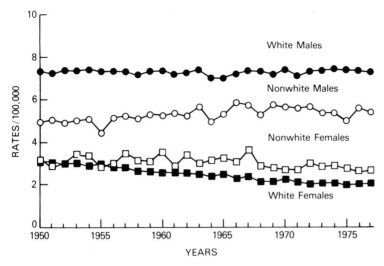

Figure 5.1. Age-adjusted mortality rates of bladder cancer.

States is about 20,000 to 30,000 new cases and 10,000 deaths/year. Bladder cancer represents a spectrum of the diseases with various natural history and etiologic factors. During the past decades, it has become apparent that there are two distinct types of bladder cancer with various natural history. The superficial tumors with low stages, low grades and normal tumor markers are slow progressing tumors. While invasive, high grades and high stages with abnormal tumor markers are included in high risk group. This group of tumors have a high rate of local invasion, regional lymphatic and distant lung metastases. The overall mortality rates of bladder cancer is shown in Figure 5.1.

The natural history of certain superficial tumors is distinct, in that they progress to invasion or distant metastases. Such tumors are usually higher grade tumor, with infiltration to lamina propria, they have lost their cell surface antigens (ABO) and have abnormal chromosomal patterns. They may also be found in association with atypia and carcinoma *in situ*. This group of superficial tumor (as opposed to slow growing, noninvading and indolent superficial tumors) invade and disseminates to lymphatic and visceral organs. The clinical distinction between these two groups of superficial bladder cancer is critical for early and appropriate therapy[26] (see Table 1.2).

ETIOLOGY

A number of agents have been suspected in causing bladder cancer. Exposure to dye stuff, leather, smoking, artificial sweeteners, nitrosamines, and tryptophan metabolism have been reported to contribute to the induction of bladder cancer. Medications, such as phenacetin, chlornaphazine, and benzidine, aniline dye, and several other dyes have been suspected in the etiology of this disease. Chronic infection and infestation with bilharzial parasite also causes mostly squamous cell cancer of the bladder. Hicks[10] has demonstrated apparent synergistic action of saccharin in the production of bladder cancer in N-methyl-N-nitrosourea-treated rats. This investigator also reported the capacity of retinoid compounds to inhibit or at least postpone the appearance of this disease in rats on a carcinogenic diet. Squire and co-workers have also reported the use of 13-*cis*-retinoic acid to inhibit the development of bladder cancer in rats for nitrosourea.

The role of cell proliferation in the initiation of the carcinogenic process is crucial. Cancer of the bladder may be induced by a variety of chemicals in laboratory animals including *N*-methyl-*N*-nitrosourea. *N*-(4-(5-nitro-2-furyl)-2-thiazolyl)formamide (FANFT), and *N*-butyl-*N*-(4-hydroxybutyl)nitrosamine (BBN).[11] Initiation consists of at least two steps, the induction of biochemical lesions in DNA and their fixation in by a round cell proliferation.

In conclusion, it appears that carcinogenesis in the bladder is a multistage phenomenon. The process may be initiated by a brief exposure of the urothelium to a carcinogen. Initiation involves a permanent alteration of the genome in the cell which prepares the potentiality for neoplastic growth. The cancer does not appear until the altered area of the genome is expressed. The neoplastic potential of initiated cells may remain unexpressed for many years until further doses of complete carcinogens or promoters convert them into tumor cells. The natural history of bladder cancer is unpredictable. In a number of patients the initial presentation is muscle invasion, and in others recurrent superficial tumors constitute the natural history of this tumor. The tumor may present in various forms.

HISTOPATHOLOGIC EXAMINATION

Epithelial tumors of the bladder constitute over 95% of malignancies of this organ. A generous biopsy, free of burned edges, is essential for histopathologic study of the tumor. Basically there are three general changes in bladder epithelium: proliferative reactions, metaplastic and neoplastic changes (Fig. 1.2). A close cooperation between pathologists and urologic surgeons is essential in complete histopathologic evaluation of the biopsy material. It is essential to know the location, pattern of growth, depth of infiltration, grade, and vascular and smaller lymphatic spread of the tumor. It is also of utmost importance to note the presence of carcinoma *in situ* in any pathologic specimen of the bladder.[27] The most common epithelial tumors are transitional cell carcinoma followed by squamous cell carcinoma and, rarely, adenocarcinoma. The nonepithelial tumors are mainly rhabdomyosarcoma in children and leiomyosarcoma in adults. The tumors of the bladder may manifest by the following histologic patterns:

1. Papillary noninvasive grade I carcinoma: this noninvasive form of the tumor is covered by thickened transitional cells with abnormal cytology and architecture.
2. Papillary carcinoma noninvasive grade II: this cancer is not invasive, but there is moderate loss of architecture and less differentiated cytology.
3. Transitional cell carcinoma grade II: this tumor is either endophytic or exophytic, and the architecture is disturbed with cellular pleomorphism and superficial invasion into the lamina propria.

4. Papillary transitional cell carcinoma grade II: this is a noninvasive papillary neoplasm with marked cellular and architectural abnormalities.
5. Transitional cell carcinoma *in situ*: the morphology of this flat neoplastic epithelium is noninvasive with varied potential to invade or metastasize.
6. Transitional cell grade III carcinoma: this is an invasive carcinoma with marked changes in architectural and cellular anaplasia.
7. Squamous cell carcinoma: the epithelium consists of squamous cells with intercellular bridges and pearl formation.
8. Adenocarcinoma: this may have various differentiations. The structure consists of tubular or glandular formation. Any adenocarcinoma of the dome of the bladder should be considered to be of urachal origin unless proven otherwise.
9. Undifferentiated carcinoma: this type of bladder cancer does not resemble the previously described tumor and is anaplastic with complete loss or architecture.
10. Occasionally a mixture of the above elements is present in the tumor. The highest grade and most invasive should be brought to the attention of the surgeon.

The various classification of transitional cell tumors of the bladder is shown in Table 5.1.

DIAGNOSIS OF BLADDER CANCER

Diagnosis of tumors of the urinary bladder depends upon a meticulous history and physical examination, as well as radiologic, laboratory, endoscopic, operative, and histopathologic findings. The clinical features of tumors of the bladder are disturbances of urination, hematuria, pyuria, pneumaturia, and mass. Although the recent advances in endoscopic and radiologic techniques may facilitate the diagnosis of this cancer, these procedures should not replace a thorough history and physical examination.

A meticulous history and physical examination should be followed by a satisfactory intravenous pyelogram (IVP) in any patient with hematuria. Urinary cytologic examination is reasonably sensitive and specific, particularly for high grade lesions and carcinoma *in situ*. Although application of routine cytology is not practical in healthy populations, in high risk patients with symptoms or history of occupational exposure to carcinogens it is helpful.

Ultrasonography (US) is well adapted to examining bladder tumors, as the fluid-filled bladder serves as a window to see not only the bladder wall, but also to examine the perivesical region.[17, 20] Intraluminal masses will result in echogenic regions within the echolucent bladder lumen. Local pelvic extension can be detected either as an extension of the bladder wall neoplasm or as a mass near the pelvic side walls. Ultrasound is also useful in evaluating the upper urinary tracts if any abnormality is suspected on the IVP.[21, 22] Transurethral ultrasonography appears to be the most accurate means of staging a bladder tumor.

Computed tomography (CT) provides complementary information to ultrasound. Instead of relying upon sound transmission, CT provides a cross-sectional radiographic image but with greatly enhanced density differentiation compared to routine radiographs.[5, 23, 28] For optimal CT examination, the bladder should be distended with a combination of air

Table 5.1
Classification of Transitional Cell Tumors of Bladder[a, b]

WHO	NBCC	AFIPF
Papilloma	Papilloma	Papilloma
Transitional cell carcinoma, grade I, stage 0	Papillary transitional cell CIS, grade 1	Papillary carcinoma, grade I, noninvasive
Transitional cell carcinoma, grade I, stage A–stage D	Transitional cell carcinoma, grade I, stage A–stage D	Papillary carcinoma, grade I, invasive
Transitional cell CIS, grade II	Flat transitional cell CIS, grade II	Transitional cell CIS, grade II
Transitional cell carcinoma, grade II, stage 0	Papillary transitional cell CIS, grade II	Papillary carcinoma, grade II, noninvasive
Transitional cell carcinoma, grade II, stage A–stage D	Transitional cell carcinoma, grade II, stage A–stage D	Papillary carcinoma, grade II, invasive
Transitional cell CIS, grade III	Flat transitional cell CIS, grade III	Transitional cell carcinoma, grade II
Transitional cell carcinoma, grade III, stage 0	Papillary transitional cell CIS, grade III	Transitional cell CIS, grade III
Transitional cell carcinoma, grade III, stage A–stage D	Transitional cell carcinoma, grade III, stage A–stage D	Papillary carcinoma, grade III, noninvasive
		Papillary carcinoma, grade III, invasive
		Transitional cell carcinoma, grade III

[a] Reproduced with permission from Gittes and Campbell's *Textbook of Urology: Tumors of the Bladder*, p. 104, edited by H. Harrison, R. Gittes, A. Perlmutler, T. Stanly, and P. Walsh. Saunders, Philadelphia, 1979.
[b] The abbreviations used are: WHO, World Health Organization; NBCC, National Bladder Cancer Cooperative; AFIPF, Armed Forces Institute of Pathology Fascicle; and CIS, carcinoma *in situ*.

and dilute contrast material. This can easily be performed after passing a Foley catheter into the bladder. Bladder distention is essential because the partially collapsed bladder wall will produce the erroneous impression of thickening of the bladder wall.[17] The patient must be scanned both supine and prone in order to search for small lesions which may be seen only when outlined by air. This technique is most useful for imaging the intravesical portion of the tumor.

Depending upon the amount of perivesical fat present, the bladder wall may be seen as a clearly defined density. In such cases the outer extent of the neoplasm may also be defined. Local pelvic metastases may be recognized in all but the most asthenic of patients. Whereas US is ineffective where bowel gas inhibits sound transmission, CT clearly identifies gas-containing bowel. Thus CT will be more useful in examining the perirectal space and greater pelvis when rectosigmoid colon and small bowel gas interferes with US. Angiography has been useful in some centers in defining the extent of bladder carcinoma, but it has not gained widespread acceptance.

The most common regional metastases are in the draining lymph nodes. The nodes draining the bladder include the internal iliac or hypogastric nodes, which are not routinely opacified on pedal lymphograms, as well as the external iliac nodes, which are demonstrated with lymphography. Metastases are seen as peripheral filling defects, usually 1 cm or more in diameter. Obstruction of lymphatic channels may be due to tumor, particularly if there has been replacement of the lymph node by a tumor metastasis. The accuracy of bipedal lymphography varies considerably and has been reported to be as high as 94%.[17,19] Once the lymphogram has been performed, an abdominal radiograph provides simple surveillance of the opacified lymph nodes.[19] Lymphography has not been universally utilized in cases of bladder carcinoma, and its exact role is not clear.[17] Both CT and US may be used to evaluate lymphatic metastases, but these modalities depend upon the presence of bulk disease and do not have the resolution for smaller-sized metastatic deposits that may be seen by lymphography.

Bone metastases are not common at presentation: however, they are seen with increasing frequency as the disease progresses. Improvement in radionuclide bone scanning agents has probably also contributed to the better recognition of bone metastases. Abnormal radionuclide bone scans should be followed by a plain radiography of any abnormal area. Bone metastases from bladder carcinomas are most commonly lytic in appearance, although blastic lesions may be seen.

TUMOR MARKERS

The major problem in the diagnosis and management of superficial noninvasive bladder cancer has been the lack of predictors to assess the potential invasiveness of such cancer. The conventional histopathologic examination of the primary or metastatic tumor rarely predicts the potential for invasion.[12] During the past several years it has become apparent that cellular differentiation in certain cancer is reflected in the presence or absence of certain cell surface antigens. In this section we review the value of multiple cell markers in superficial and invasive bladder cancer.

Cell Surface Antigens

Surface antigens identical to those which designate the ABO(H) blood groups are present on the surface of normal urothelial cells as well as cells from a variety of tissues. Davidson[6] has developed the specific red cell adherence test (SRCA) to determine the presence or absence of ABO(H) cell surface antigens. In applying the test to cancer of the cervix, they found that cells undergo malignant dedifferentiation from atypia to anaplasia and that there is a progressive loss of the ABO(H) cell surface antigen.[6] Subsequently, Decenzo applied this test to studies of stage A transitional cell carcinomas of the bladder and found that of the 13 tumors which retained the ABO(H) cell surface antigen, none progressed to invasive stages. In contrast, 8 of 9 tumors that lost the antigen ultimately did advance to invasion.[12]

Subsequent reports from our laboratory[1,7,8] and by others[3] revealed that lesions greater than stage A consistently showed absence of the ABO(H) cell surface antigen and that loss of the antigen could be correlated with advance in histologic grade.

Several investigators have demonstrated the possibility of SRCA in detecting the anaplastic potential of cancer of the cervix, stomach, pancreas, and lung. Our laboratory has applied this principle to bladder cancer and found a correlation between the presence of this cell surface

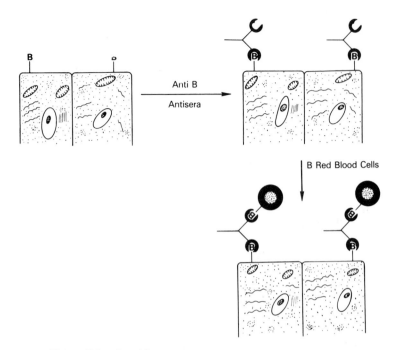

Figure 5.2. Specific red cell adherence reaction.

antigen and prognosis in stage 0, a bladder cancer. The technique of this test is simple and could be mastered in any laboratory (Fig. 5.2) (also see Chapter 6).

It is encouraging that this simple test may predict the invasive potential of superficial tumor unable to be predicted by the conventional histopathologic examination. This has also been confirmed by a number of recent studies.

CORRELATION OF THESE ANTIGENS WITH STAGE AND GRADE

In our series, seventy-six bladder tumors of various stages and grades were examined for the presence of ABO(H) cell surface antigens employing the SRCA technique. Seventy percent of the grade I lesions studied were positive for the cell surface antigen, and none of the 26 grade III tumors retained their antigens[8] (Table 5.2). When correlated with clinical stage, the tumors showed no antigens were present on those of stage B to D, while 12 of 28 stage A lesions were positive for the antigen (Table 5.3). When stage A lesions were studied and the findings correlated with recurrence and metastasis/invasion rates, the cell surface antigen was present on the initial tumor in only one lesion that recurred at an invasive stage.

PERSPECTIVE AND LIMITATIONS

The development of various techniques to detect the presence or absence of the blood group ABO(H) has been encouraging in predicting the natural history of the pathologically low grade, low stage bladder cancer that may be transformed into the high grade and high stage.

Table 5.2
Correlation of Grades and Cell Surface Antigens in 76 Patients with Bladder Cancer

Pathologic Grade	SRCA	
	Positive	Negative
I	7	3
II	15	25
III	0	26

Table 5.3
Cell Surface Antigen in 76 Patients Correlated with the Stage of Tumor

Clinical Stages	SRCA	
	Positive	Negative
A	12	16
B–D	0	48

Utilizing these markers one may predict the natural history of the bladder cancer that would not be clear otherwise. The high grade anaplastic tumor of the bladder will lose the antigen although the low grade, low stages are immunologically well differentiated. These findings by us and other investigators have important implications in the management of bladder tumor. The need for development of new markers, such as steroid receptors, needs no elaboration. We have been making every effort to develop and utilize these markers in a number of prospective and/or randomized clinical protocols. The quality control and improvements for SRCA are shown in Table 5.4.

Initially we had several false negatives, especially in patients with type O blood groups. At the present time, the prolonged (30 minutes) incubation and preparation of fresh reagents with a pH of 7.4 has dramatically diminished the false negative. However, in patients receiving radiation therapy, a conversion from a negative to a positive reaction has been demonstrated in our laboratory and has also been reported by other investigators. In light of the lack of these isoantigens on the surface of squamous metaplastic cells of the bladder, the value of this reaction is limited. This limitation of SRCA does not affect the usefulness of the test since the majority of bladder cancers in the western hemisphere are transitional cell carcinoma.

The use of immunocytochemical techniques in testing of ABO(H) antigen has been encouraging. This technique is specially rewarding in O(H) blood group where SRCA may yield false-negative results. There are other techniques, including indirect immunoperoxidase which is briefly discussed here.

Immunoperoxidase Tissue Staining

The 4- to 6-micron thick serial sections of formaldehyde-fixed tumor are deparaffinized in xylene and cleared in the usual fashion. These sections are incubated in a humid chamber for 24 hours with rabbit antihuman acid phosphatase (1:200) in 20% goat serum.

After washing, the sections are incubated for 60 minutes with goat antirabbit γ-globulin (1:200) conjugated with horseradish peroxidase in

Table 5.4
Quality Control and Improvements SRCA

Conventional H&E stain

Specificity controls
☐ Positive control
☐ Negative control
☐ Inflammatory lesions

Quality controls
☐ Fresh antisera and indicator for red cells
☐ Incubation—ulex extract (30 min)
☐ pH of TBS (7.4)

20% goat serum. The sections are washed again and exposed to diaminobenzidine containing 0.05% hydrogen peroxide for 10 minutes. All the appropriate controls, including sections exposed to normal rabbit serum are also included. Recently, peroxidase-antiperoxidase techniques have been utilized with equally reliable results[14] (Fig. 5.3).

There are a number of features that make immunoperoxidase superior to immunofluorescence, the tissue stained by immunoperoxidase is permanent and can be counterstained with routine histologic stains, allowing direct comparison of the localized markers in relation with detailed histologic features. Immunoperoxidase and avidin biotin system have proven to be more sensitive and specific in our hands.

Chromosomal Examination

Chromosomal abnormalities may be a sensitive bladder tumor marker. It appears to be of prognostic value in low grade, low stage bladder cancer to predict the rate of recurrence and invasiveness of an apparently superficial tumor, as tumors with normal chromosomes are noninvasive. Combining the SRCA and chromosome study has been reliable in our experience to predict the natural history of a superficial bladder tumor.[16] The following case illustrates the use of these modalities:

A 56-year old man was referred to National Institutes of Health (NIH) with hematuria. Physical examination, excretory urogram, and urinary cytology were unremarkable. Cystoscopic examination revealed a papillary tumor confined to the left lateral wall of the bladder. Resection of this mass revealed a grade II transitional cell carcinoma. Chromosome study showed several abnormal chromosome markers. SRCA showed the loss of cell surface antigen. Although the tumor appeared to be superficial and low grade, it was considered potentially invasive, since it carried a marker chromosome and had lost its antigen. A cystoscopic examination 12 weeks later revealed recurrence over the left lateral wall, and resection of this lesion revealed it to be stage B_2. The patient received radiation therapy in preparation for cystectomy.

This case illustrates that both SRCA and chromosomal abnormalities indicated tumor invasion, but this was not apparent from either endoscopy or biopsy. We have utilized combined cell surface antigens and chromosomal analysis to predict the natural history of bladder cancer in 20 patients in a double blind study.[16] Utilizing these two cellular changes we have studied 20 patients in order to correlate the grade,

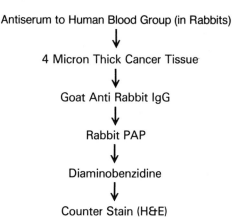

Antiserum to Human Blood Group (in Rabbits)

↓

4 Micron Thick Cancer Tissue

↓

Goat Anti Rabbit IgG

↓

Rabbit PAP

↓

Diaminobenzidine

↓

Counter Stain (H&E)

Figure 5.3. Peroxidase antiperoxidase in localization of cell membrane antigens of bladder cancer.

stage, and prognosis of these tumors to cell surface antigens and chromosomal changes in bladder cancer. These changes may not represent a specific chromosomal change similar to the Ph^1 chromosome in chronic myelocytic leukemia, nevertheless, the chromosomal changes have been proved to correlate well with grade, stage, and prognosis in the present study.

Four of the five patients with grade 1 tumor had retained their antigens. These four patients also had normal chromosomes, the remaining one patient with abnormal chromosomes also had negative SRCA. Of eight patients with grade II tumors, four had normal chromosomes, and only three patients had retained the cell surface antigens of their bladder tumors (Table 5.5). Of 7 patients with grade III cancer none had normal chromosomes, and all had lost their cell surface antigens. Therefore, the grades of tumor correlate with both chromosomal abnormalities and the loss of cell surface antigens. Although the number of patients is limited, these data indicate that SRCA and chromosomal studies may be helpful in grade I and II tumors.

All patients with stages B to D had abnormal chromosomes or had lost their antigens and although 6 of 12 patients with stage 0 or A had abnormal chromosomes, 7 had loss of cell surface antigens (Table 5.6). These data indicate the usefulness of both SRCA and chromosomes in patient with lower stage disease. However, as illustrated in the case presented it appears that if SRCA and chromosomes are abnormal in an apparently low stage (0–A) the patient should be restaged.

In contrast to the constancy of the diploid karyotype in normal tissue, malignant tumors may show a wide range of chromosomal abnormalities both in counts and structures. Also, normally the ABO antigens are shown to be more predictive of the cellular anaplasia and prognosis of the bladder cancer than the conventional histopathologic examination of the tumor alone. Therefore, these two modalities appear to have encouraging contribution in predicting the outcome of a superficial bladder cancer. Their importance in predicting the invasion of a superficial tumor is appreciated in light of only a 35 to 52% five-year survival of muscle-invading primary tumor treated with cystectomy and radiotherapy. However, if the potentially invading tumor is to be recognized

Table 5.5
Correlation of SRCA, Chromosomes, and Grade

Grade	No. of Patients	Chromosomes		Antigen	
		Normal	Abnormal	Present	Absent
I	5	4	1	4	1
II	8	4	4	3	5
III	7	None	7	None	7

Table 5.6
SRCA, Chromosomes and Stage

Stage	No. of Patients	Chromosomes		Antigen	
		Normal	Abnormal	Present	Absent
0, A	12	6	6	5	7
B, C, D	8	None	8	None	8

and treated accordingly, the patient's survival should be prolonged remarkably.

From the present limited number of patients, it appears that both cell surface antigens and chromosomal abnormalities predict the potential invasiveness of a superficial bladder cancer not otherwise detectable; combining these two modalities also increases the potential predictability of invasiveness as shown in the case presented here. The prognosis of this group of patients cannot be completely correlated with their survival at the present time because of the short follow-up. However, one may conclude that chromosomal abnormalities and presence or absence of the ABO antigens may be helpful in stage 0 and A when the conventional staging modalities, including histopathologic examination, cannot predict the anaplasia and invasiveness of a tumor. We are currently studying a larger group of patients with various stages of bladder cancer in order to further evaluate the combined role of these two markers in bladder cancer.

T Antigens

The demonstration of T antigen expression in breast carcinoma and the loss of blood group isoantigens (A, B or H antigen) in invasive transitional cell carcinoma prompted inquiry into the correlation between the carbohydrate precursor of the human blood group system M, N, and the epithelial surface blood group antigens.[14] The T antigen was identified in breast carcinomas, colon and gastric carcinomas and was left to represent a precursor of the human blood group MN glycoproteins. Expression of this antigen was noted in 17 out of 22 breast carcinomas. Those who failed to demonstrate this antigen were poorly differentiated, implying that this antigen may be further altered as the cells become more anaplastic. T antigens may be detected by red cell adherence test (Fig. 5.4).

SIMULTANEOUS DETERMINATION OF T ANTIGEN AND ABO CELL SURFACE ANTIGENS IN TRANSITIONAL CELL CARCINOMA

We have studied 17 bladder tumors in an effort to assess the role of simultaneous T antigen and ABH isoantigens. A red cell adherence

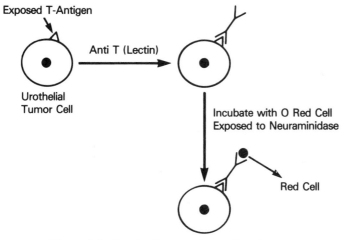

Figure 5.4. Red cell test to detect T antigen.

assay to detect T antigen or deparafinized slides of bladder carcinoma was developed. Peanut agglutinin, which has anti-T antigen properties as well as other nonspecific binding sites, is layered over the slides, washed, then covered with neuraminidase-treated red cells. Red cell adherence was noted on areas of the bladder tumor that binds plant lectin. This was compared with the SRCA for ABH antigens on the same tissue samples. Of the 17 patients, 14 demonstrated loss of their cell surface ABH antigens, 28% demonstrated expression of the onco-fetal T antigen. This would imply that T antigen may be complementary to ABH in predicting potential malignancies of bladder cancer. Also application of immunoperoxidase has improved the detection of T antigen. This antigen may be used for localization and perhaps therapy will be discussed later.

Other Laboratory Tests

Renal, hepatic and pulmonary function tests are often necessary in patients with cancer of the urinary bladder for staging and as baseline studies. However, every case should be individualized to avoid unnecessary expense and discomfort to patients.

Endoscopic Examination

The availability of various diagnostic instruments utilized in urology have rendered the preoperative diagnosis of tumors of the lower urinary tract so accurate that surgery is rarely necessary for diagnostic purposes. The diagnostic instruments utilized for diagnosis of tumors of the lower urinary tract include catheters, sounds, olivary sound, cystoscopes and panendoscopes. The passage of any instrument into the bladder must be absolutely gentle to avoid any injury. When endoscopic examination is performed properly and accompanied by biopsy of the bladder lesions, it is rare that the type and extent of the tumor cannot be detected. Complete evaluation of the bladder tumor includes location, size, structure and generous biopsy of a lesion with a bimanual examination that must be a part of evaluation of every bladder tumor.

STAGING

Cystoscopy, bladder biopsy, and bimanual examination of the bladder are essential in diagnosis and staging of bladder tumors. The formal clinical staging of bladder cancer was started by Jewett and Strong.[18] In a historical landmark analysis of 107 patients dying from bladder cancer, these investigators correlated the extent of infiltration of the primary tumor in bladder wall with a number of other clinical and pathologic findings (Table 5.7). They found that of 89 patients with perivesical fat infiltration, 58% had metastases. They also indicated that regional lymph nodes at least were grossly normal in 36% of the 52 patients with distant metastases.[18] Therefore, the risk of metastases by lymphatic or blood vessel increases with the increased depth of tumor. This landmark investigation provided some facts concerning the natural history and application of cystectomy with pelvic node dissection. There is no universally accepted classification. In addition to the staging of Jewett and Strong (Fig. 5.5), the Union Internationale Contre le Cancer (UICC) has proposed the TNM (Tumor, Node, Metastases) system (Table 5.8). The advantage of the UICC system is the distinction between clinical (T) and pathologic (P) diseases. Furthermore, the TNM staging system recognizes the clinical and pathologic carcinoma *in situ* (T_{1S}, P_{1S}) and the potential for distinction between local extent of the primary tumor (T, P) and extent of nodal and distant metastases (N, M). Comparison between these staging systems and conversion is important in order to

Table 5.7
Carcinoma of the Bladder: Relation of Depth of Invasion to Autopsy Evidence of Extravesical Extension (107 Cases)[a]

Extravesical Extension	Depth of Invasion		
	Submucosa	Muscular	Perivesical Fat
None	3	13	23
Perivesical fixation only	0	0	8
Perivesical lymphatic invasion only	0	1	6
Metastases	0	1	52
Total Number of Cases	3	15	89

[a] Adapted from Jewett and Strong.[18]

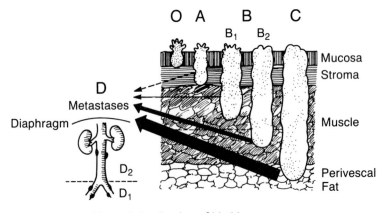

Figure 5.5. Staging of bladder cancer.

Table 5.8
Comparison of Various Staging of Bladder Cancer[a]

Extent of Disease	Jewett Marshall[18]	UICC (TNM or PNM)	
		Clinical	Pathologic
Carcinoma *in situ*	0	T_{1S}	P_{1S}
Lamina propria	A	T_1	P_1
Superficial muscle	B_1	T_2	P_2
Deep muscle	B_2	T_3	P_3
Perivesical fat	C	T_3	P_3
Invasion of adjacent organs	D_1	T_4	P_4
Regional lymph nodes (LN)	D_2	N_1	N_1
LN above aortic bifurcation	D_3	N_2	N_2
Distant metastases	M	M	M

[a] The abbreviations used are UICC: Union Internationale Contre le Cancer; TNM: T, tumor; N, nodes; M, metastases; and P, pathologic.

compare the results of treatment.[15] In clinical staging, in addition to previously mentioned modalities, hemogram, blood chemistry, and renal function tests are obtained. Although cystography, lymphangiography, arteriography, ultrasonography, and bone scan have been proposed in the clinical staging of bladder cancer, consideration of cost-effectiveness makes the routine use of these modalities debatable. Over the past several years it has become increasingly apparent that computed tomography is of value in clinical staging of this disease.

The final decision as to the treatment of bladder cancer depends on grade of the tumor in addition to the stage. Histologic grading is the evaluation of degree of anaplasia of tumor cell. Although there are a number of systems for grading bladder cancer, the most reliable and reproducible is a system of three grades. Grade I applies to tumors that have at least a degree of anaplasia compatible with diagnosis of malignancy; grade III applies to tumors with the most severe degree of cellular anaplasia; and grade II lies in between. Pathologic grading is of clinical value since it is related to the survival rate of patients. The pathologist should comment on grade, extent of muscle invasion, lymphatic and blood vessel involvement, and cell type of the tumor.

SUMMARY AND CONCLUSIONS

The clinical features of bladder cancer include hematuria, disturbance of urination, pain, mass. The initial steps in accurate diagnosis of tumors of the urinary bladder are meticulous history and physical examination including the urethra, rectal examination and palpation of the bladder *via* the anterior abdominal wall.

After careful history and physical examination, if a tumor of the bladder is suspected, an excretory urogram, hemogram and renal function tests should be obtained. If a bladder tumor is suspected, urinary cytology, excretory urography, cystoscopy, bladder biopsy with chromosome study, and red cell adherence should be performed. If histologic features reveal carcinoma of the bladder, a staging procedure including bimanual examination, a chest radiography with whole lung tomography and computed tomography of the bladder and pelvis are performed.

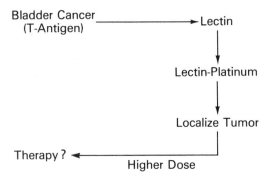

Figure 5.6. Affinity therapy of cancer by chemotherapeutic agents labeled antibody.

The value of lymphangiography in staging of the bladder cancer is not clear at the present time.

The cornerstone of the accurate diagnosis of the bladder tumor is an adequate biopsy and careful histologic examination by an expert pathologist. It is equally important to avoid unnecessary laboratory, radiologic and endoscopic manipulation when the yield is extremely low and the discomfort to the patient is high.

CURRENT PROBLEMS AND FUTURE PERSPECTIVES

The major problem at the present time is prevention of bladder tumor by eliminating the environmental causes and contributing factors. Also, we need further study in developing the predictors such as chromosomal analysis and cell surface antigens and search for other tumor markers. At the present time grading, staging, cystoscopic and bimanual examination of the bladder with biopsy of the tumor remain the cornerstone of therapeutic decision making. However, we need the means to reduce the clinical staging errors and find more reliable predictors of the natural history of a given tumor in order to avoid under- or over-treating the patients. The potential for tumor localization and chemoradioimmunotherapy may be realized with further investigation (Fig. 5.6).

REFERENCES

1. Bergman, S., and Javadpour, N. The cell surface antigen A, B, or O(H) as an indicator of malignant potential in stage A bladder carcinoma. *J. Urol. 119:*48, 1978.
2. Bryan, G. The pathogenesis of experimental bladder cancer. *Cancer Res. 37:*2813, 1977.
3. Coon, J. S., and Weinstein, R. S. Detection of ABH issue isoantigen by immunoperoxidase method in normal and neoplastic urothelium. *Am. J. Clin. Pathol. 76:*163, 1981.
4. Cummings, K. B. Carcinoma of the bladder: predictors. *Cancer 45:*1849, 1980.
5. Daily, E. T., Rosanski, R. M., Kieffer, S. A., and Dinn, W. M. Computed tomography in genitourinary pathology. *Urology 12:*95–105, 1978.
6. Davidson, I. Early immunologic diagnosis and prognosis of carcinoma. *Am. J. Clin. Pathol. 57:*715, 1972.
7. Emmott, R. C., Droller, M. J., and Javadpour, N. The ABO(H) cell surface antigens in carcinoma *in situ* and nonmalignant lesions of the bladder. *J. Urol. 125:*32, 1981.
8. Emmott, C., and Javadpour, N. Correlation of stage and grade with ABO(H) cell surface antigen in bladder cancer. *J. Urol. 121:*37, 1979.

9. Farah, R. N., and Cerny, J. C. Lymphangiography in staging patients with carcinoma of the bladder. *J. Urol. 119:*40, 1978.
10. Hicks, R. M. Carcinogenesis in the urinary bladder; a multistage process in carcinoma of the bladder. *Prog. Cancer Res. Ther. 18:*107, 1981.
11. Hicks, R. M., and Chowaniec, J. The importance of synergy between weak carcinoma in the induction of bladder cancer in experimental animals and humans. *Cancer Res. 37:*2943, 1977.
12. Javadpour, N. Biologic tumor markers in management of testicular and bladder cancer. *Urology 12:*177, 1978.
13. Javadpour, N., Hyatt, C. L., and Soares, T. Immunologic features of a carcinogen-induced murine bladder cancer *in vivo* and *in vitro* studies. *J. Oncol. Surg. 11:*153, 1979.
14. Javadpour, N. Tumor markers in urologic cancer. In *Principle and Management of Urologic Cancer,* Ed 2, p. 32, edited by N. Javadpour. Williams & Wilkins, Baltimore, 1983.
15. Javadpour, N. Natural history, diagnosis and staging of bladder cancer. In *Principle and Management of Urologic Cancer,* Ed 2, p. 293, edited by N. Javadpour, Williams and Wilkins, Baltimore, 1983.
16. Javadpour, N., Roy, J. B., Bottomly, R., and Dagg, K. Combined cell surface antigens and chromosomal studies in bladder cancer. *Urology 19:*29, 1983.
17. Javadpour, N., and Dunnick, N. R. Diagnosis of tumors of the lower urinary tract. In *Diagnosis of Genitourinary Diseases,* p. 373, edited by M. Resnick and R. Old. Thieme-Stratton, New York, 1982.
18. Jewett, H. J., and Strong, G. H. Infiltrating carcinoma of the bladder: relation of certain pathological characteristics to prognosis after extirpation. *J. Urol. 92:*668, 1946.
19. Johnson, D. E., Kaesler, K. E., Kaminsky, S., Jing, B., and Wallace S. Lymphangiography as an aid in staging bladder carcinoma. *South. Med. J. 69:*28–30, 1976.
20. Lang, E. K. The roentgenographic assessment of bladder tumors. A comparison of the diagnostic accuracy of roentgenographic techniques. *Cancer 23:*717–724, 1969.
21. McLaughlin, I. S., Morley, P., Deane, R. F., Barnett, E., Graham, A. G., and Kyle, K. F. Ultrasound in the staging of bladder tumors. *Br. J. Urol. 47:*51–56, 1975.
22. Russell, J. M., and Resnick, M. I. Ultrasound in urology. *Urol. Clin. North. Am. 6:*445, 1979.
23. Schaner, E. G., Chang, A. E., Doppman, J. L., Conkle, D. M., Flye, M. W., and Rosenberg, S. A. Comparison of computed and conventional whole lung tomography in detecting pulmonary nodules: a prospective radiologic-pathologic study. *Am. J. Roentgenol. 131:*51–54, 1978.
24. Sindelar, W. F., Bagley, D. H., Felix, E. L., Doppman, J. L., and Ketcham, A. S. Lung tomography in cancer patients. Full lung tomograms in screening for pulmonary metastases. *JAMA 240:*2060–2063, 1978.
25. Stein, B. S., and Kendall, A. R. Specific red cell adherence testing and radiotherapy. *Cancer 50:*2329, 1982.
26. Whitmore, W. F., Jr. Urothelial tumors—problems and prospects. *Semin. Urol. 1:*2–6, 1983.
27. Utz, D. C., Farrow, G. M., Rife, C. C., *et al.* Carcinoma *in situ* of the bladder. *Cancer 45:*1842, 1980.
28. Yu, W. S., Sagerman, R. H., King, G. A., Chung, C. T., and Yu, Y. W. The value of computed tomography in the management of bladder cancer. *Int. J. Rad. Oncol. Biol. Phys. 5:*135–142, 1979.

6

Cell Surface Antigens and Chromosomal Abnormalities in Bladder Cancer

Nasser Javadpour, M.D., F.A.C.S.

Perhaps the most encouraging progress in cancer immunology has been in the field of immunodiagnosis; mainly, development of specific and sensitive immunocytochemical techniques to measure and localize tumor markers in the sera and cancer cells of cancer patients. In this chapter, we will discuss the developments and utilization of multiple cell markers in bladder cancer with emphasis on more clinically established and useful markers. Nonspecific serum markers such as lactic dehydrogenase, polyamines and a number of oncofetoproteins are under study.

CELL MARKERS IN BLADDER CANCER

The major problem in diagnosis and management of a superficial noninvasive bladder cancer has been the lack of criteria to assess its potential invasiveness. The conventional histopathologic examination of the primary does not completely predict the potentiality of this cancer to invade. During the last few years it has become apparent that cellular differentiation in certain cancers is reflected in the presence or absence of certain cell surface antigens, chromosomal features and potential T antigen and tumor-associated antigens.

There are a number of cell antigens that are normally expressed on the cells of most urothelium that have been utilized as tumor markers. Among these cell antigens are[1]:

1. ABO(H) antigens.
2. T antigen.

3. Tumor-associated antigen(s).
4. DNA and RNA as detected by flow cytometry.

ABO(H) ANTIGENS IN BLADDER CANCER

Surface antigens identical to those that designate the ABO(H) blood groups are present on the surface of normal urothelial cells as well as cells from a variety of tissues. Davidsohn and co-workers[2] developed the specific red cell adherance test (SRCA) to determine the presence or absence of these cell surface antigens. In applying the test to cancer of the cervix, they found that as cells from the cervix undergo malignant dedifferentiation from atypia to anaplasia, there appears to occur a progressive loss of the ABO(H) cell surface antigens. Subsequent reports by a number of laboratories revealed that lesions greater than stage A consistently showed absence of the ABO(H) cell surface antigens and that loss of these antigens could be correlated with advance in histologic grade.[2-7] This potential ability of the cell markers to predict which early bladder tumors might be destined to invade the bladder muscle or metastases prompted the investigators to examine the association between ABO(H) cell surface and bladder cancer.[8-10]

All of the inflammatory lesions of the bladder studied so far have retained ABO(H) cell surface antigens. This is particularly important in view of the fact that inflammatory conditions such as cystitis cystica, cystitis glandularis, and squamous metaplasia are frequently seen in association with cancer and might, therefore, seriously influence interpretation of the SRCA test.[7] On the other hand, squamous metaplasia, a nonmalignant lesion, demonstrated consistent loss of the surface ABO(H) antigens. Although this is not surprising in view of previous studies that have shown the ABO(H) antigens not to be present on squamous cells from other areas of the body, it emphasized the necessity of carefully distinguishing benign squamous metaplasia from areas of carcinoma when applying these antigens to bladder lesions.

SRCA in Detection of ABO(H) Antigens

The technique of SRCA has been described before briefly.[2] Slides are deparaffinized in two 5-minute xylene washes, washed in two 5-minute absolute alcohol baths and rehydrated in three 0.05 M Tris buffer (ph 7.4) baths. Slides were then incubated with *Ulex europaeus* extract for 30 minutes of O(H) and antisera to A, B and AB for the remaining blood group. The *Ulex* extract was prepared by homogenizing 20 g of *Ulex* seeds in 100 ml buffered saline at 0 °C. This was then centrifuged at 0 °C, 7000 rpm, for 15 minutes. The supernatant was recentrifuged in like manner and kept frozen until needed. The excess *Ulex* extract was then rinsed in three 5-minute Tris buffer washes. The slides were then incubated at room temperature with O banked blood. The slides were then inverted in Petri dishes to that the buffer touched the slide, washing off untreated RBC, and read after 5 minutes. Endothelium provided a positive internal control and connective tissue and muscle provided negative internal controls. Currently, a form of immunoperoxidase may be used because it appears to be more reproducible with low false negative rates.

Peroxidase Antiperoxidase (PAP) in Detection of ABO(H) Antigens

The technique of PAP has previously been discussed.[11] Briefly, two 5- μm serial sections of formaldehyde-fixed tumor are deparaffinized in xylene. These sections are exposed to 3% hydrogen peroxide in methanol for 25 minutes. After washing 3 times with Tris solution the slides are covered with 3% normal goat serum to block the nonspecific staining. After another serial washing with Tris solution the slides are incubated with rabbit antiulex or other antisera to A or B (1:100) in a humid chamber for 60 minutes. The control slides are incubated with normal rabbit serum. After several washings with Tris solution the slides were incubated with goat antirabbit IgG (1:20) for 30 minutes in room temperature. Then the slides are washed with Tris solution 3 times and were exposed to freshly prepared peroxidase antiperidoxidase (1:50) in 1% normal goat serum for 30 minutes at room temperature. After appropriate washing the slides are covered with diaminobenzidine solution (40 mg/100 ml of Tris plus 1.75 ml of H_2O_2) for 7 minutes. Then the slides are counter-stained with hematoxylin for 60 seconds and mounted with cover slides and interpreted in a double blind fashion. The controls consist of internal controls and the slides that are treated with absorbed rabbit anti-*Ulex*, anti-A and anti-B antisera.

In a double blind study we reported that in terms of prognosis, SRCA was positive in only 1 of 8 patients with a single tumor, whereas PAP was positive in 5 of 8. In patients with recurrent tumors, all low stage, SRCA was positive in 1 of 15 while PAP was positive in 6 out of 15. In invasive lesions both PAP and SRCA were negative in all 7 patients. Thus, prognostically PAP appears to be a better predictor of prognosis than SRCA in Group O patients.[12]

The results of this study demonstrate that PAP decreases the rate of false negative results as compared to SRCA in patients with group O(H) isoantigen. We have previously reported that grade II bladder cancers have generally lost their cell surface antigen. These data also support this finding. Furthermore, it demonstrates the superiority of PAP over the SRCA technique in decreasing the false negative results.

Reports from autopsy material of normal ureters in group O patients utilizing SRCA have been found to be falsely negative in more than a third of studied specimens. Since about 45% of the population expresses the O(H) antigen, we need a more sensitive and reproducible technique than SRCA to detect this antigen. We have demonstrated that PAP correlates better with prognosis and invasiveness of bladder cancer in group O patients than SRCA in a double blind study. Furthermore, the convenience, permanence and ready availability of the PAP technique should encourage its use in conventional histopathologic laboratories.

Correlation of these Antigens with Stage and Grade

In seventy-six bladder tumors of various stage and grades examined with the SRCA technique for the presence of the ABO(H) cell surface antigen, 70% of the grade I lesions were positive for the cell surface antigen, and none of the 26 grade III tumors retained their antigens (Table 6.1). When correlated with clinical stage, the tumors showed no antigens present on those of stages B–D, whereas 12 of 18 stage A lesions were positive for the antigen (Table 6.2). When stage A lesions were studied and the findings correlated with recurrence and metastasis/invasion rates, in only one lesion (which recurred at an invasive stage) was the cell surface antigen present on the initial tumor. Therefore, it is concluded that cell surface antigens are helpful in predicting malignant potential in low grade, low stage cancer of the bladder. These antigens may offer the capability of selecting low grade, low stage bladder tumors that are destined to invade or metastasize while they are at stages curable by cystectomy.

The findings of cell surface ABO(H) antigens in a limited number of various lesions examined for these antigens are shown in Table 6.3. Squamous metaplasia in either neoplastic or non-neoplastic lesions consistently demonstrated apparent absence of the ABO(H) cell surface antigens. Conversely, cystitis cystica and cystitis glandularis were always positive for the presence of these cell surface antigens. Areas of carcinoma within lymph nodes were uniformly negative for the presence of ABO(H) antigens.

Table 6.1
Correlation of Grades and Cell Surface Antigens in 76 Patients with Bladder Cancer

Pathologic Grade	SRCA	
	Positive	Negative
I	7	3
II	15	25
III	0	26

Table 6.2
Cell Surface Antigen in 76 Patients Correlated with the Stage of Tumor

Clinical Stages	SRCA	
	Positive	Negative
A	12	16
B–D	0	48

Table 6.3
SRCA Findings in Patients with Benign Lesions and Carcinoma *In Situ*[7]

Lesions	Patients	SRCA	
		Positive	Negative
	(n)		
Cystitis cystica	8	8	
Cystitis glandularis	8	8	
Squamous metaplasia	4		4
Nodal metastases	4		4
Carcinoma *in situ*	7	1[a]	8

[a] Partial loss of cell surface antigen. This is considered as a negative.

T ANTIGEN

The changes in cell surface antigens result in the interruption of communication and interaction through the cell surface membrane. These changes reflect an alteration in the genome which modifies the biosynthetic pathways of the Golgi apparatus. The demonstration of T antigen expression in breast carcinoma and the loss of blood group isoantigens (A, B, O, or H) in invasive transitional cell carcinoma prompted inquiry into the correlation between the carbohydrate precursor of the human blood group system MN and the epithelial surface blood group isoantigens.

The T antigen has been identified in breast carcinomas, colon and gastric carcinomas and was believed to represent a precursor of the human blood group MN glycoproteins. Subsequently, a plant lectin derived from peanuts and termed peanut agglutinin was found to possess high affinity for glycoproteins containing the terminal sequence galactose (1–3)-N-acetyl-D-galastomine.[14] This concealed antigen was so termed after the Thomsen-Friedenreich phenomenon which was a result of exposure of the red blood cells to influenza viruses which contained a receptor-destroying enzyme known to be neuraminidase which released the terminal sialic acid exposing the T antigen. Expression of this antigen was noted in 17 out of 22 breast carcinomas, all of which were well differentiated. The five carcinomas that failed to demonstrate the antigen were poorly differentiated, possibly implying that the antigen may be further altered as the cell becomes more anaplastic.

Technique for Demonstration of T Antigen

A modified cell adherence assay has been utilized to demonstrate the T antigen on the cell surface membrane because of the ease and simplicity of performing the test.[12, 14] It is primarily a sandwich type reaction with the deparaffinized tissue sections as the bottom layer, the indication erythrocytes as the top layer and the specific anti-T lectin (peanut lectin) as the middle layer. Demonstration of the indicator erythrocytes implied the cells in tissue expressed the T antigen. Peanut seeds (10 gm) are soaked in H_2O_2 for 24 hours and then homogenized in 25 ml of buffered saline, this is then centrifuged for 5 minutes at 3200 rpm. The supernatant was decanted off and placed in a Beckman preparatory ultracentrifuge at 48,000 rpm for 1 hour. The supernatant is then frozen at −20 °C until needed. T antigen-activated erythrocytes are prepared by using outdated blood bank cells washed in buffered saline three times. A solution of 0.5 ml mucopolysaccharide N-acetyl-neuraminylhydrogenase (500 units/ml) plus 2.5 ml of packed erythrocytes plus 2.5 ml phosphate buffer at pH 7.4 was made and incubated at 37 °C for 4 hours. The T activated erythrocytes were stored at 2–8 °C until used. Positive and negative controls are made on each histologic section to be studied. The positive control consists of placing a solution of neuraminidase and phosphate buffer (50 units/ml) on a slide of the deparaffinized section previously described for 30 minutes. The slides are washed in three changes of phosphate buffer for 5 minutes in each change. The T-activated erythrocytes are then incubated with the slides for 30 minutes before invertions in Petri dishes containing phosphate buffer. The negative control consists of incubating the slide with peanut agglutinin for 30 minutes, then washing in phosphate buffer for 5 minutes three times. The section is then incubated with non-T-activated erythrocytes for 30 minutes. The actual test consists of a 30-minute incubation of the slide with peanut agglutinin followed by washing in phosphate buffer for 5 minutes three times. The slide is then incubated with T-activated erythrocytes for 30 minutes.

Carcinoma *in Situ*

The recognition of carcinoma *in situ* has added dimension to the dilemma in management of such lesions.[7] Predicting the ultimate natural history of carcinoma *in situ* is of utmost importance in management of this lesion.

The natural history of carcinoma *in situ* remains controversial. The high incidence of its coexistence with infiltrative tumors in the bladder and the more ominous prognosis that this situation implies have encouraged otologists toward more definitive early treatments. However, in the absence of gross lesions; carcinoma *in situ* may behave in a less aggressive fashion.

Simultaneous Determination of T Antigen and ABO Cell Surface Antigens in Transitional Cell Carcinoma

Bladder tumors have been studied utilizing combined antigens such as T antigen and ABO antigens in an effort to assess the role of combined antigens in bladder cancer. The red cell adherence assay to detect T-antigen utilizing peanut lectin which has anti-T properties as well as other nonspecific binding sites is layered over the slides, wahed, then covered with neuraminidase-treated red cells. In studying 17 patients, 14 demonstrated loss of their cell surface ABO antigens. Of the 14, 28% demonstrated expression of T antigen. This would imply that T antigen may be complementary to ABO(H) as in predicting potential malignancies of bladder cancer. Currently, these two antigens are being evaluated in bladder cancer in a prospective study, and the exact role of combined antigens in bladder cancer needs more investigation. The data from our laboratory indicates a lack of correlation of T antigen to the stage, grade and invasiveness of bladder tumor, whereas ABO(H) antigens correlate well.

Perspectives and Limitations

The development of various techniques including immunoperoxidase to detect the presence or absence of the blood group ABO(H) or T antigen has been encouraging in predicting the natural history of the pathologically low grade, low stage bladder cancer that may be transformed into the high grade and high stage. Utilizing these markers, one may predict the natural history of the bladder cancer that would not be clear otherwise. The high grade anaplastic tumor of the bladder will lose the antigen, although the low grades, low stages are immunologically well differentiated. These findings by us and other investigators have important implications in management of the bladder cancer.

Although, with attempts to perform the SRCA with O blood group, false negative results may occur. At the present time the prolonged (30-minute) incubation and preparation of fresh reagents with a pH of 7.4 have diminished the false negatives. Also in patients receiving radiotherapy, a conversion from a negative to a postive reaction has occasionally been demonstrated. In light of the lack of these isoantigens on the surface of squamous metaplastic cells of the bladder, the value of this reaction appears to be limited in squamous cell carcinoma of the bladder. This limitation of SRCA does not affect the usefulness of the test, since the majority of bladder cancers in the western hemisphere are of transitional cell origin. Another limitation of SRCA is that it is a qualitative rather than a quantitative test as are many other histopathologic tests. However, one can make this test permanent and counterstain it with eosin in order to recognize the cells that have lost their antigens in relation to the other cells in a section. It is important to realize that any given test for predicting the prognosis of cancer, including cancer of the bladder, should be most specific, sensitive, fast, inexpensive, reproducible, practical, quantitative and easy to perform with a high accuracy rate. At the present time, such a test is not available for any cancer. However, that continuous effort to improve the test and to accumulate accurate knowledge is essential in evaluating any given test, including the specific red cell adherence (SRCA) test. Currently, the (IP) and peroxidase/antiperoxidase (PAP) tests are being explored in my laboratory in an attempt to improve and to standardize this test (Fig. 6.1). The data indicate the superiority of PAP over SRCA in the detection of O(H) isoantigen.

To improve on the SRCA test, I have compared the IP test, PAP test, and the avidin-biotin system (Fig. 6.2). The SRCA test may give false-negative results with O blood group. Initial results indicate that the IP test, PAP test, and the avidin-biotin system are superior to the SRCA test for detecting the O(H) isoantigen. They may be more versatile than SRCA.

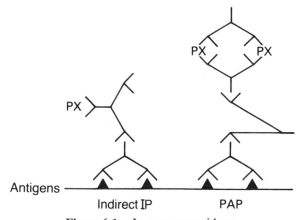

Figure 6.1. Immunoperoxidase.

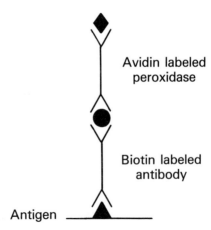

Figure 6.2. Biotin/avidin system (affinity of avidin for biotin is high).

Utilizing tumor markers such as T antigen, ABO isoantigens, and chromosomal abnormalities will help separate superficial bladder tumors with a good prognosis and low risk from superficial bladder tumors that will be invasive with a high rate of recurrence and potential for metastases. This important clinical distinction will help facilitate effective therapeutic modalities at the time of diagnosis and lead to improved prognoses for patients with superficial bladder cancer.

Currently, we consider the presence of ABO antigens as strong consideration for conservative therapy of superficial bladder cancer, although loss of these antigens will put these patients in a high risk group.

Multiple cell markers, such as ABO isoantigens, T antigen, chromosomal analysis and flow cytometry, can distinguish the patients with high or low risk superficial bladder cancer and guide the clinician in selecting appropriate therapy when these markers are considered with grade, stage, and other clinical findings. They do not perform cystectomy in these patients solely on the basis of loss of cell surface antigens, but they consider this loss as another parameter of future recurrence and invasiveness.

Potentiality for Radioimmunodetection (RID) Radioimmunotherapy (RIT) in Bladder Cancer

There are a number of cell surface antigens that are normally expressed on the cells of most urothelium or urothelial cancer. The antigens that are expressed on bladder cancer cells are T antigen and tumor-associated antigens. These antigens are concealed from the normal transitional cell of the bladder and expressed during carcinogenesis. T antigen has been detected on bladder cancer utilizing a specific red cell adherence test[15] or immunoperoxidase in bladder cancer. It appears attractive to attempt to label a γ-emitting radioactive material to the T antigen or other tumor-associated antigen for the purpose of RID or perhaps chemo- or radioimmunotherapy of metastatic bladder cancer. These approaches are attractive because of the lack of reliable techniques to localize the lymphatic involvements, in terms of diagnosis[16] and prognosis. Furthermore, the advent of monoclonal antibodies have provided additional encouragement in this field.[5,17]

With the advent of monoclonal antibodies one may prepare large amounts of pure antibodies for diagnostic and therapeutic purposes.

Combined Cell Surface Antigens and Chromosomal Analysis

Chromosomal abnormalities also appear to be sensitive bladder tumor marker. Chromosomal changes appear to be of prognostic value in low grade, low stage bladder cancer in predicting the rate of recurrence and invasiveness of a clinically superficial tumor. Tumors with normal chromosomes are usually noninvasive. The combination of the SRCA, chromosome testing, and computed tomography has been of value in staging and determining the natural history of bladder cancer. In a prospective study of 20 patients with bladder cancer in which cell surface antigens and chromosomal analysis were employed, the preliminary conclusion was that chromosomal analysis and the presence or absence of ABO antigens have good correlations with grades and stages of these tumors and are the most reliable markers for bladder cancer at the present time.

TUMOR-ASSOCIATED ANTIGEN

Tumor-specific antigens have been demonstrated on a variety of animal tumors. Evidence that human tumors contain tumor-specific antigens comes from many sources including the increased incidence of cancer in immune deficiency states, the *in vitro* demonstration of cellular and humoral immune responses to tumor antigens, positive skin-test reactivity of patients of autologous tumor extracts, and a variety of circumstantial clinical suggestions. Much has been learned about the basic immunobiology of the immune response to tumors in animals and humans. Many hypotheses exist to explain the continued growth of the tumor in the face of an active immunological response against it. Immunological tests have been developed to a variety of tumor-associated antigens that may be of use in the immunodiagnosis and immunoevaluation of patients with cancer. Attempts to utilize the immune response for the treatment of malignant tumors are in their earliest stages. However, there are many suggestions that this approach may be of value in the future. There is evidence that human bladder cancer may have tumor-associated antigen.

Acute phase proteins such as plasminogen, hepatoglobulin, immunoglobulin have been reported to be associated with transitional carcinoma of the bladder. They are also seen in inflammatory lesions of the bladder and, therefore, are not specific. Oncofetoproteins such as CEA and HCG have also been reported to be elevated in bladder cancer, but they are not consistent enough to serve as tumor markers.

Other protein markers include urinary polyamines, urinary fibrin degradation products, urinary aminoisobutyrate, urinary β-glucuronidase and urinary tryptophan metabolic products have been occasionally found in bladder cancer but they are not specific.

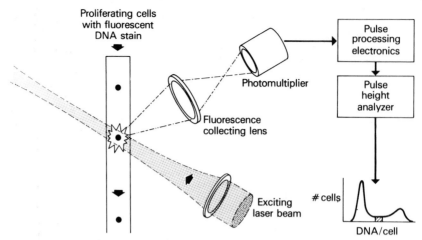

Figure 6.3. Flourescence flow cytometer.

FLOW CYTOMETRY FOR DNA AND RNA

The flow cytometry is based on passing the urinary sediments from patients with bladder cancer through a focused Argan laser beam in single file. Prior to this testing, the urinary sediments are stained with acridine orange which caused DNA to be fluorescent green and RNA to be red (Fig. 6.3). In a study of 48 patients with papilloma of the urinary bladder, Klein and co-workers[18,19] have concluded that for patients at risk developing tumor of the bladder, a combination of DNA and RNA flow cytometry appears to offer greater diagnostic sensitivity than flow cytometry based on CNA content alone.

In following 97 patients with history of low grade, low stage bladder cancer utilizing flow cytometry these authors[19] have also concluded that flow cytometry is a sensitive, quantitative method of detecting abnormal cells in bladder irrigation specimens. Therefore, it appears that flow cytometry of DNA and RNA will play a more important role in diagnosis and follow-up of patients with bladder cancer in the future.

FUTURE PERSPECTIVES

The role of cell surface antigens in superficial bladder cancer with low grade and low stage is encouraging. Utilization of immunoperoxidase in detecting cell surface antigens specially in O blood group has yielded a low false-negative, making this test more attractive and reproducible. Furthermore, application of chromosomal studies with T antigen detection has provided additional parameters in diagnosis and management of bladder cancer. Flow cytometry also appears to be useful in the follow-up of patients with low grade, low stage superficial bladder cancer. Utilizing multiple markers specially ABO(H) when detected with immunoperoxidase or PAP technique and chromosomal abnormality will predict the natural history of a superficial bladder cancer as to the future recurrence, invasiveness and potential for prognosis.

It is appropriately emphasized that cell markers should be related to other parameters such grade, stage, multiplicity in time and space, recurrence and available therapeutic options. It is our experience that when superficial bladder tumors lose their ABO(H) and have abnormal chromosomes, they are highly at risk for recurrence, invasion and metastases.

REFERENCES

1. Bergman, S., and Javadpour, N. The cell surface antigen ABO(H) as an indicator of malignant potential in stage A bladder carcinoma. Preliminary report. *J. Urol. 119:*49, 1978.
2. Davidsohn, I. Early immunologic diagnosis and prognosis of carcinoma. *Am. J. Clin. Pathol. 57:*715, 1972.
3. Coon, J. S., and Weinstein, R. Variability in the expression of the O(H) antigen in human transitional epithelium. *J. Urol. 125:*301, 1981.
4. Coon, J. S. Weinstein, R. S. Detection of the ABH tissue isoantigen by immunoperoxidase methods in normal and neoplastic urothelium. *Am. J. Clin. Pathol. 76:*163, 1981.
5. Diamond, B. A., Dale, E. Yelton, B. A., and Scharff M. D. Monoclonal antibodies— a new technology for producing serologic reagents. *N. Engl. J. Med. 304:*1344, 1981.
6. Emmott, R. C., Javadpour, N., Bergman, S. M., and Soares T. Correlation of the cell surface antigens with stage and grade in cancer of the bladder. *J. Urol. 121:*37, 1979.
7. Emmott, C., Droller, M., and Javadpour, N. Studies of ABO(H) cell surface antigen specificity: Carcinoma *in situ* and nonmalignant lesions of the bladder. *J. Urol. 125:*35, 1981.
8. Lange, P. H., Limas, C., and Fraley, E. E. Tissue blood group antigens and prognosis in low stage transitional cell carcinoma of the bladder. *J. Urol. 119:*52, 1978.
9. Lippert, M., and Javadpour, N. Detection of cell surface antigen in renal pelvic and ureteral tumors. *Urology 22:*366, 1983.
10. Stein, B. S., and Kendall, A. R. Specific red cell adherence testing and radiotherapy. *Cancer 50:*23–29, 1982.
11. McAlpine, R., and Javadpour, N. Comparison of specific red cell adherence and immunoperoxidase in detection of ABO(H) antigens in normal urothelium—a double blind study. *Urology* April, 1984.
12. Vafier, J., Javadpour, N., Worsham, G. F., and O'Connell, K. A double blind comparison of T antigen and ABO(H) cell surface antigen in bladder cancer. *Urology* (In press).
13. Javadpour, N. Cell surface antigen in bladder cancer. *J. Urol. 129:*439, 1983.
14. Howard, D. R., and Batsakis, J. G. Cytostructural localization of a tumor-associated antigen. *Science 210:*201, 1980.
15. McAlpine, R., and Javadpour, N. T-antigen in bladder cancer as detected by specific red cell adherence test and immunoperoxidase. *J. Surg. Oncol.* (In press).
16. Javadpour, N. The role of radioimmunodetection in urologic cancer. In *Radioimmunoimaging and Radioimmunotherapy*, pp. 385–393, edited by S. Burchiel and B. Rhodes. Elsevier New York, 1983.
17. Milstein, C., Adetugbo, K., Cowan, N. J., *et al.* Somatic cell genetics of antibody-secreting cells: Studies of clonal diversification and analysis by cell fusion. *Cold Spring Harbor Symp. Quant. Biol. 41:*793–803, 1977.
18. Klein, F. A., Melamed, M. R., Whitmore, W. F., Herr, H. W., and Sogani, P. C. Characterization of bladder papilloma by 2 parameters DNA/RNA flow cytometry. In *Proceeding of 1982 American Urological Association, Abstract 73.*
19. Klein, F. A., Herr, H. W., Whitmore, W. F., and Melamed, M. R. Flow cytometry in follow-up of patients with low stage bladder tumors. *Proceedings of 1981 American Urological Association, Abstract 548.*

7

Multicentricity in Carcinoma of the Urinary Bladder

Fernando Algaba, M.D.
Eduardo Zungri, M.D.
José Vicente, M.D.
Francisco Solé-Balcells, M.D.

When we talk about carcinoma of the urinary bladder we include diverse pathologic entities with different biology and only two common facts: that of being malignant epithelial tumors and that they originate in the vesical mucosa. Therefore, when we refer to any of their characteristics, such as multicentricity, we have to consider the histologic types because they all behave differently.

The information used in this chapter is based on findings from 72 patients with transitional cell carcinoma, 11 patients with true squamous cell carcinoma, 13 cases of adenocarcinoma of the bladder (primary and secondary) and 14 patients in which the embedment of the whole specimen from cystectomy showed areas of carcinoma *in situ*. We would like to point out that a systematic or random biopsy of normal vesical mucosa has not been carried out in all these cases since the methodical introduction of this practice in our institute dates from 1981.

Histologic Types of Bladder Cancer

The epithelium of the urinary bladder is designated as transitional because it is considered to be an intermediate (or transitional) variant between the stratified squamous epithelium and simple squamous epithelium. Its morphological and functional peculiarities, however, justify the more precise term of urothelium.[1]

In 1954, Mostofi[2] clearly established the potentialities of bladder urothelium—transformation into squamous epithelium and glandular epithelium; if we add to this the foci of squamous cells which is found in the trigone of 46% of normal female bladders and in 7% of normal male bladders,[3] as well as the existence of epithelial mucoproducing areas,[4] the histologic types of bladder carcinoma will be clearly understood.

Ninety percent of bladder carcinomas are transitional,[6] 6–7% are squamous cell carcinomas, 1–2% are vesical adenocarcinomas and the remaining 1–2% are poorly differentiated carcinomas.[6, 7]

Growth Patterns in Urinary Bladder Cancer

Independently from the histologic type, three types of growth patterns may be recognized: the exophytic variant (mostly papillary but occasionally more polyploid), the plano- or planophytic variant (without much excrescence towards the vesical lumen and with a wide implantation base), and the mixed type (combination of the two patterns.)[8]

Seventy percent of bladder tumors are papillary and noninfiltrating, 10% are planoinfiltrating and 20% are exophytic and infiltrating,[7] so that plano- or solid tumors are almost always infiltrating at the time of diagnosis, whereas papillary and exophytic tumors are usually of superficial type.

Correlation Between Histologic Types and Growth Patterns

TRANSITIONAL CARCINOMA

There is a close correlation between cellular malignant grade, degree of spread, and macroscopic growth pattern.

Ninety-four percent of grade I transitional carcinomas are superficial[8] and only 6% are, or will be, infiltrating tumors, especially recurrent malignancies.[9]

Grade II transitional carcinomas are infiltrating in 52% of the cases; grade III are infiltrating in 82% of the cases[8] and usually exhibit a planophytic growth pattern.

SQUAMOUS CELL CARCINOMA

Seventy percent of all true squamous cell carcinomas show muscular invasion at the time of diagnosis.[10] They are often undifferentiated solid tumors.[11]

ADENOCARCINOMAS

Primary vesical adenocarcinomas are divided into two groups: those of urachal origin and those of urothelial origin. Urachal tumors recognize a vesical origin in 90% of the cases and are mostly frequently located in the bladder dome and the anterior wall (87% of the cases). Owing to their peculiar histologic type urachal adenocarcinomas are always intraparietal and have a solid pattern.[12]

Adenocarcinomas of urothelial origin can be classified as signet ring type and well differentiated type. Primary signet ring cell adenocarcinomas (linitis plastica of the bladder) are more common on the posterior wall and are infiltrating, papillary forms being exceptional.[13] Well differentiated adenocarcinomas may range from papillary to solid tumors, although they are often solid and infiltrating.[11, 14]

UNDIFFERENTIATED CELL CARCINOMAS

These are all solid and infiltrating tumors regardless of their having fusiform and/or giant cells.[11]

CARCINOMA *IN SITU*

This variant deserves a special mention because it is a form of bladder carcinoma with marked anaplasia and a tendency to evolve into invasive undifferentiated carcinoma.[15] Carcinoma *in situ* shows a planophytic growth pattern.

Correlations Between Carcinogenesis, Growth Patterns and Histologic Type

It is already well known that some carcinogenic factors are specific for each histologic type,[16] but the correlation between carcinogen, growth pattern in a same variant and histologic type (basically transitional carcinoma) is not clear.

Theoretical aspects of bladder carcinogenesis suggest that there are either two different routes for bladder carginogens (by blood-planophytic tumors, or by urine-exophytic tumors) or different tumor responses according to the level of the target cell (intermediate-exophytic, basal-*in situ*-planophytic) with differences in the vascular submucosal response.[17–19]

MULTICENTRICITY IN URINARY TRACT TUMORS

The concept of multicentricity in carcinoma of the urinary bladder cannot be restricted to vesical mucosa, because the entire urinary tract is formed by the same type of epithelium (with slight variations) and also because the great majority of bladder carcinogens or their metabolites are transported to the bladder by the urine[20] especially all those which are responsible for transitional carcinoma.

Concept of Multicentricity

As the word suggests, multicentricity means the presence of several foci of neoplastic growth. Although the concept is simple, identifying true multicentricity may be difficult because this phenomenon is not always synchronous. For that reason the differential diagnosis with recurrences caused by residual tumors should be considered (tumor persistence). In other respects the criterion of multicentricity is usually established macroscopically (except for carcinoma *in situ*), thus apparent multiple neoplastic foci may have been microscopic neoplastic areas that surrounded the initial tumor and were not detected by the endoscopist at the time of removal of the primary tumor.[21] To avoid diagnostic misinterpretations it is necessary to define a series of criteria of multicentricity, being as strict and realistic as possible.

Criteria for the Diagnosis of Multifocal Tumors

SYNCHRONIC VESICAL MULTICENTRICITY

If at the time of endoscopic diagnosis of a bladder carcinoma diverse areas of neoplastic growth are identified, they should be considered as different and independent foci when macroscopic and microscopic findings of the intertumoral mucosa are normal (Fig. 7.1).

ASYNCHRONIC VESICAL MULTICENTRICITY

We should be sure that the following criteria are applied: (1) certainty of a total resection or removal of the previous tumor; (2) negativity of the standard biopsies of the macroscopically normal mucosa, and (3) the appearance of a new tumor must take place at least 1 month after

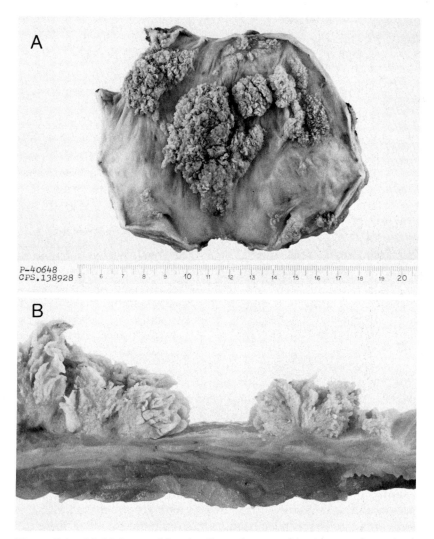

Figure 7.1. Multiple transitional cell carcinoma with absence of neoplastic lesions (macro- and microscopically) in the intertumor areas.

the diagnosis of the previous tumor.[22] The last criterion is questionable because endoscopic follow-up examinations are not usually carried out before 3 months after resection.

EXTRAVESICAL MULTICENTRICITY

The criteria are not so well defined and only depend on the proximity or distance from the bladder mucosa. If the neoplastic areas are far from the bladder (renal pelvis, calyces, lumbar and pelvic ureter, distal urethra) they can always be considered as independent foci, unless there is a widespread carcinoma *in situ*. If the neoplastic foci are near to the bladder (terminal ureter and prostatic urethra) the characteristics of the neighboring vesical mucosa should be evaluated before diagnosing multicentricity.

HYPOTHESIS OF MULTIFOCAL TUMORS

The theories on urothelial multicentricity can be systematized as follows:

Multicentricity Caused by Urothelial Disease

According to this theory (field change) the change is multiclonal[23] and secondary to the continuous action of a carcinogenic agent.[24, 25]

Multicentricity by Dissemination Starting from a Focus

In this case the tumor would be a monoclonal expression and multicentricity could be due either by lateral intraepithelial migration of the neoplastic cells, or by the implantation of tumor cells detached spontaneously, or during diagnostic or therapeutic manipulations,[23, 26] especially if vesical mucosa has been previously damaged.[27–29] For this reason intravesical chemotherapy can reduce the number of further recurrences.[29, 30]

However, the acceptance of implantation of neoplastic cells and their possible growth and clinical manifestation is not fully explained if cell kinetics are taken into account. In general about 25 cell replications are needed to reach a 0.03-cm mass, which is the minimum necessary in order to be seen, and the timing of these events has been approximately estimated as 4 years,[31] whereas development of new foci (first recurrence) usually occurs 1 or 2 years after the diagnosis of the first tumor.[22]

Obviously there are many unknown factors but every day new carcinogenic links are identified such as the *in vitro* growth-stimulating factors of endothelial cells[32] that are present in recurrent bladder cancers and absent in those bladder tumors that do not recur. All of these facts will contribute to a more comprehensive understanding of the biology of human bladder cancer.

MULTICENTRICITY IN TRANSITIONAL CELL CARCINOMA

Vesical Multicentricity

SYNCHRONIC VESICAL MULTICENTRICITY

We have studied 72 consecutive cases of transitional cell carcinoma with a mean follow-up period of 24.7 months. Twenty-five cases (34.7%) were multifocal at the beginning, 80% of them being superficial tumors. These findings are in accordance with those reported by Heney *et al.*[33] Systematized multiple biopsies were carried out in 16 of these 25 cases and in three of them (18.8%) concomitant sites of carcinoma *in situ* were detected; cellular dysplasia was noticed in one case (6.2%).

Sixty-eight percent of these multiples tumors recurred. Comparison of some characteristics of single tumors with multiple tumors reveals that the latter accounted for a higher incidence of associated carcinoma *in situ* and rate of recurrence (Table 7.1).

ASYNCHRONIC VESICAL MULTICENTRICITY

Forty-four (61.1%) of 72 cases have recurred. Recurrences usually occurred within approximately 15 months after complete excision of the initial tumor. Twenty-three (52.3%) of these 44 cases had a second recurrence within an average of 10.6 months after the first recurrence. Five cases (11.4%) had more than two recurrences. The chronologic relapses of our series is somewhat faster than in other studies, in which the average time has been 31 and 13 months for the first and second recurrences, respectively.[22]

The following characteristics of the primary tumor have been correlated with further recurrence: (1) the already aforementioned initial multicentricity; (2) the size of the tumor (1 cm with a 2% recurrence rate *versus* 5 cm with a 21% recurrence rate)[22]; (3) the grading, although the incidence is similar for grades II and III in our series (Table 7.2); (4) the staging which in our opinion is not easy to correlate as infiltrating tumors are managed with radical surgery with no possibility of follow-up as far as recurrences are concerned, and (5) chromosome anomalies.[34, 35]

Table 7.1
Transitional Cell Carcinoma. Comparison Between Single and Multiples Tumors

Tumors	No. Cases	Staging		Grades		Association *in situ*	Recurrences
		PA–P$_1$	P$_2$–P$_3$	II	III		
Single	47/72	37/47	10/47	31/47	16/47	2/30	27/47
	(65.3%)	(78.7%)	(21.3%)	(66.0%)	(34.0%)	(6.7%)	(57.4%)
Multiple	25/72	21/25	4/25	15/25	10/25	3/16	17/25
	(34.7%)	(84%)	(16%)	(60%)	(40%)	(18.8%)	(68%)

Table 7.2
Transitional Cell Carcinoma. Asynchronic Multicentricity According to the Histologic Grade[a]

Initial tumor	No. Cases	Recurrences	No. Recurrences	Mortality	Cystectomy
Grade II	46	30/46 (65.2%)	15/46 (32.6%)	1/46 (2.2%)	
Grade III	26	14/26 (53.8%)	7/26 (26.9%)	1/26 (3.8%)	4/26 (15.4%)

[a] None of the cases included in this study were diagnosed grade I because excessive atypia was found on histologic examination.

EXTRAVESICAL MULTICENTRICITY

Synchronic Extravesical Multicentricity

In our series of 72 cases of transitional cell carcinoma, one case of pyelocalyceal carcinoma synchronic to the bladder cancer was detected (on the right side, grade II, P_1). There was no case of ureteral tumor. In a larger series Hvidi and Feldt-Rasmussen[36] reported up to 4% of simultaneous bladder carcinomas in primary tumors of the renal pelvis and 2% in primary ureteral tumors.

Asynchronic Extravesical Multicentricity

Out of the 72 cases only 1 pyelocalyceal tumor occurred 13 months after the diagnosis of bladder cancer.

In a retrospective study of 188 cases of carcinoma of the upper urinary tract there were 16.5% of cases with concomitant or previous bladder cancer,[37] but as we do not record the overall number of bladder tumor cases treated over this period, we do not know the percentage of bladder cancer cases that develop a tumor in the upper urinary tract. Seven (8.6%) of 81 cases of bladder cancer presented with upper urinary tract tumors that developed after the vesical tumor had been diagnosed.[38]

This asynchronic extravesical multicentricity can be explained by the same aforementioned causes; however, many experimental[39] and clinical studies have shown a certain correlation between upper urinary tract tumors and ureteral reflux. In the series of Martinez-Piñeiro et al.,[38] 71.4% of tumors in the upper urinary tract occurred in patients with ureteral reflux, and also 80% of patients with ureteral reflux and upper urinary tract tumors had undergone multiple surgical resections. These facts together with the average latent period (2–3 years) elapsed between the diagnosis of the bladder cancer and the pyeloureteral tumor[37] suggest the possible implantation of neoplastic cells that have flowed back from the vesical tumor.[26] Nevertheless, the incidence of recurrence of prostatic urethral tumors in patients who have undergone a simultaneous resection of the prostate gland is similar to that of patients who have not undergone prostatic resection.[40] These events are in disagreement with the experimental pattern of cell implantation in humans as well as with the hypothesis on the role of ureteral reflux and subsequent implantation of malignant cells in the upper urinary tract.

MULTICENTRICITY IN SQUAMOUS CELL CARCINOMA

We have reviewed 11 cases of true squamous cell carcinoma of the urinary bladder. These were all single and infiltrating at the time of diagnosis. Some extensive studies have found 6.2–10% of multifocal tumors.[10, 41]

Squamous cell carcinomas had a solid macroscopic appearance, wide implantation base and did not appear limited to a certain area of the urinary bladder. They may occur in any location, but were most frequent on the lateral walls (63.6%), vesical cupulae and posterior wall. One case (9%) was intradiverticular. None of them presented other tumors in the rest of the urinary tract and, as they were infiltrating and were managed with radical surgery, data on vesical asynchronic multicentricity was not available.

MULTICENTRICITY IN ADENOCARCINOMAS

Seven (53.8%) of 13 cases of adenocarcinoma of the urinary bladder were secondary to invasion of an immediate vicinity tumor (rectosigmoid neoplasm in five cases (71.4%) and prostatic cancer in two cases (28.6%)). There were five primary adenocarcinomas of the bladder (38.5%) and one case of undetermined origin (7.7%). None of our cases arose from an extrophic bladder.

MULTICENTRICITY IN URACHAL ADENOCARCINOMAS

Urachal adenocarcinomas of the urinary bladder are difficult to diagnose because histogenetic features may be inconspicuous at the time of clinical symptoms.

Three of our five cases (60%) were located on the vesical cupulae (Table 7.3), but only one of them (20% of the total) can be strictly considered of urachal origin according to diagnostic criteria such as displacement of the urothelium, predominant intramural growth and possible involvement of the Retzius' space.

In a group of 74 cases of urachal adenocarcinomas reported by Beck et al.[12] only one case (1.4%) relapsed after partial surgery, but it was not classified as tumor recurrence.

As a consequence multicentricity in urachal adenocarcinomas of the

Table 7.3
Primary Bladder Adenocarcinomas

Origin	No. Cases	Multiple	Vesical Cupulae
Urachal	1/5 (20%)		1
Urothelial	4/5 (80%)	1/4 (25%)	2

bladder is practically nonexistent and therefore certain conservative surgical approaches could be justified. The problem, however, lies in the difficulty of establishing a preoperative believable diagnosis.

MULTICENTRICITY IN UROTHELIAL ADENOCARCINOMAS

One of our four cases (25%) of primary bladder adenocarcinomas showed synchronic multicentricity. This percentage is similar to that reported in other series whose incidence of multicentricity varied from 20–50% with an average rate of 34.2%.[14,42,43]

Extravesical multicentricity was not observed in our series. A coincident bladder tumor was not found in the only primary pyelocalyceal adenocarcinoma diagnosed at our institution.[44]

MULTICENTRICITY IN CARCINOMA *"IN SITU"*

Carcinoma *in situ* of the urinary bladder was first described by Melicow[45] in 1952. Since then much data has been compiled regarding its biology but its precise natural history is still unknown. The present information available, however, justifies the acceptance of carcinoma *in situ* as a true clinical entity.

MULTICENTRICITY OF THE LESIONS *IN SITU*

Studies with multiple biopsies in areas of apparently normal bladder mucosa show a high incidence of positive histopathologic results. Again, multicentricity of the bladder biopsies does not correspond necessarily with multifocal lesions, because it is possible that an extensive area of carcinoma *in situ* has undergone the biopsies at different levels. Criteria of true multicentricity can only be established in those cases in which a complete and exhaustive examination of all vesical mucosa has been carried out (cystectomy specimen mapping) (Fig. 7.2).

Table 7.4 refers the incidence of multifocal lesions in 14 cystectomy specimens following mapping bladder changes of carcinoma *in situ*. The lesions *in situ* were relatively extensive and involve different vesical areas as has been reported in other studies.[46]

Three (21.4%) of the 14 cases were not associated with a macroscopic bladder tumor but underwent cystectomy because of uncontrollable clinical symptoms. Two of these three cases (66.6%), however, already showed microinvasive foci and intramuscular invasion. The remaining 11 cases (78.6%) were associated with macroscopic tumors, and in only three cases (27.3%) carcinoma *in situ* areas showed foci of microinvasion.

Table 7.4 summarizes the clinicopathologic characteristics of isolated carcinomas *in situ*[47] and those associated with a macroscopic tumor.[48] The three cases of isolated carcinomas *in situ* showed multifocal and generalized lesion with extension towards the ureters included in the surgically removed cystectomy specimen in two cases (66.6%); intraep-

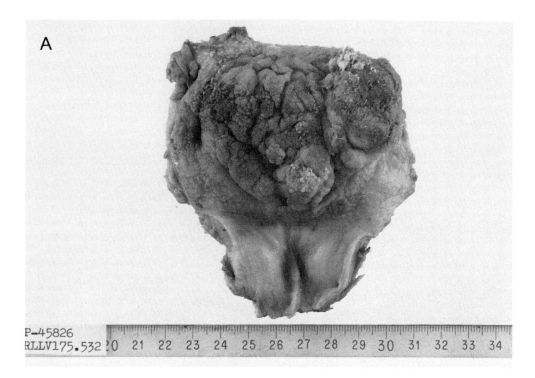

P-45826
RLLV175.532 20 21 22 23 24 25 26 27 28 29 30 31 32 33 34

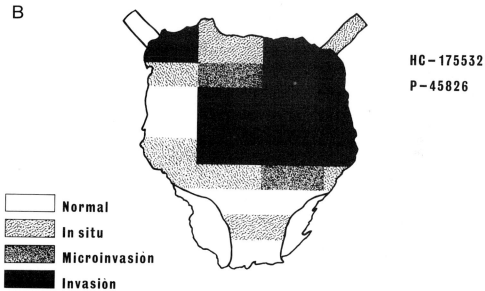

HC – 175532
P – 45826

☐ **Normal**
▨ **In situ**
▧ **Microinvasión**
■ **Invasión**

Figure 7.2.   Study of a total cystectomy specimen by mapping. Areas of multiple carcinoma *in situ* in urethra and left ureter are evident.

ithelial neoplastic changes in the prostatic urethra were also found in two cases (66.6%).

Eight (72.7%) of 11 cases with carcinoma *in situ* associated with a macroscopic bladder tumor showed multiple lesions. Three cases (27.3%) presented with ureteral spread; this percentage is slightly lower than that reported by Utz and Farrow[49] who observed up to 56.8% of

Table 7.4
Study by Mapping in Carcinoma "*in situ*" of the Bladder

	No. Cases	Microinvasion Plus Invasion	Multicentricity	
			Vesical	Ureteral
Isolated Carcinoma *in situ*	3/14 (21.4%)	2/3 (66.6%)	3/3 (100%)	2/3 (66.6%)
Carcinoma *in situ* and macroscopic tumor	11/14 (78.6%)	3/11[a] (27.3%)	8/11 (72.7%)	3/11 (27.3%)

[a] Microinvasion in areas *in situ*.

ureteral involvement. Neoplastic foci in the prostatic urethra were detected in four cases (36.3%); this percentage is slightly superior to that reported by other authors, *i.e.* 15% in the experience of Koss et al.,[46] and lower than others, *i.e.* 61.9% in the series of Utz and Farrow.[49]

Out of the four cases with prostatic urethral lesions, in one case (25%) extension of the lesion *in situ* to the paraurethral prostatic ducts was noticed. This facts does not appear to worsen the prognosis unless extension to the prostatic glands occur.[50]

Relationship Between Carcinoma *In Situ* and Histologic Types of Bladder Tumors

CARCINOMA *IN SITU* AND TRANSITIONAL CELL CARCINOMA

Transitional cell carcinoma is usually the tumor associated with carcinoma *in situ* of the urinary bladder. The incidence of this association varies between 10%[51] and 30%.[52]

Multiple biopsies of normal bladder mucosa were carried out in 46 of 72 cases with transitional cell carcinoma. Carcinoma *in situ* was demonstrated in five cases (10.7%), all cases coinciding with a grade III tumor infiltrating the muscle in three of the five cases (60%) and being multiple in three other cases (60%). In accordance with Cooper *et al.*[53] we also noticed a greater correlation between carcinoma *in situ* and the macroscopic tumor grade rather than the tumor staging. Nevertheless, almost all authors agree in accepting a greater infiltrating capacity for those tumors associated with carcinoma *in situ* than for those not associated with it.[54]

CARCINOMA *IN SITU* AND SQUAMOUS CELL CARCINOMA

In 3 of our 11 cases with squamous cell carcinoma changes of dysplasia-carcinoma *in situ* were found in the epithelium adjacent to the tumor. Although the incidence was 27.2% a systematic study of the nontumor areas was not carried out.

In several series of patients with squamous cell carcinoma there is reference to the presence of squamous metaplasia without atypia (25–72% of the cases).[55, 56] This finding, however, has a doubtful prognostic value if it is not accompanied by cellular atypia.

None of our cases showed intraepithelial changes in the nontumor mucosa, but a systematized study of the whole bladder mucosa was not performed. Adenocarcinoma *in situ* as a definite pathologic condition has not been recognized.[56]

PREVENTION OF MULTICENTRICITY

Controversy regarding the pathogenesis of asynchronic multicentricity extends itself to the theoretical bases of intravesical chemotherapy. Faced with this dilemma the current methodology does not supply a reliable answer and it is even feasible that a combination of the therapeutic protocols suggested by each hypothesis should be recommended.[57]

Another subject under discussion is the pathogenetic role of ureteral reflux in the development of pyeloureteral tumors in patients with previous urinary bladder carcinoma. As has been mentioned above, ureteral reflux has been diagnosed in 71.4% of the cases with recurrent tumors in the upper urinary tract; however, only 22.7% of the patients with ureteral reflux and bladder cancer developed a tumor in the upper urinary tract.[38] In our opinion only an accurate and controlled study would justify the usefulness of anti-reflux surgical procedures to prevent this possibility in patients with urinary bladder tumors.

Multicentricity is one of the most common and typical characteristics of bladder cancer, although the intrinsic mechanism of multifocal lesions is still unknown. Some factors closely related with multicentricity are being recognized, such as the identification of intraepithelial cellular changes (carcinoma *in situ*), so a wider range of knowledge is being established which will contribute to a better diagnostic approach and beneficial therapy for our patients.

REFERENCES

1. Melicow, M. M. The urothelium: a battleground for oncogenesis. *J. Urol. 120*:43–47, 1978.
2. Mostofi, F. K. Potentialities of bladder epithelium. *J. Urol. 71*:705–714, 1954.
3. Wiener, D. P., Koss, L. G., Sablay, B., and Freed, S. Z. The prevalence and significance of Brunn's nests, cystitis cystica and squamous metaplasia in normal bladders. *J. Urol. 122*:317–321, 1979.
4. Koss, L. G. *Diagnostic Cytology and Its Histopathologic Bases*, pp. 711–716, Ed. 3, Vol. 2. Lippincott, Philadelphia, 1979.
5. Olsson, C. A., and White, R. W. Cancer of the bladder. In *Principles and Management of Urologic Cancer*, pp. 337–376, edited by N. Javadpour. Williams & Wilkins, Baltimore, 1979.
6. Corwin, S. H., Tassy, F., Malament, M., and Grady, H. G. Signet ring cell variant of mucinous adenocarcinoma of the bladder. *J. Urol. 106*:697–700, 1971.
7. Mostofi, F. K., and Dorris, C. J. Pathology of urologic cancer. In *Principles and Management of Urologic Cancer*, p. 55, edited by N. Javadpour. Williams & Wilkins, Baltimore, 1979.
8. Friedell, G. H. Current concepts of the aetiology, pathogenesis and pathology of bladder cancer. *Urol. Res. 6*:179–182, 1978.
9. Greene, L. F., Hanash, K. A., and Farrow, G. M. Benign papilloma or papillary carcinoma of the bladder? *J. Urol. 110*:205–207, 1973.

10. Johnson, D. E., Schoenwald, M. B., Ayala, A. G., and Miller, L. S. Squamous carcinoma of the bladder. *J. Urol. 115:*542–547, 1976.
11. Koss, L. G. Tumors of the urinary bladder. In *Atlas of Tumor Pathology, fascicle 11*, pp. 46–54. Armed Forces Institute of Pathology, Washington, 1975.
12. Beck, A. D., Gaudin, H. J., and Bonham, D. G. Carcinoma of the urachus. *Br. J. Urol. 42:*555–562, 1970.
13. Gonzalez, E., Fawler, M. R., and Venable, D. D. Primary signet ring cell adenocarcinoma of the bladder (linitis plastica of the bladder): report of a case and review of the literature. *J. Urol. 128:*1027–1030, 1982.
14. Jones, W. A., Gibbons, R. P., Correa, R. J. Jr., Cummings, K. B., and Mason, J. T. Primary adenocarcinoma of bladder. *Urology 15:*119–122, 1980.
15. Koss, L. G., Tiamson, E. M., and Robbins, M. A. Mapping cancerous and precancerous bladder changes. A study of the urothelium in ten surgically removed bladders. *JAMA 227:*281–286, 1974.
16. El-Bolkainy, M. N., Chu, E. W., Ghoneim, A. S., and Ibrahim, A. S. Cytologic detection of bladder cancer in rural Egyptiane population infested with schistosomiasis. *Acta Cytol. 26:*303–310, 1982.
17. Sarma, K. P. Genesis of papillary tumours: histological and microangiographic study. *Br. J. Urol. 53:*228–236, 1981.
18. Melicow, M. M. Reflections on bladder neoplasia: exophytic papillary urothelial tumors *versus* planophytic carcinoma *in situ*. *Urology 20:*440–445, 1982.
19. Frith, C. H., Wiley, L. D., and Shimohara, Y. Sequential morphogenesis of urinary bladder tumors in Balb/c mice given 2-acetylaminofluorene. *J. Urol. 128:*1071–1076, 1982.
20. Paulson, D. F. Carcinogenesis in urogenital sites. *Invest. Urol. 16:*77–86, 1978.
21. Friedell, G. H., Parija, G. C., Nagy, G. K., and Soto, E. A. The pathology of human bladder cancer. *Cancer 45:*1823–1831, 1980.
22. Cutler, S. J., Heney, N. M., and Friedell, G. H. Longitudinal study of patients with bladder cancer: factors associated with disease recurrence and progression. In *Bladder Cancer, A.U.A. Monographs*, Vol. 1, pp. 37–46, edited by W. W. Bonney and G. R. Prout, Jr., Williams & Wilkins, Baltimore, 1982.
23. Weinstein, R. S. Intravesical dissemination and invasion of urinary bladder carcinoma. In *Bladder Cancer, A.U.A. Monographs*, Vol. 1, pp 29–33, edited by W. W. and G. R. Prout, Jr., Williams & Wilkins, Baltimore, 1982.
24. Melicow, M. M. The role of urine in a patient with a bladder neoplasm. *J. Urol. 127:*660–664, 1982.
25. King, C. M. The origins of urinary bladder cancer. In *Bladder Cancer, A.U.A. Monographs*, Vol. 1, pp. 15–25, edited by W. W. Bonney and G. R. Prout, Jr., Williams & Wilkins, Baltimore, 1982.
26. Weldon, T. E., and Soloway, M. S. Susceptibility of urothelium for neoplastic cell implantation. *Urology 5:*824–827, 1975.
27. Goslin, J. A., Dixon, J. S., and Dunn, M. The structure of the rabbit urinary bladder after experimental distension. *Invest. Urol. 14:*386–389, 1977.
28. Page, B. H., Lenison, V. B., and Curwen, M. P. The sites of recurrence of noninfiltrating bladder tumours. *Br. J. Urol. 50:*237–242, 1978.
29. Soloway, M. S., Nissenkorn, I., and MacCallum, L. Urothelial susceptibility to tumor cell implantation: comparison of cauterization with *N*-methyl-*N*-nitrosourea. *Urology 21:*159–161, 1983.
30. Soloway, M. S., and Murphy, W. M. Experimental chemotherapy of bladder cancer—systemic and intravesical. *Semin. Oncol. 6:*166–183, 1979.
31. Melicow, M. B. Bladder tumors Quo Imus?. In *Progress in Surgical Pathology*, pp. 17–26, edited by C. M. Fenoglio and M. Wolff, Masson, New York, 1982.
32. Chodak, G. W., Scheiner, C. J., and Zetter, B. R. Urine from patients with transitional cell carcinoma stimulates migation of capillary endothelial cells. *N. Engl. J. Med. 305:*869–874, 1981.
33. Heney, N. M., Nocks, B. N., Daly, J. J., Prout, G. R. Jr., Newall, J. B., Griffin, P. P., Perrone, T. L., and Szyfelbein, W. A. Ta and T_1 bladder cancer: location, recurrence and progression. *Br. J. Urol. 54:*152–157, 1982.
34. Javadpour, N. Chromosomes in urologic cancers. In *Recent Advances in Urologic Cancer* (Libertino's series of International Perspectives in Urology), Vol. 2, p. 31.

Williams & Wilkins, Baltimore, 1982.

35. Martorana, G., Giberti, C., Ferrari, M., Coui, P., Ottagio, L., and Pescatore, D. Cytogenetic analysis of transitional cell carcinoma of the bladder. Clinical implications. *Eur. J. Urol. 9:*28–31, 1983.

36. Hvidi, V., and Feldt-Rasmussen, K. Primary tumours in the renal pelvis and ureter with particular attention to the diagnostic problems. *Acta Chir. Scand. (Suppl.) 433:*91–101, 1973.

37. Sole-Balcells, F., and Zungri, E. Les tumeurs de la voie excréto-urinaire haute. *Journées urologiques du Necker*, pp. 93–105. Masson et Cie., Paris, 1981.

38. Martinez-Piñeiro, J. A., Pertusa, C., Torrenteras, J., and Armero, A. H. Tumeurs urothéliales du haut appareil urinaire apparaissant après le traitement d'un carcinome de vessie. *Journées Urologiques du Necker.* pp. 22–29. Masson et Cie., Paris, 1981.

39. Edwards, L., Rosin, D., Leaper, D., Swedan, M., Trott, P., and Vertido, R. The induction of cystitis and the implantation of tumours in rat and rabbit bladders. *Br. J. Urol. 50:*502–504, 1978.

40. Laor, E., Grabstald, H., and Whitmore, W. F. The influence of simultaneous resection of bladder tumors and prostate on the recurrence of prostatic urethral tumors. *J. Urol. 126:*171–172, 1981.

41. Rundle, J. S. M., Hart, A. J. L., McGeorge, A., Smith, J. S., Malcolm, A. J., and Smith, P. M. Squamous cell carcinoma of bladder. A review of 114 patients. *Br. J. Urol. 54:*522–526, 1982.

42. Jacobo, E., Loening, S., Schmidt, J. D., and Culp, D. A. Primary adenocarcinoma of the bladder: a retrospective study of 20 patients. *J. Urol. 117:*54–56, 1977.

43. Nocks, B. N., Heney, N. M., and Daly, J. J. Primary adenocarcinoma of urinary bladder. *Urology 21:*26–29, 1983.

44. Galindo, L., Algaba, F., and Solé-Balcells, F. Adenocarcinomas pielo-caliciales. *An. Fund. Puig. 6:*161–176, 1976.

45. Melicow, M. M. Histological study of vesical urothelium intervening between gross neoplasm in total cystectomy. *J. Urol. 68:*261–278, 1952.

46. Koss, L. G., Nakanishi, I., and Freed, S. Nonpapillary carcinoma *in situ* and atypical hyperplasia in cancerous bladders. Further studies of surgically removed bladders by mapping. *Urology 9:*442–455, 1977.

47. Farrow, G. M., Utz, D. C., Rife, C. C., and Greene, L. F. Clinical observations on sixty-nine cases of *in situ* carcinoma of the urinary bladder. *Can. Res. 37:*2794–2798, 1977.

48. Althausen, A. F., Prout, G. R., Jr., and Daly, J. J. Noninvasive papillary carcinoma of the bladder associated with carcinoma "*in situ*". *J. Urol. 116:*575–580, 1976.

49. Utz, D. C., and Farrow, G. M. Management of carcinoma *in situ* of the bladder: the case for surgical management. *Urol. Clin. North Am. 7:*533:541, 1980.

50. Chibber, P. J., McIntyre, M. A., Hindmarsh, J. R., Hargreave, T. B., Newsam, J. E., and Chisholm, G. D. Transitional cell carcinoma involving the prostate. *Br. J. Urol. 53:*605–609, 1981.

51. Catalona, W. J. Bladder carcinoma. *J. Urol. 123:*35–36, 1980.

52. Schade, R. O. K., and Swinney, J. Precancerous changes in bladder epithelium. *Lancet 2:*943–946, 1968.

53. Cooper, P. H., Waisman, J., Johnston, W. H., and Skinner, D. G. Severe atypia of transitional epithelium and carcinoma of the urinary bladder. *Cancer 31:*1055–1060, 1973.

54. Wolf, H., and Højgaard, K. Prognostic factors in local surgical treatment of invasive bladder cancer, with special reference to the presence of urothelial dysplasia. *Cancer 51:*1710–1715, 1983.

55. Richie, J. P., Waisman, J., Skinner, D. G., and Dretler, S. P. Squamous carcinoma of the bladder: treatment by radical cystectomy. *J. Urol. 115:*670–672, 1976.

56. Daly, J. J. Carcinoma *in situ* of the urothelium. *Urol. Clin. North Am. 3:*87–105, 1976.

57. Schulman, C. C. Quimioterapia intravesical en tumores superficiales de vejiga. *Arch. Esp. Urol. 36:*32–40, 1983.

8

Cytology in the Detection and Follow-Up of Urothelial Tumors

William M. Murphy, M.D.
Alexander W. Miller, M.D.

Cytology is a valuable procedure in the detection and follow-up of patients with urothelial malignancies. Urine collection is rapid, inexpensive, noninvasive, and can be performed in the office or clinic; cytologic preparation and evaluation requires <24 hours; and malignant cells can often be detected in urinary samples long before tumors are visible in histologic specimens or on endoscopic examination. Although the method has been used for over 100 years, the potential value of urinary cytology has only recently been widely recognized in the United States. The relatively hostile environment of urine for cellular preservation, the subtle cellular abnormalities of low grade papillary transitional cell tumors, the unrealistic expectations of diagnostic yield among many cytopathologists, and the lack of cellular criteria specifically relating to urothelial neoplasms have discouraged many in the past. Recent developments in our understanding of specimen collection and preparation as well as the recognition of cytologic criteria specific for urothelial neoplasms have rekindled interest in the study of urothelial cells. Technological advances in computer assisted evaluation may offer new insights into the carcinogenic process and will undoubtedly add to the consistency and reliability with which cytologic diagnoses are made.

URINARY SPECIMENS

Various methods have been proposed for the collection, preservation, and processing of urinary samples.[1,2] The exact procedure used has been influenced by multiple factors including the previous education and current experience of laboratory personnel, the volume of material received, and the cost of supplies and equipment. Specimens suitable for urinary cytology include random voided urine and catheterized samples with and without lavage. Early morning and 24-hour collections may contain more cells but yield inferior preparations and should be avoided. Many pathologists prefer bladder washing in an attempt to obtain more and better preserved cells but in a recent evaluation of paired cystoscopic urine and bladder washing specimens collected from the same patients at the same time, we found no consistent differences in cellular yield or preservation.[3] Malignant cells were present slightly more often in bladder washings but in almost 14% of instances appeared only in the urine. Although bladder washings are a valuable source of diagnostic cells, patients should not be instrumented solely for the purpose of collecting cytologic specimens. Overall, randomly voided urine remains the most appropriate type of specimen for detection and follow-up of urothelial malignancies.

Urine is a relatively hostile environment for cells and many pathologists have recommended the addition of alcohol (usually 50% v/v) in an effort to prevent sample deterioration prior to processing.[4] While this may be beneficial in the preparation of direct smears, it has not been useful when membrane filters were employed.[2] Indeed, the degenerative effects of urine have rarely been studied and the scanty available data indicate that the major deleterious effects occur while cells are within the bladder rather than after they are voided.[5] For most purposes, fresh urinary samples can be kept refrigerated for several hours prior to further processing without diminishing the diagnostic yield. If long delays are anticipated, polycarbonate filter preparations covered with Carbo wax have been successfully used. Fresh urinary sediment stained with toluidine blue can be examined as a rapid screening procedure but the yield has been relatively low and all suspicious specimens must be reexamined after permanent slides have been prepared.[2] Air dried cells lack fine nuclear detail and are not optimal for the cytologic interpretation of urothelial malignancies.

Urothelial cells may be recovered by centrifugation and direct smearing, cytocentrifugation or membrane filtration and all methods can yield adequate results for the determination of high grade malignancies if carefully performed. Some methods, *e.g.* membrane filters with modified Papanicolaou staining, display finer nuclear detail than others and are better for distinguishing the more subtle abnormalities of low grade urothelial tumors and their precursors.

DIAGNOSTIC CYTOLOGY

The greatest value of the cytologic method in the diagnosis of urothelial cancer is achieved when cellular evaluation is expressed in terms compatible with histologic classification schemes. Currently, there are five classifications in widespread use (Table 8.1).[6-10] As indicated by Table 8.1, the level at which cytologic abnormalities occur varies among classifications so that a grade I neoplasm in the World Health Organization (WHO) classification would be composed of atypical cells whereas a grade I Bergkvist tumor would contain relatively normal cells arranged in multiple layers on a fibrovascular stalk and a grade I Ash lesion might be composed of normal cells arranged in normal layers on a papillary stalk (a papilloma in the WHO scheme). For the histopathologist, it is the delicate fibrovascular stalk rather than the cells that defines low grade papillary neoplasms. Not surprisingly, accurate cytologic correlation for low grade papillary lesions is difficult and depends upon recognition of subtle cellular abnormalities requiring high quality preparations. For the purpose of this discussion, the cytologic analysis of urothelial malignancies will be expressed in terms of our slight modification of the WHO histologic classification (Table 8.2), a scheme wherein papilloma is defined as a papillary tumor covered by normal urothelium, transitional cell carcinomas grade I and II are all papillary and transitional cell carcinomas grade III are almost all invasive.[11] Flat, noninvasive, nonpapillary grade III neoplasms are designated carcinoma *in situ* or, if the malignant cells do not occupy the full thickness of the epithelium, severe dysplasia/carcinoma *in situ* (SD/CIS).

Urinary samples have commonly been evaluated using criteria developed for other organs, *e.g.* uterine cervix. While this approach has been satisfactory for high grade urothelial cancers, it has not been entirely applicable to low grade lesions. Indeed, some have indicated that cells from grade I papillary carcinomas so closely resemble normal elements that they cannot be accurately assessed in urinary specimens.[12,13] Even where data concerning the cytology of low grade lesions exist, cytopathologists have often registered disappointment that the cytohistologic correlations were not equal to their expectations.[14-17] Cytologic criteria for the recognition of low grade urothelial neoplasms have been mentioned in the literature[18-20] but detailed descriptions of the cellular

Table 8.1
Cytologic Correlation with Histologic Classifications[a]

Classification	Level of Cytologic Atypia
WHO	TCC I
Bergkvist	TCC II
Ash	TCC I-II
Dukes	Papilloma
AFIP	TCC I-II

[a] The abbreviation used is: TCC, transitional cell carcinoma.

Table 8.2
Classification of Urothelial Carcinoma at BMH/UTCHS[a]

Papilloma-exophytic, inverted
Transitional cell carcinoma
    Grade I
    Grade II
    Grade III
Carcinoma *in situ*/severe dysplasia
Squamous cell carcinoma
Undifferentiated carcinoma
Mixed carcinoma

[a] The abbreviations used are: BMH, Baptist Memorial Hospital; and UTCHS, University of Tennessee Center for Health Sciences.

features have not appeared. Over the past several years we have developed criteria for the recognition of cells comprising the entire spectrum of transitional cell carcinomas as well as flat, dysplastic lesions. These criteria evolved from a detailed examination of the morphological features of developing urothelial carcinoma in experimental model systems with subsequent application to clinical material.[21,22] It was our goal to define the cytologic features of cells comprising all grades of transitional cell carcinoma (TCC) and to categorize them according to accepted histologic terminology. We soon realized, however, that the cytologic criteria were not sufficiently refined to reliably distinguish all TCC-Is from TCC-IIs nor in many cases to separate transitional cell from adenocarcinoma. Since the differentiation of grade I from grade II lesions in histologic specimens often depends upon preservation of the superficial cell layer, cellular crowding, and the number of mitoses rather than the pattern of nuclear chromatin or the characteristics of the nuclear borders, it was not always possible to exactly correlate cytologic and histologic grades. In view of this, we settled on the cytologic nomenclature "low grade" and "high grade neoplasm." In this system, cells designated "low grade neoplasm" correlate with the histological lesions called TCC-I and some, but not all, TCC-IIs. The designation high grade neoplasm correlates with TCC-III and CIS. We further attempted to distinguish cells comprising papillary tumors from those in dysplasia. For the purpose of this classification, dysplasia describes a flat, noninvasive lesion which can be distinguished from reactive/reparative epithelium but is composed of cells of lesser degrees of cytologic atypia than CIS or SD/CIS. Cytologic specimens were interpreted using the following nomenclature:

Negative for malignancy (includes reactive cells),
Dysplastic cells,
Abnormal cells, suspicious for malignancy,
Malignant tumor cells consistent with origin in:
    Low grade neoplasm,
    High grade neoplasm,
    Adenocarcinoma,
    Squamous cell carcinoma,
    Undifferentiated malignant tumor,
    Nonepithelial neoplasm.

The diagnostic criteria for urothelial neoplasms have been previously published.[21-24] High grade neoplasms (some TCC-IIs, all TCC-IIIs and SD/CIS) are composed of large, pleomorphic cells with increased N:C ratios and amphophilic cytoplasm (Fig. 8.1). Their nuclei have irregular borders and coarsely clumped, irregularly distributed chromatin. Nucleoli are prominent. The cells are numerous and occur singly as well as in loose clusters and often lie in a background of necrotic debris and inflammation. Low grade neoplasms (TCC-Is and some TCC-IIs) comprise cells which are larger than normal basal and intermediate urothelial cells (Fig. 8.2). They have eccentric nuclei, increased N:C ratios and homogeneous slightly cyanophilic cytoplasm. The nuclei of these cells have one or two well defined indentations which appear as notches

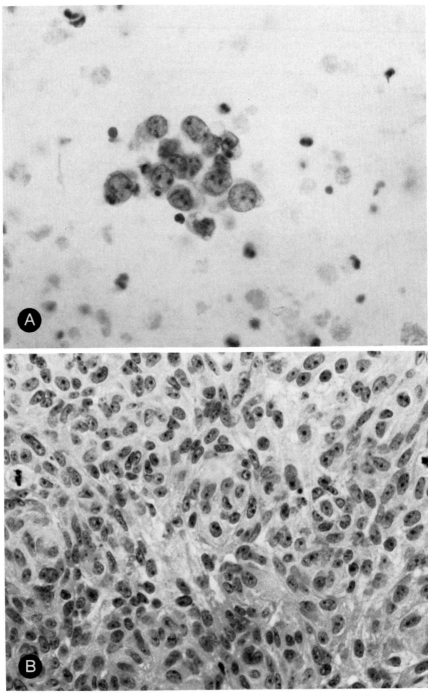

Figure 8.1. *A*, high grade neoplastic cells from a transitional cell carcinoma, grade III. (EA50 × 180) *B*, the TCC-III from which the cells in *A* exfoliated (H&E × 112).

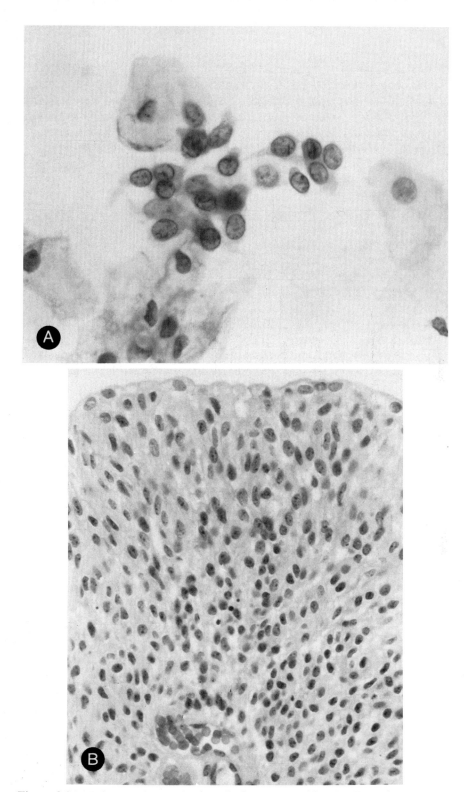

Figure 8.2. *A*, low grade neoplastic cells from a transitional cell carcinoma, grade I. Note the increased N:C ratios, irregularities of the nuclear borders, and eccentric nuclei (EA50 × 180). *B*, the TCC-I from which the cells in *A* exfoliated (H&E × 112).

CYTOLOGY IN DETECTION OF UROTHELIAL TUMORS   105

when viewed on edge and creases when oriented "*en face.*" Their chromatin is more granular than normal but still fine and evenly distributed. Nucleoli are absent or small. The cells are often numerous and may be arranged in tight papillary aggregates but aggregation itself is not a reliable diagnostic feature. Superficial urothelial cells (umbrella cells) comprise a morphologically distinct, highly differentiated layer of epithelium which apparently does not enter into the carcinogenic process and recognizable superficial cells are not considered in the cytologic diagnosis of malignancy (Fig. 8.3). Squamous cell carcinomas are often well differentiated, keratinizing neoplasms which are recognized in cytologic samples by the presence of fiber-like cells with eosinophilic, often refractile cytoplasm and abnormally oriented, usually degenerated, nuclei (Fig. 8.4). Small, more polygonal cells with increased N:C ratios and cyanophilic or amphophilic cytoplasm containing irregular degenerated or pyknotic nuclei with dense chromatin can also be observed. The cells usually occur singly but may aggregate into loose clusters. In contrast, the cells of squamous metaplasia are polyhedral and often wafer-like with variable cytoplasmic tones but low N:C ratios. Their nuclei, when not pyknotic, have evenly distributed finely granular chromatin without prominent nucleoli. The cellular appearances of adenocarcinomas in urinary cytology are extremely variable and, in many cases, cannot be distinguished on morphological grounds from transitional cell carcinomas (Fig. 8.5). The distinctive features of adenocarcinomas include clusters of cells which do not usually form rosettes or lumina but have translucent, amphophilic cytoplasm and eccentric

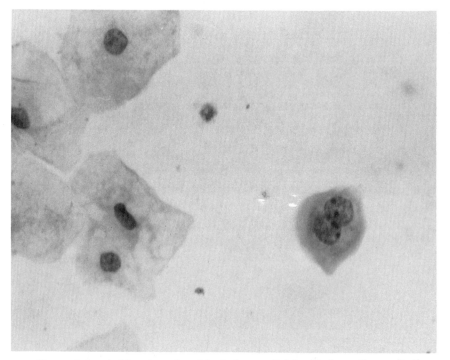

Figure 8.3. A binucleated polyhedral superficial cell from the urothelium. Compare to the adjacent wafer-like squamous cells from the skin (EA50 × 180).

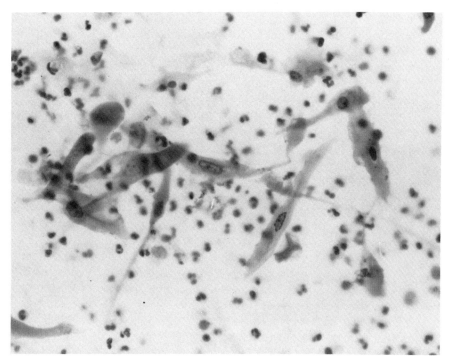

Figure 8.4. Fiber-like cells from a well differentiated squamous carcinoma of the urinary bladder (EA50 × 112).

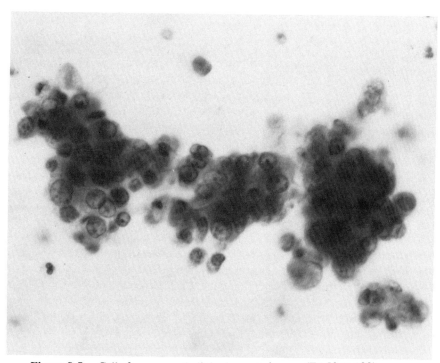

Figure 8.5. Cells from a urothelial adenocarcinoma (EA50 × 180).

CYTOLOGY IN DETECTION OF UROTHELIAL TUMORS   107

nuclei. Their N:C ratios vary with the amount of intracytoplasmic secretion product. The nuclei of recognizable adenocarcinoma cells are round with regular borders and peripherally concentrated chromatin having areas of nuclear clearing associated with large nucleoli. The cells of undifferentiated carcinomas resemble those of lymphomas in that they occur as numerous isolated elements having scanty cytoplasm. They tend to be larger with more coarsely clumped and irregularly distributed nuclear chromatin, however. Urine is a poor culture medium and mitoses are uncommon among all types of urothelial malignancies.

The diagnostic accuracy of urinary cytology depends upon the cytologic criteria and histologic classification used, the experience and expectations of the pathologist, the quality of cytological preparations, and the patient population being evaluated. Given adequate samples, almost all high grade tumors whether transitional, glandular, squamous, invasive or *in situ* can be reliably detected cytologically.[12,25] Exceptions occur only where tumor cells are in the upper collecting system, kidney, or prostate gland; are covered with fibrin and necrotic debris (usually following surgery); are deep within muscular walls; or are otherwise unavailable to the urine or washing solution.

Low grade neoplasms are more difficult to detect cytologically and various experiences have been reported.[26-28] One of the most carefully conducted series involved a urologic clinic population.[17] Freshly voided urine was processed onto polycarbonate membrane filters and the results were correlated with the Ash histologic classification scheme, a four-grade system where papillomas (WHO) are included with grade I neoplasms. All samples were analyzed by a single cytopathologist using consistent cellular criteria. Overall, a diagnostic yield of 34% for grade I and 75% for grade II neoplasms was achieved. The sensitivity and specificity of urinary cytology in this study were 67 and 95%, respectively. Many cancers were accurately predicted by urinary cytology even though they were initially undetected cystoscopically and histologically. Recently, we have completed a long-term study of patients from our institution who were entered into a surveillance protocol of the National Bladder Cancer Collaborative Group-A (NBCCG-A).[21] In contrast to the Mayo clinic study summarized above, our patients were highly selected in that all had a history of bladder cancer. These individuals were followed at regular intervals with cystoscopy, urinary cytology, and tumor resections as well as selected site mucosal biopsies. Recognizing from previous work that the reliability of urinary cytology can be fully realized only after prolonged patient observation, positive cytohistological correlations were recorded if carcinoma appeared in tissue samples taken within 2 years of a positive cytologic diagnosis. A typical case is summarized in Table 8.3. Urinary samples were processed onto cellulosic membrane filters, examined by a single pathologist without knowledge of the clinical or pathologic data, and correlated with our modification of the WHO histologic classification (Table 8.2), a three-grade system where papillomas are considered separately from grade I neoplasms. The diagnostic yield for TCC-I and II was 70 and 98%, respectively. The overall sensitivity and specificity of positive or suspicious cytologic diagnoses were both 90%. This level of accuracy cannot be

Table 8.3
Typical Case of Bladder Cancer[a]

Date	Cystoscopy	Cytology	Histology	Treatment
5/75	T	ND	TCC-III; CIS	
8/75	T	Positive	TCC-II	XRT
12/75	Negative	ND	Dysplasia	
3/76	Negative	Negative	Dysplasia	
7/76	Negative	Positive	Denuded	
10/76	Negative	Positive	SD/CIS	
2/77	Suspicious	Dysplasia	ND	
5/77	Negative	Dysplasia	TCC-I	
8/77	T	Positive	TCC-III	
11/77	T	Positive	TCC-III	CDDP
4/78	T	Negative	Normal	CDDP

[a] The abbreviations used are: T, tumor; TCC, transitional cell carcinoma; CIS, carcinoma *in situ*; XRT, x-ray therapy; SD, severe dysplasia; CDDP, *cis*-diamminedichloroplatinum; ND, not done.

achieved without a false positive rate in the range of 10% nor should such high yields be expected in unselected patient populations. These studies highlight the value of urinary cytology in the detection of low grade urothelial neoplasms, however, and should promote greater confidence in the use of urinary cytology among practicing cytopathologists.

The observations cited above apply primarily to the diagnosis of urothelial carcinomas in the urinary bladder. Sarcomas of the urinary tract are rare and specific cytologic criteria for their recognition have not been developed. Although urine drains both the kidneys and male reproductive organs, urinary cytology has not been of consistent value in the detection or follow-up of renal, prostatic or seminal vesicle neoplasms. Metastatic carcinomas involving the urinary bladder can be detected in urinary samples but the variety of histological types and the paucity of reports precludes generalizations in this area. Carcinomas of the female genital tract are often detected in cytologic specimens but such patients usually have large tumors causing symptoms related to the primary organ and urinary cytology is not a standard procedure in the evaluation of these individuals.

PITFALLS AND CONFOUNDING FACTORS

As in all diagnostic pathology, accurate assessment of the urinary specimen cannot be achieved without the recognition of certain confounding factors and limitations to the method.[11] Among the foremost of these is the interpretation of tumors of the urethra, ureters, and renal pelves. Although lined by transitional epithelium, these areas comprise cells which are normally larger than their urinary bladder counterparts and are often arranged in crypts. The resulting exfoliated or avulsed cells may appear in papillary aggregates and have slightly eccentric nuclei with slightly increased N:C ratios which may lead the cytopathologist to consider a low grade neoplasm (Fig. 8.6). This pitfall can be avoided by knowledge of the source of the specimen and the requirement for significant nuclear abnormalities before a diagnosis of cancer is

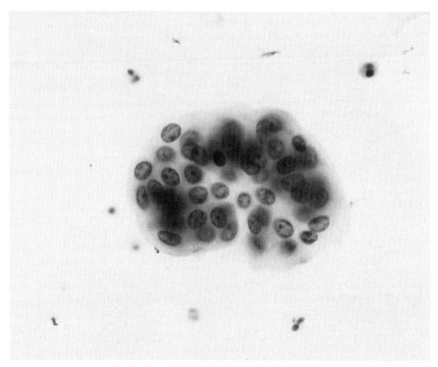

Figure 8.6. Urothelial cells from a renal pelvic washing. Despite the papillary aggregation, the normal arrangement of a superficial layer covering uniform basal and intermediate cells is preserved (EA50 × 180).

rendered. Catheterization of the urinary bladder and especially the ureters and renal pelves may be followed by exfoliation of papillary aggregates of large cells with nuclear features of malignancy. In the absence of appropriate information, such cells may be erroneously interpreted as malignant. Knowledge of previous instrumentation is essential for the accurate diagnosis of urothelial carcinoma in cellular samples. Superficial (umbrella) urothelial cells may resemble mildly dysplastic cells of the uterine cervix. More importantly, they may react to various stimuli so that their nuclei are often large with coarsely granular chromatin and prominent nucleoli. Their N:C ratios remain low, however, and these cells should not be interpreted as malignant regardless of their nuclear features. Superficial cells are highly differentiated and often have tetraploid elements which apparently do not enter into the neoplastic process and should not be considered in the cytologic evaluation of malignancy. Urothelial abnormalities associated with calculi can be distinguished from those of high grade carcinoma but may be a confounding factor in the differential diagnosis of low grade neoplasms (Fig. 8.7). Cells emanating from the area of stones may occur in papillary aggregates but usually have vacuolated cytoplasm and nuclei with regular borders and evenly distributed chromatin. Nucleoli may appear in every cell. In most cases, the clinician is aware of the possibility of a urinary stone and this information should be imparted to the cytopathologist. Any patient with bladder outlet obstruction may deliver urine containing papillary aggregates. These aggregates probably ema-

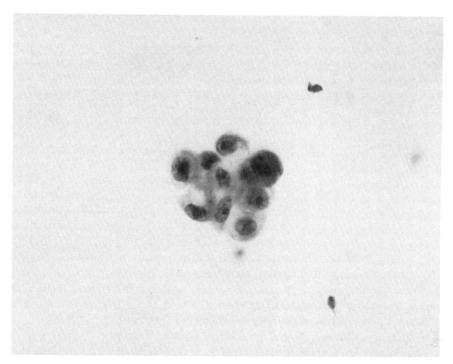

Figure 8.7. Reactive/reparative urothelial cells from a patient with a ureteral stone. Despite the papillary aggregation and slight irregularities of the nuclei, the N:C ratios are low; cytoplasmic vacuoles are conspicuous; and each nucleus contains a prominent nucleolus (EA50 × 180).

nate from the epithelial undulations resulting from trabeculation of the bladder and are usually composed of an inner core of uniform intermediate and basal cells covered by superficial cells. Although papillomas may yield similar aggregates, the presence of normal urothelial cells within the cluster should militate against a diagnosis of malignancy. Occasionally, specimens labeled "urine" are received from patients having ileal conduits. While the specimen is indeed urine, it does not come from the bladder and the cellular background is not one of urothelial cells. Degenerated mucosal cells from the small intestine may suggest a low grade carcinoma but a detailed examination of the cellular constituents of the aggregates will usually prevent a misinterpretation. Ileal conduits are frequently colonized by *Candida* species and this may be an important clue to the origin of such specimens. Very rarely, seminal vesicle cells may appear in urinary specimens. These cells often have all of the nuclear features of malignancy but also contain lipofuscin pigment. While melanoma may be suspected, the absence of a confirmatory clinical history should lead to sufficient caution to prevent an error.

CARCINOMA *IN SITU*

Carcinoma *in situ* is currently characterized by most clinicians and pathologists as a noninvasive nonpapillary transitional cell neoplasm of high cytologic grade; squamous cell CIS has not been defined.[29-31] CIS of the urothelium differs both biologically and morphologically from CIS of the uterine cervix and direct extrapolations should be avoided. The term does not refer to either flat or papillary epithelial lesions of moderate degrees of cytologic atypia (dysplasia or papillary TCC-I and II) although these lesions may be strictly speaking "*in situ.*" Our knowledge in this area continues to evolve and many points of controversy remain.

Detection and follow-up of urothelial CIS is best accomplished through urinary cytology (Fig. 8.8). The lesions are composed of loosely cohesive cells which readily exfoliate into the urine and are easily identified morphologically. It should be emphasized that while malignant tumor cells readily appear in urinary specimens from untreated patients, there are no reliable morphological features which will allow the cytopathologist to determine the presence or absence of invasion. In most cases, the cells emanating from carcinoma *in situ* are identical to those of other high grade neoplasms. Occasionally, one may see a uniform population of single or loosely aggregated malignant cells with scanty cytoplasm and uniformly distributed, coarsely granular chromatin similar to those described for uterine cervical CIS.[32] We have not seen an example of the large cell or so-called "pagetoid" type of CIS in cytologic material but one would expect cells with relatively low N:C ratios, cyanophilic cytoplasm, and nuclei with irregularly clumped chromatin and very large nucleoli.

UROTHELIAL DYSPLASIA

The subject of urothelial dysplasia is highly controversial and is perhaps best approached at present by describing our own experience rather than attempting to integrate the widely variable opinions expressed in the literature.[33,34] We define dysplastic lesions as flat, noninvasive areas of urothelium composed of cells very similar to those of papillary TCC-I. They differ chiefly in that dysplastic cells are less abundant in urinary specimens, occur in small but loose clusters, are smaller with lower N:C ratios and have more finely granular chromatin than cells of papillary TCC-I (Fig. 8.9). Dysplastic cells differ from reactive/reparative elements such as might be found in patients with renal calculi in that the latter have vacuolated cytoplasm, low N:C ratios and centrally placed nuclei with smooth borders and prominent nucleoli. Since endoscopic localization of dysplastic lesions is currently not possible and the presence of dysplasia is considered to be a risk factor in the development of invasive urothelial carcinoma, cytologic studies offer the best method for detection and follow-up. The application of the cytologic method to urothelial dysplasia is in its formative stages and only preliminary results can be reported at this time. In a study of 1550 consecutive urinary specimens received in the cytology laboratory over a 5-year period, we identified dysplastic cells as the most serious abnormality in 77 (5%). These 77 specimens were from 50 patients, the records of 48 of whom were available for evaluation (Table 8.4). The

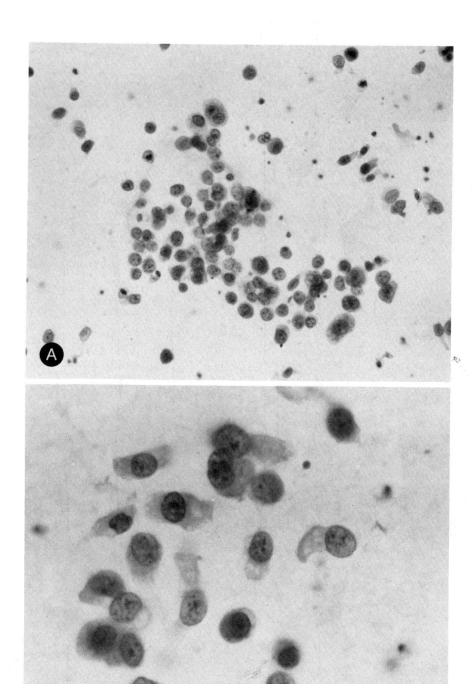

Figure 8.8. *A*, abundant malignant cells from a patient with carcinoma *in situ* (EA50 × 72). *B*, high magnification of *A*. Cells exfoliating from CIS usually resemble those illustrated in Figure 8.1*A*. These cells are smaller and more uniform with less conspicuous nucleoli but have coarsely granular chromatin and eccentric nuclei with high N:C ratios (EA50 × 180).

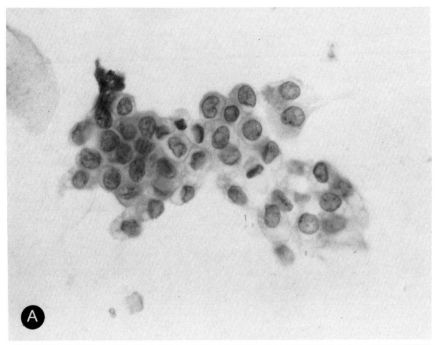

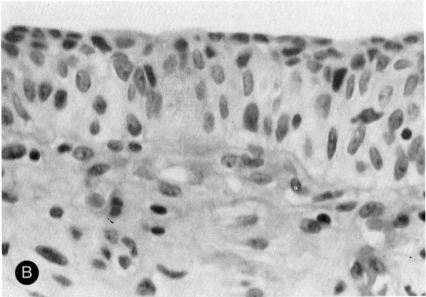

Figure 8.9. *A,* dysplastic urothelial cells. The cells of urothelial dysplasia are morphologically similar to those of TCC-I and in many cases the two lesions can not be distinguished in cytologic samples. Dysplastic cells tend to occur in tighter clusters and have lower N:C ratios than those of TCC-I; compare with Figure 8.2*A* (EA50 × 180). *B,* dysplasia of urothelium (H&E × 180).

patients represented a heterogeneous group from various clinical services. Examination of the records revealed that 60% were being followed for cancer but that not all neoplasms were urothelial. Not surprisingly, 27% had neither neoplasia nor its precursors. Most of these suffered from bladder outlet obstruction or calculi. In contrast, when dysplastic cells were identified in the highly selected group of patients entered into the NBCCG-A surveillance protocol, 26 of 35 patients (74%) had either dysplasia or grade I transitional cell carcinoma as their most severe histologic abnormality[21] (Table 8.5). It is important to note that almost 25% of patients with dysplastic cells in their urinary specimens had transitional cell carcinomas grade I in their bladders, indicating that the cytologic finding of dysplasia may herald the presence of recurrent papillary tumors. Whether the morphologic resemblance of dysplastic cells in flat areas to those in papillary lesions means that both are neoplastic or that both are benign is a matter of current investigation. To date, most of the evidence favors the latter hypothesis.

DRUG-RELATED CHANGES

Among the myriad chemotherapeutic agents in current use in the United States, only three have exhibited significant effects on urothelium: cyclophosphamide (Cytoxan), triethylenethiophosphoramide (thiotepa), and mitomycin C (MMC).[35-37] All are alkylating agents whose mechanism of action is not completely understood but which have been shown *in vitro* to prevent DNA replication by binding nucleic acids. Whether this actually occurs in humans depends on multiple factors including the mode of administration of the drug, its activation, the exposure time, the effective dose to tumor cells and the growth rate and

Table 8.4
Patients with Urothelial Dysplasia

Condition	Clinical Records		Histologic Specimens	
	No.	%	No.	%
Cancer	29	60.5	25	73.6
Bladder	20	41.7	20	58.9
Urethra	2	4.2	2	5.9
Prostate	6	12.5	2	5.9
Cervix	1	2.1	1	2.9
Dysplasia	5	10.4	5	14.7
Hyperplasia	1	2.1	1	2.9
Benign prostatic hyperplasia	4	8.2	1	2.9
Urethral stricture	2	4.2		
Renal stones	2	4.2		
Others	5	10.4	2	5.9
Total patients:	48	100.0	34	100.0

Table 8.5
Dysplastic Cells in Urinary Cytology

Histology	Patients	Specimens
TCC-I	9	11
Dysplasia	17	28
Normal	8[a]	14[a]
Denuded	1	2
Total	35	55

[a] Dysplasia on previous biopsies: two patients, five specimens.

environment of the tumor. Cyclophosphamide is used to treat a variety of benign diseases and nonurothelial malignancies. It is administered systemically and its active form is concentrated in the urine where it can be in contact with urothelial cells for prolonged periods. A major complication is denuding and hemorrhagic cystitis manifested either clinically or by the appearance of large cells with increased N:C ratios and hyperchromatic, partially degenerated nuclei in the urine[38] (Fig. 8.10). Although previously considered to be benign alterations of normal urothelium, over 20 cases of high grade urothelial carcinoma among patients treated with cyclophosphamide have been reported.[39] Most of the patients had other malignancies but at least two individuals had been treated for benign conditions such as rheumatoid arthritis.[40] The appearance of abnormal cells in patients after cyclophosphamide therapy may indicate serious urothelial disease and should be noted so that appropriate action can be taken.

Mitomycin C and thiotepa are given topically *via* catheter specifically for the treatment and/or prophylaxis of superficial bladder tumors. The drugs remain in contact with urothelium for variable periods usually not exceeding 2 hours before they are voided. Most clinical reports indicate a 30–50% response when measured at a single point in time by cystoscopic examination alone.[41,42] Although the recurrence rate is decreased, most studies have not shown significant long-term effects when adequate controls were used.[43]

The morphologic effects of MMC and thiotepa have been studied in

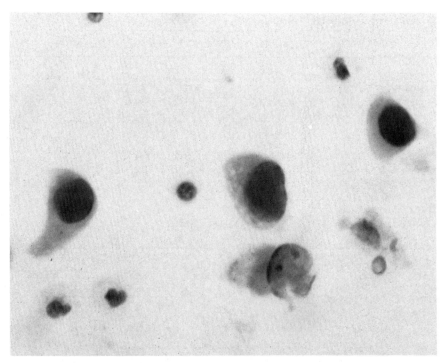

Figure 8.10. Large cells with degenerated "smudged" nuclei are characteristic of cyclophosphamide effect. Like other drug related changes, however, the morphologic features of these cells are not diagnostic (EA50 × 283).

both experimental animals and in humans. Both drugs cause increased exfoliation and denudation without increased degeneration of urothelial cells within 24–48 hours of the first instillation. These changes may persist for several weeks. Subsequent instillations do not increase exfoliation further but apparently suppress the growth of bladder tumors so that fewer cells appear in urinary samples.[37,44] This is especially important in the follow-up of carcinoma *in situ*, where abundant tumor cells in untreated cases are an important diagnostic clue. Vacuolization and multinucleation occur more often after topical chemotherapy than after catheterization alone but neither change is specific for the drugs. Cells with bizarre nuclei such as those reported after Cytoxan treatment are rare and, when present, are easily distinguished from malignant cells by experienced observers (Fig. 8.11). The changes seen with these topical chemotherapeutic agents are virtually confined to superficial cells both histologically and cytologically. Although cytology is essential in adequate follow-up of patients treated with topical chemotherapy, we have recently seen instances where nests of malignant cells have apparently been overgrown by normal urothelium so that both cystoscopy and cytology were unremarkable.

Our studies indicate that whereas thiotepa and MMC may inhibit tumor growth and prolong the disease-free interval, neither prevents the eventual occurrence of tumors in susceptible individuals.[45] This probably relates to the slow growth rate of most superficial bladder cancers, even CIS, rather than to deficiencies in the drugs themselves. Since

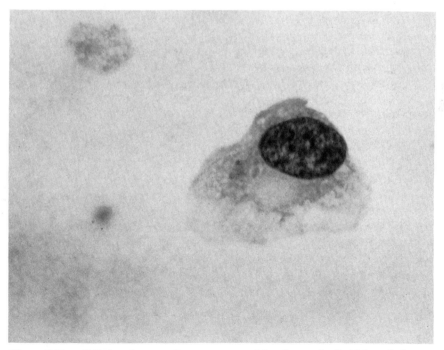

Figure 8.11. Cellular changes after treatment with mitomycin C. Although the nucleus has many of the features of malignancy, it occupies a very large cell so that the N:C ratio is low. The polyhedral shape indicates that this cell is from the superficial layer of urothelium.

alkylating agents must be incorporated into DNA to exert a biological effect on tumors and most bladder tumor cells are not in the S phase of DNA replication during the brief period that they are in contact with the drug, it is not surprising that eventual tumor growth is not prevented. Evidence from animal studies indicates, however, that thiotepa and MMC may inhibit the progression of bladder cancers from low grade and superficial to high grade and invasive.

AUTOMATED CYTOLOGY

The vagaries of cytologic examination of urothelial malignancies may be obviated in the future with the introduction of automated systems for tumor analysis. Currently, two such systems are nearly ready for clinical application. Perhaps the most promising of these is the flow-through system in which single cell suspensions of urothelial cells stained with fluorescent dyes are propelled past a laser beam which creates measurements of various parameters of DNA content as well as cell and nuclear size.[46,47] Cellular features such as RNA content, DNA content, N:C ratios, ploidy, and even variation in textural qualities can be determined. Large numbers of cells can be evaluated and numerous samples can be examined relatively rapidly. The technique is potentially valuable in screening selected populations as well as in follow-up of patients with superficial bladder tumors where changes in urothelial cells are subtle. While not yet ready for clinical use, this technique has already indicated that hyperploidy may be an important risk factor in patients with low grade urothelial neoplasms. Flow-through systems have the disadvantage that results are expressed in computerized scattergrams and the cells cannot be easily reexamined by conventional light microscopic techniques.

The Taxonomic Intracellular Analytic System (TICAS) is perhaps the most elaborate and certainly the most expensive of automated techniques.[48,49] Although it can be used in a very simple form to identify cells for subsequent visual analysis, TICAS is a very sophisticated imaging system designed to scan cells spread on glass slides and integrate the data obtained in a computer. Nuclear densities, nuclear sizes, cytoplasmic sizes and nuclear:cytoplasmic ratios can be identified as well as irregularities in nuclear borders and the relative frequency of occurrence of these features. Preparations can be subsequently examined by light microscopy. The system is slow, however, and not particularly suitable for screening large numbers of cells or groups of individuals. At present, the major disadvantages of automated systems are the initial expenses of equipment and the necessity for laboratory personnel dedicated to the instruments.

SCANNING ELECTRON MICROSCOPY

Experimental studies have indicated that scanning electron microscopy can be useful in the detection of the earliest surface changes manifested by neoplastic cells.[50,51] The technique has been successfully applied to urinary samples and may be useful in determining the biological nature of selected urothelial tumors. At present, scanning electron microscopy is time consuming and relatively expensive, factors which will limit its usefulness in routine diagnostic cytology.

SUMMARY

Urinary cytology in urothelial neoplasia is a complicated problem which can best be approached by multiple examinations of patients over rather long periods. Cytologic results must be understood in light of two persistent problems. The first concerns histogenesis and the terminology used to reflect the biologic potential of certain bladder tumors. Low grade papillary tumors frequently "recur" but uncommonly invade and rarely metastasize. They are associated with a long patient survival which approaches that in the normal population[52] and have been called "carcinoma" more to emphasize the biologic potential of the urothelium as a whole than to indicate the nature of any one papillary tumor. These low grade lesions are composed of cells with characteristic, but only slight to moderate, morphological abnormalities. Almost all retain normal blood group antigens and have diploid chromosomal modes and other biochemical characteristics of normal cells.[53-55] When these cells line delicate fibrovascular stalks, the resulting lesion is easily recognized cystoscopically and has been called carcinoma grade I and/or II on histologic examination. Similar cells occurring in flat, noninvasive areas of urothelium have been recognized and partially characterized. Although our studies indicate that there are morphological differences between the cells lining the stalks and those in flat areas, there are many similarities and these are reflected by occasional misinterpretations of dysplasia for TCC-I and *vice versa* in cellular samples.

The second major problem in the study of bladder cancer concerns the determination of the true state of the urothelium at any one point in time. Assuming that we are unwilling to obtain this information by removing and serially sectioning the bladder, we must rely upon cystoscopy, biopsy, urinary cytology, and clinical follow-up. Unfortunately, none of our methods of investigation is sufficiently refined to accurately determine the state of the urothelium in every situation. Small papillary tumors, especially when situated in the dome or the anterior wall, as well as flat dysplastic and carcinomatous lesions, are difficult to identify endoscopically. Biopsies may miss the lesions and, even when collected from the appropriate areas, may be denuded of urothelium. Topical chemotherapy may flatten papillary stalks, rendering them cystoscopically invisible or pseudodysplastic on biopsy. When cells with the morphologic features of bladder cancer are identified in urinary specimens, four possible situations might exist:

1. Tumor is present—cystoscopically recognized and confirmed by biopsy,
2. Tumor is present—not recognized cystoscopically but confirmed on selected site or random biopsies,
3. Tumor is present—not recognized cystoscopically and either not biopsied or not confirmed on biopsy,

4. Tumor is not present.

The first two possibilities yield positive cytohistologic correlations at the same point in time. The last two possibilities yield negative cytohistologic correlations at that point in time and the accuracy of the cytology can only be determined with follow-up including additional cystoscopic and histologic evaluations.

The recognition of cellular elements with morphologic features specific for urothelial neoplasia and dysplasia has expanded the role of urinary cytology in the detection and follow-up of patients with bladder cancer. These benefits have been achieved at an acceptable but not insignificant cost in unconfirmed positive diagnoses. A thorough understanding of the uses and pitfalls of the cytologic method in patients with bladder cancer is important if the method is to be properly used and caution is advisable while experience is being gained.

REFERENCES

1. De Voogt, H. J. Rathert, P., and Beyer-Boon, M. E. *Urinary Cytology,* pp. 7–15. Springer-Verlag, Berlin, 1977.
2. Holmquist, N. D. *Monographs in Clinical Cytology.* Vol. 6, *Diagnostic Cytology of the Urinary Tract,* pp. 69–76. Karger, Basel, 1977.
3. Murphy, W. M., Crabtree, W. N., Jukkola, A. F., Soloway, M. S. The diagnostic value of urine *versus* bladder washing in patients with bladder cancer. *J. Urol. 126:*320, 1981.
4. Koss, L. Ꮆ. *Diagnostic Cytology and its Histopathologic Bases.* Ed. 3, pp. 1179. Lippincott, Philadelphia, 1979.
5. Crabtree, W. N., and Murphy, W. M. The value of ethanol as a fixative in urinary cytology. *Acta Cytol. 24:*452, 1980.
6. Bergkvist, A., Ljungqvist, A., and Moberger, G. Classification of bladder tumors based on the cellular pattern: preliminary reports of a clinicopathological study of 300 cases with a minimum follow-up of 8 years. *Acta Chir. Scand. 130:*371, 1965.
7. Dukes, C. E. In *Neoplastic Disease at Various Sites,* Vol. 2, *Tumors of the Bladder,* p. 107, edited by D. M. Wallace. Livingstone, Edinburgh, 1959.
8. Friedman, N. B., and Ash, J. E. Tumors of the urinary bladder. In *Atlas of Tumor Pathology.* Armed Forces Institute of Pathology, Washington, 1959.
9. Koss, L. G. Tumors of the urinary bladder. *Atlas of Tumor Pathology II,* Series 2. Armed Forces Institute of Pathology, Washington, D.C., 1975.
10. Mostofi, F. K., Sorbin, L. H., and Torloni, H. Histological typing of urinary bladder tumors. *International Classification of Tumors 19,* WHO, Geneva, 1973.
11. Murphy, W. M. Current topics in the pathology of bladder cancer. *Pathol. Annual 18:*1, 1983.
12. Esposti, P. L., and Zajicek, J. Grading of transitional cell neoplasms of the urinary bladder from smears of bladder washings. *Acta Cytol. 16:*529, 1972.
13. Koss, L. G.: *Diagnostic Cytology and its Histopathologic Bases.* Ed. 3, pp 767. Lippincott, Philadelphia, 1979.
14. Friedell, G. H., Hawkins, I. R., Ahmed, S. W., and Schmidt, J. E. The role of urinary tract cytology in the detection and clinical management of bladder cancer. In *AUA Monograph,* Vol. 1, *Bladder Cancer.* pp. 49–62, edited by W. W. Bonney. Williams & Wilkins, Baltimore, 1982.
15. Harris, M. F., Schwinn, C. P., Morrow, J. W., Gray, R. L., and Browell, B. M. Exfoliative cytology of the urinary bladder irrigation specimen. *Acta Cytol. 15:*385, 1971.
16. Kern, W. H. The cytology of transitional cell carcinoma of the urinary bladder. *Acta Cytol. 19:*420, 1975.
17. Rife, C. C., Farrow, G. M., and Utz, D. C. Urine cytology of transitional cell neoplasms. *Urol. Clin. North Am. 6:*599, 1979.

18. Crabbe, J. G. S. Cytology of voided urine with special reference to "benign" papilloma and some of the problems encountered in the preparation of the smears. *Acta Cytol.* 5:233,1961.

19. Hicks, R. M., and Chowaniec, J. Experimental induction, histology and ultrastructure of hyperplasia and neoplasia of the urinary bladder epithelium. *International Review of Experimental Pathology Vol. 18*, p. 199, edited G. W. Richter and M. A. Epstein. Academic Press, London, 1978.

20. Kalnins, Z. A., Rhyne, A. L., Morehead, R. P., and Carter, B. J. Comparison of cytologic findings in patients with transitional cell carcinoma and benign urologic diseases. *Acta Cytol. 14*:243, 1970.

21. Murphy, W. M., Soloway, M. S., Jukkola, A. F., Crabtree, W. N., and Ford, K. S. Urinary cytology and bladder cancer—the cellular features of transitional cell neoplasms. *Cancer* (In press).

22. Murphy, W. M., and Irving, C. C. The cellular features of developing carcinoma in murine urinary bladder. *Cancer 47*:514, 1981.

23. Murphy, W. M., and Soloway, M. S. Developing carcinoma (dysplasia) of the urinary bladder. *Pathol. Annual 17*:197, 1982.

24. Murphy, W. M., and Webb, J. N. Pathology of bladder cancer. In *Bladder cancer*: UICC Technical Report Series Vol. 60, Chap. 1, edited by P. Skrabanek and A. Walsh Geneva, 1981.

25. Koss, L. G. *Diagnostic Cytology and its Histopathologic Bases*, Ed. 3, pp. 749–811. Lippincott, Philadelphia, 1979.

26. De Voogt, H. J., and Wielenga, G. Clinical aspects of urinary cytology. *Acta Cytol. 16*:349, 1972.

27. Foot, N. C., Papanicolaou, G. N., Holmquist, N. D., and Seybolt, J. F. Exfoliative cytology of urinary sediments. A review of 2829 cases. *Cancer 11*:127, 1958.

28. Prall, R. H., Wernett, C., and Mims, M. M. Diagnostic cytology in urinary tract malignancy. *Cancer 29*:1084, 1972.

29. Daly, J. J. Carcinoma *in situ* of the urothelium. *Urol. Clin North Am. 3*:87, 1976.

30. Farrow, G. M., Utz, D. C., Rife, C. C., and Greene, L. F. Clinical observations on sixty-nine cases of *in situ* carcinoma of the urinary bladder. *Cancer Res. 37*:2794, 1977.

31. Melamed, M. R., Voutsa, N. G., and Grabstald, H. Natural history and clinical behavior of *in situ* carcinoma of the human urinary bladder. *Cancer 17*:1533, 1964.

32. Voutsa, N. G., and Melamed, M. R. Cytology of *in situ* carcinoma of the human urinary bladder. *Cancer 16*:1307, 1963.

33. Murphy, W. M., Nagy, G. K., Rao, M. K., Soloway, M. S., Parija, C. G., Cox, C. E., and Friedell, G. H. "Normal" urothelium in patients with bladder cancer. *Cancer 44*:1050, 1979.

34. Murphy, W. M., and Soloway, M. S. Urothelial dysplasia: a review. *J. Urol. 127*:849, 1982.

35. Forni, A. M., Koss, L. G., and Geller, W. Cytological study of the effect of cyclophosphamide on the epithelium of the urinary bladder in man. *Cancer 17*:1348, 1964.

36. Mishina, T., and Watanabe, H. Mitomycin C bladder instillation therapy for bladder tumors. In *Mitomycin C.: Current Status and New Developments*, pp. 193–204, edited by S. K. Carter, S. T. Crooke. Academic Press, New York, 1979.

37. Murphy, W. M., Soloway, M. S., and Finebaum, P. J. Pathologic changes associated with topical chemotherapy for superficial bladder cancer. *J. Urol. 126*:461, 1980.

38. Koss, L. G. *Diagnostic Cytology and its Histopathologic Bases*, Ed. 3, pp. 739–743. Lippincott, Philadelphia, 1979.

39. Pearson, R. M., and Soloway, M. S. Does cyclophosphamide induce bladder cancer? *Urology 11*:437, 1978.

40. Plotz, P.H., Klippel, H. J., Decker J. L., Grauman, D., Wolfe, B., Brown, B.C., and Rutt, G. Bladder complications in patients receiving cyclophosphamide for systemic lupus erythematosus or rheumatoid arthritis. *Ann. Intern. Med. 91*:221, 1979.

41. Nocks, B. N., Nieh, P. T., and Prout, G. R., Jr. A longitudinal study of patients with superficial bladder carcinoma successfully treated with weekly intravesical thiotepa. *J. Urol. 122*:27, 1979.

42. Soloway, M. S. The management of superficial bladder cancer. *Cancer 45*:1856, 1980.

43. Byar, D., and Blackard, C. Comparisons of placebo, pyridoxine, and topical thiotepa

in preventing recurrence of stage 1 bladder cancer. *Urology 10:*556, 1977.

44. Murphy, W. M., Soloway, M. S., and Lin, C. J. Morphologic effects of thiotepa on mammalian urothelium: Changes in abnormal cells. *Acta Cytol. 22:*550, 1978.

45. Murphy, W. M., and Soloway, M. S. The effect of thiotepa on developing and established mammalian bladder tumors. *Cancer 45:*870, 1980.

46. Collste, L. G., Devonec, M., Darzynkiewicz, Z., Traganos, F., Sharpless, T. K., Whitmore, W. F. Jr., and Melamed, M. R. Bladder cancer diagnosis by flow cytometry: Correlation between cell samples from biopsy and bladder irrigation fluid. *Cancer 45:*2389, 1980.

47. Devonec, M., Darzynkiewicz, Z, Kostyrka-Claps, M. L., Collste, L., Whitmore, W. F., and Melamed, M. R. Flow cytometry of low stage bladder tumors: correlation with cytologic and cystoscopic diagnosis. *Cancer 49:*109, 1982.

48. Koss, L. G., Bartels, P. H., Sychra, J. J., and Wied, G. L. Diagnostic cytologic sample profiles in patients with bladder cancer using TICAS system. *Acta Cytol. 22:*392, 1978.

49. Wied, G. L., Bartels, P. H., Bahr, G. F., and Oldfield, D. G. Taxonomic intracellular analytic system (TICAS) for cell identification. *Acta Cytol. 12:*180, 1968.

50. Domagala, W., Kahan, A. V., and Koss, L. G. The ultrastructure of surfaces of positively identified cells in the human urinary sediment. *Acta Cytol. 23:*147, 1979.

51. Jacobs, J. B., Arai, M., Cohen, S. M., and Friedell, G. H. Early lesions in experimental bladder cancer: 2. Scanning electron microscopy of cell surface markers. *Cancer Res. 36:*2512, 1976.

52. Barnes, R. W., Dick, A. L., Hadley, H. L., and Johnston, O. L. Survival following transurethral resection of bladder carcinoma. *Cancer Res. 37:*2895, 1977.

53. Fulker, M. J., Cooper, M. D., Tanaka, T. Proliferation and ultrastructure of papillary transitional cell carcinoma of the human bladder. *Cancer 27:*71, 1971.

54. Levi, P. E., Cooper, E. H., Anderson, C. K., Path, M. C., and Williams, R. E. Analyses of DNA content, nuclear size and cell proliferation of transitional cell carcinoma in man. *Cancer 23:*1074, 1969.

55. Newman, A. J. Jr., Carlton, C. E. Jr., and Johnson, S. Cell surface A, B or O(H) blood group antigens as an indicator of malignant potential in stage A bladder carcinoma. *J. Urol. 124:*27, 1980.

9

Immunobiology and Immunotherapy of Bladder Cancer

Alvaro Morales, M.D., F.R.C.S.(C), F.A.C.S.

IMMUNITY IN BLADDER CANCER

Considerable efforts have been directed toward the elucidation of immune reactions against experimental as well as human tumor systems. A tremendous impetus in this area was provided by the conclusive demonstration of tumor-associated antigens (TAA) and tumor-specific transplantation antigens (TSTA) in animal models. The availability of syngeneic animals allowed the performance of experiments in which immunological responses to histocompatibility antigens could be eliminated and this leads to the clear demonstration that tumors induced by chemical carcinogens exhibit individually specific TSTA.

Although the antigenicity of human bladder cancer has not been conclusively demonstrated, there are experimental and clinical studies suggesting the presence of TAA in these neoplasms. Various investigators have identified TSTA in carcinogen-induced vesical tumors of rats and mice. Early studies demonstrated specific cytotoxic activity of human peripheral blood lymphocytes against bladder cancer cell lines.[1] More recent investigations, employing assays of indirect cytotoxicity[2] and mixed lymphocyte culture,[3] have indicated that recognition of TAA can be demonstrated in some patients with a recent history of transitional cell carcinoma of the urinary bladder. It must be emphasized, however, that the nature and the specificity of the effector cells in human studies have not been thoroughly investigated. Nevertheless, these findings, taken as a whole, suggest that urothelial tumors possess antigens capable of eliciting a specific cellular immune response. Humoral immunity in transitional cell carcinoma (TCC) has been suggested by studies demonstrating cytotoxicity by sera of patients with bladder cancer.[4] In these and other studies the factor in serum was found to be antibody and it was believed that there exists an arming of effector cells with antibody for the generation of antibody-dependent cytotoxicity. Further support for the presence of tumor-specific antigens (TSA) was based on the demonstration of antigen-antibody reactions between sera from patients with TCC and TCC cultured cell lines.[5] Despite the numerous studies aimed at determining the presence of TSA in bladder cancer, no individual test or technique has been established to apply to clearly defined clinical questions in the diagnosis or treatment of bladder cancer.

The importance of assay systems demonstrating tumor specificities was greatly diminished with the discovery, a decade ago, of the natural killer (NK) activity. NK was initially identified when it was noted that individuals without a history of cancer exhibited cell-mediated immune responses against tumor cells, a property initially believed to be restricted to previously immunized subjects. Nowadays NK cells, together with macrophages, are recognized as the first line of defense against tumor development and progression. Considerable efforts are being made at finding ways to enhance the population of NK cells as a means of cancer therapy. It is commonly recognized that alterations in NK activity reflect an individual's ability to mount a response against cancer and that monitoring of NK activity may be useful in the follow-up of patients receiving immunotherapy.[6,7] The usefulness of NK monitoring is still in a developmental phase; initial studies, however, suggest that established and progressive neoplasms have a detrimental effect on NK activity. This has been demonstrated in animals[8] and in patients harboring bladder cancer (Fig. 9.1). Studies are being conducted[9] to separate the tumor-selective cytotoxicity displayed by the lymphocytes from

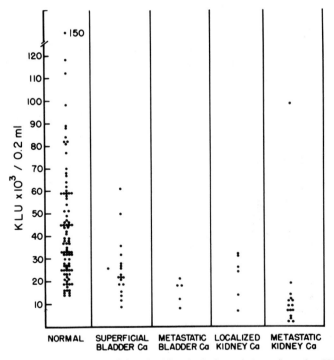

Figure 9.1. Natural cytotoxicity (in kinetic lytic units) against the K562 cell line shown by normal individuals and patients with tumors of the urinary tract. NK cell activity is inversely proportional to the stage of the disease.

patients with transitional cell carcinoma of the bladder from the spontaneous or NK cell-mediated cytotoxicity which can be demonstrated in peripheral blood lymphocytes from almost any normal individual.

Nonspecific immune reactions such as skin testing with a variety of antigens or *in vitro* testing for general evaluation of an individual's immunological integrity have been used for many years and are believed to have some prognostic value, particularly when immunotherapy is being used. The role of AB and H(O) and other antigenic markers in the human blood group system is discussed in Chapter 6.

IMMUNOTHERAPY OF BLADDER CANCER

Animal Models

A sound approach to the clinical immunotherapy of malignant disease must be based on experimental studies of the immunobiology of cancer is general and the immune responsiveness of the bladder in particular. Two experimental studies are of particular significance to individuals interested in immune modulation for therapy of vesical neoplasms. In 1966, Coe and Feldman,[10] in elegant experiments, clearly demonstrated that the bladder is an ideal organ for the development of delayed hypersensitivity reactions. Their studies showed that previously immunized guinea pigs exposed to an antigenic challenge exhibited particularly strong delayed hypersensitivity reactions in the skin and in the bladder, while the responses were much less significant in kidney, muscle, or testes. This important observation, however, was largely ignored during the immunotherapy renaissance of the early 1970s. Equally important were the series of experiments of Zbar and his group[11] which clearly and conclusively established the basis for successful nonspecific activity immunotherapy, principles which probably can be applied to all forms of experimental and clinical categories of immunotherapy (i.e. active, passive, adoptive). These workers, employing a hepatoma model in guinea pigs and treatment with *Myocobacterium bovis* demonstrated the following basic principles for optimal results in immune modulation in cancer:

1. Tumors respond better when confined to the parent organ or when their microscopic spread is limited to the regional lymph nodes;
2. The tumor burden must be small. The diameter and mass of the tumor appear to be a critical factor in response;
3. Direct contact between the tumor cells and the vaccine is essential; and
4. The dose of the immunizing agent must be adequate. In the case of *M. bovis*, effectiveness was confined in a range of 10^6–10^8 viable organisms injected into the transplanted tumor.

Active nonspecific immunotherapy has been more commonly used in the clinical setting for practical and ethical reasons. In experimental systems, however, active specific immunotherapy has been widely used. In these cases an enhancement of the host's immune response is achieved by its exposure to antigenic elements of the tumor. These antigens may be administered to the animal in the form of live or irradiated tumor cells or subcellular components. In experimental bladder cancer, chemically induced tumors have been found to be immunogenic and amenable to immune prophylaxis by vaccination with whole tumor cells[12] or their extracts.[13] A typical amputation-challenge experiment to demonstrate immune protection obtained with live cells is shown in Fig. 9.2. Administration of live tumor cells has no practical clinical use; therefore, nonviable tumor cells or subcellular components have been tried in tumor models. Inactivated tumor cells, however, are not easily diluted or concentrated before use and may transmit viral antigens and small numbers of viable cells with the potential for establishing new tumors. On the other hand, administration of tumor extracts for protection against supralethal doses of neoplastic cells have been found effective in a variety of animal tumors[14] including experimental vesical neoplasms.[11]

Bladder cancer can consistently be produced in a variety of experi-

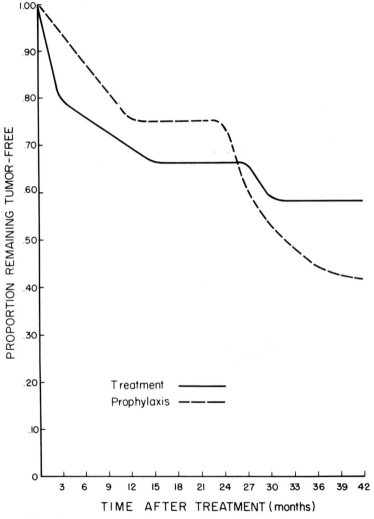

Figure 9.2. These curves indicate that there is a progressive decline in the tumor-free population after completion of treatment with BCG. The figures suggest that periodic boosting of immunity may improve the results.

mental animals by feeding *N*-(4-(5-nitro-2-furyl)-2-thiazolyl)formamide (FANFT). Studies using chemically induced tumors may help in the understanding of the biological behavior of their human counterparts because of the similarities they share: chemical etiology, prolonged latent period and histological appearance. The use of various carcinogens, particularly FANFT, has permitted the development of autochthonous and transplantable bladder tumors which have been useful in the development of clinical immunotherapy protocols.

A bladder tumor induced by FANFT administration into C3H mice produced the MBT-2 cell line initially employed at the National Cancer Institute (NCI). The development of a tumor cell line and the availability of tissue culture cells from this tumor constituted a definite asset for studies on the immunobiology of bladder cancer. Initial studies with the *in vivo* line demonstrated the MBT-2 tumor to be immunogenic by Javadpour and his co-workers.[12] The availability of an *in vitro* cell line, furthermore, provided a fairly uniform cell population, a relatively abundant source of cells free of overt microbial contamination and necrotic material, and permitted the extraction of antigens on multiple occasions. Moreover, the development of low grade passenger infections resulting in the appearance of cellular neoantigens could be partially circumvented by cryopreservation of tumor cells obtained within a limited number of passages by these investigators.[12]

A wealth of information on the immunobiology of bladder cancer has been obtained by detailed study of the MBT-2 tumor and immunotherapy protocols have been refined and improved by observations made on the biological behavior of this experimental neoplasm. Important data in the context of developing immunotherapy for bladder cancer was obtained however, without the use of an experimental tumor: Bloomberg et al.[16] reported a marked inflammatory reaction in the bladder of healthy dogs after intravesical instillation of bacillus Calmette-Guérin (BCG); the cellular infiltrates in the reaction were mostly histiocytes and macrophages. This observation, together with the studies of Coe and Feldman[10] and those of Zbar and his group,[11] provided the basis for effective immunotherapy protocols for vesical neoplasms. The MBT-2 tumor, furthermore, has permitted comparative studies of various nonspecific immune modifiers[17-19] to be carried out and the information obtained from this and other chemically induced tumors should be used for improving the effectiveness and decreasing the side effects of currently available agents. As a valid example are the interesting studies of Shapiro et al.[20] which have shown the effectiveness of intravesical BCG in preventing tumor takes in a disrupted bladder mucosa. It is believed that such tumor implants occur clinically after transurethral resections and it appears that this occurrence may be eliminated by postoperative instillations of the vaccine.

Clinical Experience

Bladder cancer is a major cause of death in the elderly population; it is estimated that over 40,000 new cases are diagnosed in North America every year. Fortunately, the large majority of these tumors are diagnosed early and are, therefore, potentially curable. Endoscopic surgery remains the primary and most effective treatment of early bladder cancer. The high incidence of recurrence and the multiplicity of these neoplasms, however, have created a need for the development of new agents with activity against noninfiltrating vesical neoplasms. Various chemotherapeutic agents have been used in the treatment of early disease with variable success (see Chapter 14). Superficial bladder cancer appears to be ideally suited for immunological intervention; since, with the possible exception of cutaneous neoplasms, no other tumor so well fulfills the criteria for immunotherapy as superficial bladder cancer.[11] In addition, studies cited earlier[10,16] have shown that the bladder develops very marked immune responses to a variety of antigens. These characteristics of the bladder and the numerous *in vitro* studies utilizing human bladder cancer lines have provided a solid experimental basis for the design of treatment strategies with immune modifiers in the prophylaxis of recurrence and the treatment of superficial lesions. Although some of these therapeutic approaches have met with considerable success, immunotherapy has been a dismal failure in the treatment of locally advanced and metastatic transitional cell carcinoma of the bladder. These disappointing results, however, were predictable on the basis of available experimental data.

Three general forms of clinical immunotherapy are currently available: active, passive and adoptive, and each one of these can be specific or nonspecific. Most of the immunotherapeutic experience in bladder cancer is limited to nonspecific active immunotherapy. Perhaps the only form of active, specific immunotherapy which has been used in bladder cancer was the hydrostatic technique of Helmstein.[1,21] The hypothesis was suggested that the tumor necrosis caused by pressure on the tumor would generate an antigenic stimulus which would mount a specific immune response against the tumor. This was never proven and the technique is seldom used nowadays.

Vitamin A and its natural and synthetic derivatives, the retinoids, have been known to be effective in the prevention of cancer.[22] These compounds are included in the discussion of immunotherapy of vesical neoplasms because administration of retinoids has been found to enhance both humoral and cell-mediated immune responses. In fact recent reports indicate that both natural and antibody-dependent cytotoxicities as well as macrophage activity can be stimulated by analoges of vitamin A. Trials are being conducted to determine the effectiveness of these drugs in the prevention of recurrent bladder tumors.

Keyhole limpet hemocyanin (KLH) has been used for many years in the assessment of immune reactivity by delayed cutaneous hypersensitivity. A decade ago, Olsson *et al.*[23] found decreased cutaneous responses in patients with bladder cancer and later on they used KLH in an attempt to prevent recurrence of superficial tumors. Although they found a significant reduction in the number of recurrences in those patients receiving and reacting to KLH, conclusive evidence was not presented in the study. Additional investigations with KLH, unfortunately, were not pursued by this or any other group of investigators.

Further compounds used as immune modifiers include levamisole and polyinosinic and polycyticylic acids (Poly I:C). Levamisole was reported to be ineffective in the prevention of recurrences in a randomized trial of patients with various stages of superficial and invasive bladder cancer.[24] Poly I:C is an interferon inducer and it was hoped that it would, indirectly, promote and enhance immune responses in humans. Although evidence was found for the effectiveness of poly I:C as an interferon inducer, its systemic administration proved to be ineffective in the treatment of TCC.[25] It is possible that regional instead of systemic administration of poly I:C may be more effective if higher local levels of interferon are produced.[26] Intralesional and systemic interferon has been found effective in small studies[26]; larger trials will be necessary to determine its activity. Other compounds such as transfer factor and bacterial preparations, including *Corynebacterium parvum* have been used with little success.[26]

The notable exception to the disappointing role of immunotherapy in urological malignancies has been the effectiveness of BCG in superficial bladder cancer. Successful destruction of a metastatic vesical melanoma by intratumoral, transurethral injection of BCG in a patient previously immunized with the vaccine has been reported.[27] This single observation was in keeping with the experimental data indicating that the bladder responds promptly and strongly to antigenic challenge.[10] Furthermore, it provided clinical support to the observations of Bloomberg et al.[16] and the model for BCG immunotherapy of Zbar et al.[11] The following year, Morales and his group[28] reported their preliminary experience with systemic and intravesical administration of BCG in patients with superficial bladder cancer. The results showed that the vaccine exhibited significant activity against noninfiltrating TCC of the bladder. Further nonrandomized studies by Morales et al.[29] also showed that BCG was effective in the treatment of residual tumors and of carcinoma *in situ*.[30] The protocol employed in these studies was essentially the same.[29] The BCG vaccine used was the Pasteur strain produced by Institute Frappier of Montreal. The vaccine was administered intradermally and intravesically. For the intradermal route, 5 mg were given. The anterior aspect of a thigh received multiple punctures with a Heaf gun; a small amount of the BCG suspension was spread over the area of punctured skin and allowed to dry. The vaccine was reapplied until it was all used. The area was dressed and left undisturbed for 24 hours. For the intracavitary administration, the patient was prepared for routine bladder catheterization under sterile conditions. A solution of 120 mg BCG in 50 ml of saline was instilled into the bladder and the catheter was removed immediately afterwards. The patient was instructed to retain the medication for not less than 2 hours and to lie alternately in the prone and supine positions at 15-minute intervals. The intradermal and intravesical administrations of the vaccine were repeated weekly for 6 weeks. Alternate thighs were used for the intradermal applications. Particular effort was made to start treatment within 10 days after the cystoscopy and biopsies on the assumption that the disrupted epithelium would facilitate localization of the bacterial antigens in the bladder and promote the inflammatory reaction detrimental to the tumor.

Clinical studies on intracavitary BCG therapy for bladder cancer were activated at our institution 10 years ago. Ninety-three patients have entered the trials and have been treated with a standard protocol.[29] The mean follow-up of these patients is 51 months. It has been found that the vaccine is highly active against superficial bladder cancer. It was noted, however, that after 12–24 months there is a decline in the tumor-free population (Fig. 9.2) which reaches a plateau about 3 years after completion of therapy. From this large and long experience it has been concluded that prolonged treatment as proposed by others (see below) is a valid improvement in therapy since the declines observed in the tumor-free populations with the short protocol may be eliminated by periodic immunizations. Shortly after treatment the endoscopic and histological appearance of the bladder shows marked inflammation which usually subsides within a few weeks (Figs. 9.3 and 9.4). In none of the 93 patients followed for up to 8 years has there been any evidence of permanent functional or structural damage to the bladder.

The National Cancer Institute saw merit in this approach and supported randomized controlled trials in which the above protocol was strictly duplicated, including the same strain of BCG. The results of three studies are now available. Lamm and associates[31] reported on 51 patients randomized into transurethral resection alone *versus* transurethral resection plus BCG. In this study the incidence of recurrence was statistically significantly smaller in the BCG group as compared to endoscopic surgery alone. Pinsky *et al.*[32] reported similar results also in a randomized prospective study in which transurethral resection of the

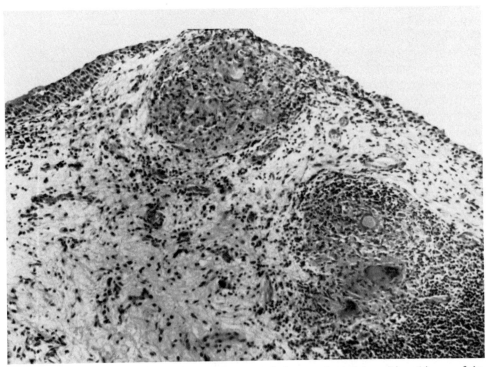

Figure 9.3. Chronic granulomatous inflammation observed in a biopsy of the bladder after BCG treatment. Note the multinucleated giant cells within the granulomata.

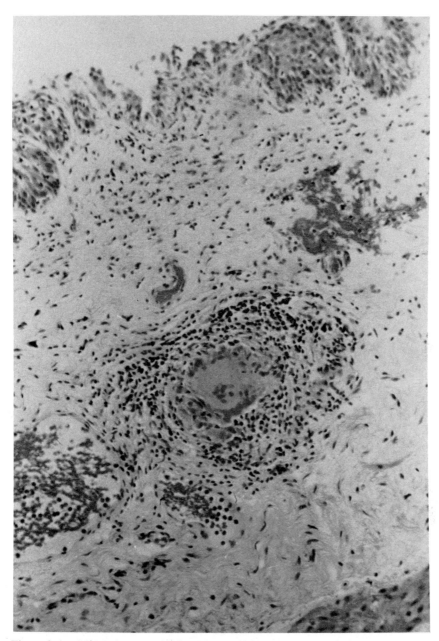

Figure 9.4. Microphotograph of a characteristic granuloma after BCG therapy. The granuloma is located in the submucosa and consists of a multinucleated giant cell surrounded by an inflammatory infiltrate.

tumor(s) was compared to transurethral resection plus BCG. In a subsequent report from Lamm et al.[33] a longer follow-up of their original patients continued to support their initial experiences but, in addition, 10 patients with infiltrating TCC who were not candidates for cystectomy and were treated with intravesical and intradermal immunizations of BCG were rendered disease-free. This is the only report available in the literature demonstrating that the vaccine may be effective in stage

B disease. Such an approach, however, must be taken cautiously and should be reserved only for patients not amenable to more orthodox treatments; the results, nevertheless, are encouraging.

The results of a pilot study reported by Morales[30] on the treatment of carcinoma *in situ* of the bladder were clearly confirmed in a controlled study.[34] These authors found that the majority (65%) of patients had complete resolution of the *in situ* tumors following administration of the vaccine. These authors, however, have cautioned about the presence of TCC *in situ* in the prostatic ducts distal ureters which does not seem to be favorably affected by BCG immunotherapy.

Brossman[35] has used a modified protocol for BCG immunotherapy of superficial bladder cancer. He employs a different strain (Tice) of the vaccine at higher doses, for a longer period (2 years) and does not use the intradermal route. In addition to these modifications to the original protocol, this study is of interest because it represents the first comparative work of BCG against a well known chemotherapeutic agent: thiotepa. The results of this trial were clearly superior for the BCG group when the vaccine was used for prophylaxis of recurrence as well as for the treatment of carcinoma *in situ*.

Complications arising from intravesical BCG therapy have been self-limiting and minor in the large majority of cases when the initial protocol has been used.[28-33] Brossman,[35] however, reported a much higher incidence of side effects attributable to the vaccine. He found bladder irritability in every patient and systemic toxicity in 28% of the 39 patients receiving BCG. These differences can be readily explained by the respective discrepancies between the protocols of Morales *et al.*[28] and of Brossman: low (1.2×10^6) *versus* high (6×10^6) doses of viable organisms, short (6 weeks) *versus* long (2 years) duration of treatment and source of the vaccine (Frappier *versus* Tice). It is important to note that systemic infection with BCG responds rapidly to a short course of isoniazide. Since isoniazide interferes with the immunogenicity of the vaccine, it has not been advocated to use antituberculous medication to prevent complications from BCG therapy.

Prolonged treatment for up to 2 years has been found to be more effective despite the potential increase in the number and severity of side effects.[35] Our initial experience with longer treatment supports the concept that periodic boosting of immunity by administration of BCG improves the overall results of treatment.[36]

Our current protocol for prophylaxis and treatment of superficial bladder cancer, therefore, has been modified. We employ 120 mg (1.2×10^9 viable) organisms for intravesical instillation one time weekly for 6 weeks and then one time monthly for 1 year. The use of intradermal immunizations no longer appears mandatory although their need has not been conclusively deemed unnecessary.

The experience with BCG immunotherapy of bladder neoplasms has not been universally satisfactory. Flamm and Grot[37] noted no beneficial effect from BCG treatment, not a surprising result in view of the small amounts of the vaccine used by these investigators: one or two treatments at half the recommended strength of the vaccine. Equally disappointing were the results noted by Robinson and Rigby.[38] These authors used the proper amounts of BCG but unfortunately they chose a strain (Glaxo) of recognized low immunogenicity. This study brought into sharp focus an important fact which is frequently overlooked by clinicians designing protocols with BCG: there are multiple strains of variable viability and immunogenicity (in fact there is no absolute homogeneity among batches of the same strain!). Multiple studies have repeatedly shown that there are strains of BCG exhibiting high and low quality for experimental cancer therapy (as opposed to immunization for tuberculosis). Modified protocols are doomed to failure unless such crucial factors as strain of the vaccine, route of administration and frequency of immunizations are carefully chosen on the basis of previous experimental or clinical studies. A recent report has suggested that megadoses of oral BCG are effective in the treatment of superficial vesical neoplasms.[39] These results are very preliminary but, if supported by controlled studies, would facilitate treatment and eliminate some of the annoying bladder symptoms noted with intracavitary instillations. Little is known about the effectiveness of killed BCG or the bacterial cell walls; these are intriguing possibilities because some of the cellular components retain immunogenicity but do not have the ability to replicate and produce systemic infections.

FUTURE PROSPECTS

The availability of adequate experimental models of bladder cancer with marked similarities to the human neoplasms has greatly facilitated our understanding of the biological behavior of the latter. Vigorous research with experimental neoplasms is being pursued at various centers and the beneficial results are beginning to appear in the form of effective modifications of current clinical studies. A better understanding of the tumor-host interactions is rapidly developing thanks to the available experimental tumor systems. The immunobiology of bladder cancer is one of the most extensively investigated among human cancers and this interest by urologists and basic scientists alike has translated into one of the few examples of successful clinical immunotherapy. However, much has to be learned about the mechanisms of action of BCG and other biological immune response modifiers. The elucidation of such mechanisms will offer enormous possibilities in the treatment of cancer.

Current approaches to bladder cancer immunotherapy are crude, unsophisticated and largely empirical. There is an obvious urgency for improvement of the available protocols and an unquestionable need for comparative studies to determine the individual merits of immune modifiers and chemotherapeutic agents alone and in combination. The dismal response of metastatic bladder cancer to our present armamentarium may be improved by such combined approaches. To expect immunotherapeutic successes where surgery, chemotherapy, and radiation have previously failed is beyond reasonable expectations. The proper and well timed combination of these modalities may prove to be a worthwhile and fruitful endeavor.

REFERENCES

1. O'Toole, C., Helmstein, K., Perlman, P., and Moberger, G. Cellular immunity to transitional cell carcinoma of the urinary bladder. III. Effects of hydrostatic pressure therapy. *Int. J. Cancer 16:*413–426, 1975.
2. Morales, A. *In vitro* generation of cytotoxic lymphocytes by tumor extracts of transitional cell carcinoma. *Natl. Cancer Inst. Monogr. 49:*173–174, 1978.
3. Herr, H. W., Bean, M. A., and Whitmore, W. F. Mixed leukocyte culture reactivity of lymph node cells regional to transitional cell carcinoma of the bladder. *Natl. Cancer Inst. Monogr. 49:*177–181, 1978.
4. Elhilali, M. M., and Nayak, S. K. Immunologic evaluation of human bladder cancer: *in vitro* studies. *Cancer 35:*419–431, 1975.
5. Elliott, A. Y., Dambrovskis, E. E., and Fraley, E. E. Transitional cell cancer: fluorescent antibody binding to tumor cells *in vitro*. *Natl. Cancer Inst. Monogr. 49:*199–201, 1978.
6. Pross, H. F., and Baines, M. G. Studies on human natural killer cells. I. *In vivo* parameters affecting normal cytotoxic function. *Int. J. Cancer 29:*383–390, 1982.
7. Morales, A., and Ottenhof, P. C. Clinical application of a whole blood assay for human NK cell activity. *Cancer 52:*667–670, 1983.
8. Pang, A. D. S., and Morales, A. The effect of tumor burden on the modulation of natural killer (NK) cell activity. Abstract No. 71. Presented at the 78th Annual Meeting of the American Urological Association, Las Vegas, April 17–21, 1983.
9. Vilien, M., Troye-Blomberg, M., Perlmann, P., Wolf, H., and Rasmussen, F. Human spontaneous lymphocyte mediated cytotoxicity against malignant and normal tissue target cell lines tested in autologous and allogeneic combination by the microcytotoxicity assay. *Cancer Immunol. Immunother. 14:*137–144, 1983.
10. Coe, J. E., and Feldman, J. D. Extracutaneous delayed hypersensitivity, particularly in the guinea pig bladder. *Immunology 10:*127–135, 1966.
11. Zbar, B., Bernstein, I. D., Bartlett, G. L., Hanna, M. G., and Rapp, H. J. Immunotherapy of cancer: regression of intradermal tumors and prevention of growth of lymph node metastases after intralesional injection of living *Mycobacterium bovis. J. Natl. Cancer Inst. 49:*119–130, 1972.
12. Javadpour, N., Hyatt, C. L., and Soares, T. Immunologic features of a carcinogen-induced murine bladder cancer: *in vivo* and *in vitro* studies. *J. Surg. Oncol. 11:*153–159, 1979.
13. Morales, A., Djeu, J., and Herberman, R. B. Immunizations by irradiated whole cells or cell extracts against an experimental bladder tumor. *Invest. Urol. 17:*310–313, 1980.
14. Meltzer, M. S., Leonard, E. J., Hardy, A. S., and Rapp, H. J. Protective tumor immunity induced by potassium chloride extracts of guinea pig hepatomas. *J. Natl. Cancer Inst. 54:*1349, 1975.
15. Soloway, M. S. Intravesical and systemic chemotherapy of murine bladder cancer. *Cancer Res. 37:*2918–2929, 1977.
16. Bloomberg, S. D., Brossman, S. A., Hausman, M. S., Cohen, A., and Battenberg, J. D. The effect of BCG on the dog bladder. *Invest. Urol. 12:*423–427, 1975.
17. Lamm, D. L., Reichert, D. F., Harris, S. C., and Lucio, R. M. Immunotherapy of murine transitional cell carcinoma. *J. Urol. 128:*1104–110, 1982.
18. Pang, A. S. D., and Morales, A. Immunoprophylaxis of a murine bladder cancer with high dose BCG immunizations. *J. Urol. 127:*1006–1009, 1982.
19. Pang, A. S. D., and Morales, A. Chemoimmunoprophylaxis of an experimental bladder cancer with retinoids and BCG. *J. Urol. 130:*166–170, 1983.
20. Shapiro, A., Ratliff, T. L., Oakley, D. M., and Catalona, W. J. Reduction of bladder tumor growth in BCG treated mice; its correlation to NK cell activity and interferon levels. Abstract No. 55. Presented at the American Urological Association 77th Annual Meeting, Kansas City, May 16–20, 1982.
21. Helmstein, K. Treatment of bladder carcinoma by a hydrostatic pressure technique. *Br. J. Urol. 44:*434, 450, 1972.
22. Sporn, M. B., Dunlop, N. M., Newton, D. L., and Smith, J. M. Prevention of chemical carcinogenesis with vitamin A and its synthetic analogs. *Fed. Proc. 35:*1332–1338, 1976.

23. Olsson, C. A., Chute, R., and Rao, C. N. Immunological reduction of bladder cancer recurrence rate. *J. Urol. 111:*173–176, 1974.

24. Smith, R. B., deKernion, J., Lincoln, B., Skinner, D. G., and Kaufman, J. J. Preliminary report of the use of levamisole in the treatment of bladder cancer. *Cancer Treat. Rep. 62:*1709–1714, 1978.

25. Herr, H. W., Kemeny, N., Yagoda, A., and Whitmore, W. F. Poly I:C immunotherapy in patients with papillomas or superficial carcinomas of the bladder. *Natl. Cancer Inst. Monogr. 49:*325, 1978.

26. Shapiro, A., Kadmon, D., Catalona, W. J., and Ratliff, T. L. Immunotherapy of superficial bladder cancer. *J. Urol. 128:*891–894, 1982.

27. deKernion, J. B. Golub, S. H., Gupta, R. K., Silverstein, M., and Morton, D. L. Successful transurethral intralesional BCG therapy of bladder melanoma. *Cancer 36:*1662–1667, 1975.

28. Morales, A., Eidinger, D., and Bruce, A. W. Intracavitary bacillus Calmette-Guérin in the treatment of superficial bladder tumors. *J. Urol. 116:*180–183, 1976.

29. Morales, A., Ottenhof, P., and Emerson, L. Treatment of residual noninfiltrating bladder cancer with bacillus Calmette-Guérin. *J. Urol. 125:*649–651, 1981.

30. Morales, A. Treatment of carcinoma *in situ* of the bladder with BCG. A phase II trial. *Cancer Immunol. Immunother. 9:*69–71, 1980.

31. Lamm, D. L., Thor, D. E., Winters, W. D., Stoydill, V. D., and Radwin, H. M. BCG immunotherapy of bladder cancer: inhibition of tumor recurrence and associated immune responses. *Cancer 48:*82–88, 1981.

32. Pinsky, C. M., Camacho, F. J., Kerr, D., Braun, D. W., Whitmore, W. F., and Oettgen, H. F. Treatment of superficial bladder cancer with intravesical BCG. In *Immunotherapy of Human Cancer*, pp. 309–313, edited by W. D. Terry and S. A. Rosenberg. Elsevier North Holland, New York, 1982.

33. Lamm, D. L., Thor, D. E., Stogdill, V. D., and Radwin, H. M. Bladder cancer immunotherapy. *J. Urol. 128:*931–935, 1982.

34. Herr, H. W., Pinsky, C. M., Whitmore, W. F., Oettgen, H. F., and Melamed, M. R. Effect of intravesical BCG on carcinoma *in situ* of the bladder. *Cancer 51:*1323–1326, 1983.

35. Brossman, S. A. Experience with bacillus Calmette-Guérin in patients with superficial bladder carcinoma. *J. Urol. 128:*27–30, 1982.

36. Morales, A. Long-term results and complications of intravesical BCG therapy for cancer. Presented at the 78th Annual Meeting of the American Urological Association. Abstract No. 344.

37. Flamm, J., and Grot, F. Adjuvant local immunotherapy with bacillus Calmette-Guérin (BCG) in the treatment of urothelial carcinoma of the urinary bladder. *Wien Med. Wochenschr 131:*501–503, 1981.

38. Robinson, M. R. G., and Rigby, C. C. Intravesical BCG therapy for Ta and T1 bladder tumors: histopathology and toxicity. In Bladder Cancer Principles of Combination Therapy, pp. 287–295, edited by R. T. D. Oliver, W. F. Hendry, H. J. G. Bloom. Butterworths, London, 1981.

39. Netto N. R., and Lemos, G. C. A comparison of treatment methods for the prophylaxis of recurrent superficial bladder tumors. *J. Urol. 129:*33–34, 1983.

10

Superficial Bladder Tumors

Kevin J. O'Connell, M.D.

Historically, the first bladder tumor was reported by Scluelardo in 1718.[1] Impetus to preautopsy diagnosis of bladder cancer was made by the introduction of the cystoscope by Nitze in 1879; and, in spite of significant advances in cytology and radiology, its fiber optic descendant remains the primary diagnostic instrument.[12] Since that time urologists have been fascinated and frustrated by transitional cell carcinoma which represents 90–95% of bladder carcinoma.

Painless hematuria is the most common presenting symptom and occurs almost 90% of the time.[9] Passing of tissue, persistent microscopic hematuria, suprapubic discomfort, and serendipitous observations account for most of the remainder of localized tumors. Papillary tumors occur originally most commonly around the orifices. Approximately 30% will be multiple at first observation and less than 3 cm in diameter.[12] Transitional cell carcinoma will be newly diagnosed in approximately 30,000 patients and will kill approximately 10,000 each year. The vast majority of the newly discovered patients will have localized disease (82%).

Most urologists prefer to think of bladder cancer staging in Marshall's revision of Jewett's staging because the TNM system is cumbersome for discussion but is needed in scientific reporting for comparisons. We will consider superficial tumors to be those diagnosed carcinoma *in situ* (CIS), O, and A in Marshall-Jewett, and TIS, Ta and T_1 in the TMN system.

Eighty percent of patients newly diagnosed will be over the age of 50; however, increasingly, recognition is being made of patients considerably younger being diagnosed as transitional cell carcinoma.[14] Originally these patients were believed to have nonrecurrent tumor; however, follow-up studies have revealed a recurrence rate of 14% as well as a documented progression to an invasive tumor.

Cystoscopically the lesions may be: (1) frondular, resembling seaweed waving to and fro in the pulse of the irrigating fluids; (2) pedunculated, short stubby base sometimes said to resemble a raspberry; or (3) a more cauliflower appearance, which might suggest more anaplasia. Ulcerative lesions, or sheet-like lesions, are usually extremely anaplastic and infiltrative and suggest a poor prognosis.

The biopsy, of course, is the definitive diagnostic tool and occasionally minor biopsy may be performed in the clinic without the use of regional or general anesthesia. However, an experienced endoscopist should balance the risk of significant bleeding *versus* a swift diagnosis. Occasionally it seems easier to fulgurate a small lesion rather than biopsy it; however, we believe appropriate biopsies should be taken to clearly document the disease rather than have a patient carry a malignant diagnosis based only on an observation. For a fulgurated benign lesion, we believe it also appropriate to perform random biopsies on both seemingly inflammatory and normal appearing areas to document any "field defect" which may be occuring and possibly alerting us to recommend earlier follow-ups, intravesical chemotherapy, or possibly leading to earlier cystectomy.

Papanicolaou popularized the use of cytology for cervical smears as a means for determining early cervical cancer. This technique was then investigated in urinary sediment and did show that exfoliated cells from transitional cell tumors could be detected in the urine. Clinical investigators in the 1960s showed that it was of little value in detecting low grade tumors and therefore not useful in mass screening. It has been used in screening individual workers subjected to carcinogens and is part of a follow-up of bladder tumor patients but it has not replaced the timely follow-up cystoscopy. Cytologies will occasionally be positive before visual tumor is present. It is well to remember when this occurs that transitional cells, and therefore transitional cell tumors, are not confined to the bladder but may be in the collecting system of the kidney, ureter, prostatic urethra, and some of the prostatic ducts.

Of the patients treated with local fulguration or resection, 70% will have a recurrence within 2 years. There are a number of theories to explain this phenomenon. The first theory is that the urothelium has been exposed to a carcinogen and areas exposed the most, *i.e.* the trigone especially around the orifices, exhibit the earliest manifestations (the first tumor). Later tumor sites are not yet ripe and subsequent tumors manifest themselves later. The second theory is that the bladder defenses are weakened by surgery, and the cells free floating in the urine then implant. A third theory is that, as the bladder collapses after each micturition, the dome contacts the trigone, the common area of primary, and the tumor implants.

Soloway et al.,[25] reporting in 1978 on 42 patients having random biopsies at the time of their initial biopsy and/or fulguration, found 33% had abnormal histology in normal appearing sites and 5% had carcinoma *in situ* or carcinoma.

In patients with repeat cystoscopic exams the overall incidence of abnormal histology was 77%, with 30% being severe atypia, carcinoma *in situ*, or frank carcinoma.

Epidemiologically, in the United States, men are more commonly diagnosed with bladder tumor with a male/female ratio of 2/1 and a black/white ratio of 1/4.[9] Some national studies seem to indicate an increase in the incidence of bladder cancer. The extent that earlier or more complete diagnosis, more sophisticated evaluations, aging populations and/or industrial pollutants contribute to this potential increase is unknown. Recent studies in Iceland indicate that female incidence of bladder cancer is increasing slightly faster than the male incidence.[20] This observation is noted in spite of the fact that, except for the fishing industry, industrial chemical carcinogens are extremely low. Cigarette smoking and coffee drinking have been very common in Iceland since World War II. Exposure to nitrates in food has been common for many years.

Prognostic factors reviewed by Lutzeyer *et al.*[11] in 315 patients studied revealed recurrences in 52%, 69%, and 77% in those with stages Ta, T_1, and T2 disease and 63%, 67%, and 71% of those with grades 1, 2, and 3, respectively. Recurrences in this study were found to be 45% after primary tumor but 84% after a second tumor. Recurrence was noted at a higher grade or stage in 19%, 34%, and 46% of those with grades I, II, and III disease, respectively. The interval between primary tumor and progression to a higher stage is dependent on the stage and grade of the primary. Stage T_a grade I showed progression in 2 years, stage T_1 grade II in 14 months; and T_2 grade III in less than 1 year. Increasing grades of tumor revealed increasing rate of abnormal histologic findings in other sites as being 61, 89 and 84% for grades I, II and III, respectively.

Eisenberg, as reported by Soloway et al.,[25] commented on progression of lesions from cystitis cystica and glandularis to atypia and papillary hyperplasia to carcinoma *in situ*. They noted a 26% incidence of proliferative lesions adjacent to papillary tumors and a 60% incidence associated with invasive cancers. This type of information suggests that segmental cystectomy may be advisable only in very selected patients. When the urothelium is becoming particularly unstable early cystectomy might be considered.

ETIOLOGY

Almost 100 years ago, it became apparent that aniline dye workers were experiencing a higher rate of bladder cancer than expected.[9] Work in this area revealed that a variety of aromatic amines were the carcinogens involved. These compounds consist of a benzene ring with an amino radical attached. Intact animal models produced bladder tumors with oral administration of 2-napthylamine, but superficial bladder application or oral administration with a diverted urinary stream did not produce bladder cancer.

In humans, Melicow[15] noted that when two-stage cystectomies were common, and the two stages were separated by a significant time interval, there was a significant reduction and occasional disappearance of bladder cancer in the bladder separated from the urine stream. This suggests that a metabolic product is necessary for the development of cancer and that the carcinogen is not necessarily from the distant past. The tumor is the result of an ongoing exposure which is potentially reversible. Present information suggests that any aromatic amine with a hydroxy radical in the *ortho* position has carcinogenic potential.

Some of these carcinogens are endogenous, being produced in the metabolic breakdown of the amino acid tryptophan. These carcinogens then enter the nicotinic acid pathway where pyridoxine is a necessary coenzyme. This fact had led to some experimental work evaluating pyridoxine deficiency as a potential cause of bladder cancer.

Cigarette smoking is associated with a 2–5 times greater risk for bladder cancer. Cigarette smoking seems to block carcinogen metabolic pathway in the nicotinic acid pathway similar to a pyridoxine deficiency.[15]

Coffee drinking has been suggested but not proven as a potential hazard.[15] Phenacetin abuse, artificial sweeteners, irradiation and chemotherapeutic agents (cyclophosphamide (Cytoxan)) have also been associated with bladder cancer.

At present clear etiological agents for the vast majority of transitional cell tumors cannot be made, but clear association can be made for certain industrial exposures, cigarette smoking and phenacetin abuse. The small populations who have had Cytoxan cystitis or pelvic radiation may also experience an added risk. The association of coffee drinking and artificial sweeteners with cancer is less clear.

TREATMENT

Since a significant number of patients have recurrence in spite of adequate resection, adjuvant therapies have been advanced. They include oral and intravesical chemotherapy, external and intracavitary radiation, immunotherapy, surgery and others. The most popular, are intravesical agents which theoretically subject the superficial tumors to a relatively tumoricidal concentration of the agent without simultaneously exposing sensitive organ systems. At the same time potentially premalignant and microscopic malignancies are also treated.

Intravesical Chemotherapy

SUPERFICIAL CHEMOTHERAPY

In 1961 Jones and Swinney[9a] reported on the use of thiotepa in superficial bladder tumors. Since that time a search has been conducted for the ideal intravesical chemotherapeutic agent. Considering our present experience the following properties would need to be considered:

1. Complete destruction of the tumor,
2. Limited number of applications,
3. Lack of recurrence,
4. Lack of local side effects,
5. Lack of systemic side effects,
6. Lack of carcinogenic effects, and
7. Reasonable cost.

A number of intravesical regimens have been and are being studied. Thiotepa, which is the best known and most widely used intravesical chemotherapeutic agent, has been reported by the National Bladder Cancer Collaborative Group as having a complete response rate of 47%.[18]

SUPERFICIAL BLADDER TUMORS   139

THIOTEPA

Thiotepa (Triethylenethisophosphoramide) is probably the best known and most widely used superficial intravesical chemotherapeutic agent used against superficial bladder tumors.[19] Clinical experience with this drug exceeds 15 years, first being introduced by Jones and Swinney[9a] in 1961. Thiotepa, an alkalating agent, causes cellular changes similar to those found after radiation. Thiotepa acts by the substitution of an alkyl group to an x-receptor through a sulfur, nitrogen or oxygen ion which reacts by replacing a hydrogen ion. Although the clinical experience has been extensive there still lacks universal agreement on efficacy and regimen. In 1977 Byar and Blackard[4] and the Veteran's Administration group reported on comparisons of placebo, pyridoxine, and intracavitary thiotepa in superficial bladder tumors in 121 patients. Pyridoxine was selected because of the appreciable incidence of abnormalities of tryptophan metabolism in patients with bladder cancer. It has been thought that pyridoxine could correct these abnormalities. In those patients who did not have their first recurrence within 10 months, thiotepa significantly reduced the recurrence rate and pyridoxine was significantly better than placebo. Nocks et al.,[19] reporting in 1979, noted that monthly intravesical instillations of thiotepa did not demonstrate a significant difference in preventing recurrences of bladder carcinoma. Those patients who were successfully treated previously with weekly (8 weeks) administrations of thiotepa have greater tumor-free periods. A slightly better response rate was noted at the 60-mg doses in terms of fewer patient recurrences, increase in intervals free of tumor, and diminished frequency of new tumor formation.

Schulman et al.[25] reporting in 1982 compared thiotepa and epipodophyllotoxin (VM26) combining 4 weekly instillations followed by 11 monthly instillations. There was no significant difference between the groups with respect to time of first recurrence.

Thiotepa reduced the overall recurrence as compared to the prestudy rate and other treatment group rates.

Generally it is the consensus that the value of thiotepa is not clearly documented. However, it does seem to reduce recurrence posttransurethral resection (TUR). The most effective dose is not yet known. Using higher doses can cause severe bone marrow depression, and deaths have been reported. The most effective dosage, timing, and frequency have yet to be defined as well as what other additional agents would be beneficial.

MITOMYCIN C

Mishina et al.[16] in 1975 reported on their experience with 50 patients with mitomycin C treatment of superficial bladder tumors. Mitomycin C, like thiotepa, is an alkylating agent with potential myelosuppressive effects. Mitomycin C is believed to inhibit deoxyriboneleic acid neurosynthesis. It is this action which is believed to inhibit tumor growth. Mitomycin C is considered to be minimally absorbed, possibly because of the high molecular weight (334) of mitomycin C when compared to thiotepa. Most reports indicate no clinical evidence of systemic effects but there are reports of palmar rashes, and one report of systemic rash.

These reports have been questioned as to the possibility of patients contaminating themselves with mitomycin C and the rashes representing a local effect. Approximately 20% of the patients complain of local bladder irritations.

Results from mitomycin C seem to be promising with complete response rate of 45% and partial response rate of 35% for an effective rate of 80% in tumors less than 1 cm in a study of 169 patients. This high rate of response seems to be reproduceable. Braken et al.[2] reporting in 1980 found the minimal effective dose of mitomycin C was 30 mg. Frequency protocols have not yet been clearly established.

There are some significant drawbacks to mitomycin C. First, it is significantly more expensive than thiotepa. Second, mitomycin C has a carcinogen potential which is not well understood. Its questionable long-term effect on unstable carcenogenic-sensitive urothelium causes great concern. Third is the report that morphologic alterations produced by thiotepa and mitomycin C in murine ureothelium may denude urothelial surface without altering neoplastic potential.

DOXORUBICIN

Doxorubicin (14-hydroxydaunomycin), (Adriamycin)) is a water soluble glycoside antibiotic agent which has been shown to have an antitumor effect.[1] Its mechanism seems to be blocking cell progression from G2 to mitosis.

Doxorubicin is commonly administered intravenously when treating leukemia, lymphoma, and certain solid tumors. It has been used with mixed success as adjuvant therapy in some urologic tumors. Doxorubicin has been used in superficial bladder tumors. Dosages of 80–100 mg have been instilled intravesically either within the immediate postoperative period or 1 month postoperatively. Results have been mixed with one report noting no reduction in recurrence, others noting best results against carcinoma in situ.

All articles note no systemic reactions to doxorubicin. Side effects seem to be localized to the bladder with pain limited to 24 hours. Systemic reactions such as stomatitis, nausea, and myocardial infarction are not being reported. Plasma levels of doxorubicin postcatheterization are less than 5 ng/ml, suggestive of minimal to no absorption.

Attempts to potentiate doxorubicin by detergent have been reported as effective with a 10% aqueous solution of Tween 80 but not effective with urokinase. Tween 80 seems to increase the permeability of cell membranes resulting in an enhancement of the cellular uptake of the doxorubicin.

Results of doxorubicin though promising have been on small populations. Clear recommendations regarding indicated dosage, frequency, etc. cannot be made. One report indicates that a single dose postoperatively can significantly reduce recurrence.

EPODYL

Epodyl (triethylene glycol diglycidyl ether) is probably the most common intravesical anticancer agent in Europe. Well differentiated tumors respond best to Epodyl. Complications include frequency 50%, dysuria 35%, urgency 28%, small capacity bladder 20%, and bone marrow depression 4%. Small capacity bladders can be so severe that cystectomies are necessary.[21]

OTHER CHEMOTHERAPY

Cisplatin is the single most active agent for treating advanced metastatic bladder cancer. A recent report (1982)[1a] indicates it is ineffective controlling superficial bladder cancer.

Oral Agents

METHOTREXATE

In an effort to provide more frequent and longer setting cytotoxic levels of chemotherapy, attempts have been made to have patients take methotrexate 50 mg by mouth weekly. This provides 24–36 hours of cytotoxic levels per week. Initial results suggest it will not irradicate tumors, but might reduce recurrences. The studies reported are on multiple primaries, and therefore difficult to compare to other reports.

ASCORBIC ACID

Laboratory studies have suggested that ascorbic acid will prevent the metabolism of certain precarcinogins to the carcinogins and therefore prevent recurrence of tumors.[22a]

Immunotherapy

BCG VACCINE

Morales et al.[17] in 1976 noted that antigenicity of bladder might allow immunotherapy to eradicate superficial bladder tumors. Successful BCG therapy would be dependent on (1) ability of the patient to develop immune response, (2) adequate BCG dose, (3) dose contact between BCG and tumor, (4) relatively small tumor load, and (5) minimal side effects.

Morales et al.[17] studied 9 patients and noted that all became responsive to tuberculin. Other reports noted a positive prognostic sign with PPD conversion during therapy. Brosman[3] noted no correlation with recurrence of tumor with *Candida* or *Trichophyton* antigens but patients who were negative to PPD pre-BCG therapy remained negative and seemed to have more recurrences than those who went from negative to positive. BCG has been used with melanoma and kidney cancer, but presently seems to be most promising with bladder cancer. Various studies have used different strains of BCG as well as different innoculums and protocols. Intradermal innoculum to generate response as well as to enhance response has been reported. Both intravesical injection cystoscopically as well as intravesical innoculation have been attempted.

The bladder has some anatomical advantages in that multiple innoculations, observations, and biopsies can be performed with comparative ease. The papillary nature of the tumors also allows a high contact area between the innoculum and tumor in conjunction with a relatively low tumor load.

Side effects to BCG therapy include dysuria (95%) and frequency (85%) which lasted 48 hours. Mild hematuria was seen in 34% and fever in 21%. High fevers (2/57 per Lamm[10] are not commonly reported. One case of anaphalaxis associated with intravesical injection has been reported. Lamm[10] reported one case of hydronephrosis secondary to severe cystitis which resolved in 1 week.

Lamm[10] reported that patients who demonstrate the more aggressive tumors, those with the absence of AB(H) antigens, had less frequent reoccurence after BCG therapy than those patients with less aggressive AB(H) positive tumors.

Lamm[10] noted that 4 of 6 patients who had recurrences after thiotepa therapy responded to BCG therapy. Current literature suggests that BCG immunotherapy may provide a significant addition to our armamentarium for superficial bladder tumors. This therapy at present continues to be on protocol use.

OTHER IMMUNOTHERAPY

A review of immunotherapy of superficial bladder cancer has been performed by Shapiro.[24] Transfer factor polyinosinic acids, OK432, levamisole showed little or no improvement in recurrence rates. Only one report of keyhole limpet hemocyanin is available and is inconclusive.

Interferon showed interesting preliminary reports but further investigation will be needed.

IMMUNO MARKERS

Work with monocyte chemotaxis reveals no difference in normal patients and patients with superficial bladder tumors but significant difference was seen in patients with invasive bladder tumors.

An unspecific immune response (dinitrochlorobenzene skin test) revealed that patients with a positive skin test had a better prognosis than those with a negative test for various tumors including lung, breast and bladder.

MARKERS

Approximately 15% of patients with superficial tumors will eventually develop invasive lesions in spite of localized conservative therapy. Unfortunately the alternative is a cystectomy which is disfiguring, costly, painful, dangerous and engenders a significant alteration in the patient's body image. The decision to recommend a cystectomy cannot be taken lightly. The timing of the procedure is also important as a delay of 6 months to a year while another modality of conservative treatment is attempted may allow distant metastases for which we have at this time no dependable therapy. For this reason surface antigens have been investigated as possible indicators of impending aggressiveness of the tumor.

It is postulated that morphologically similar cells may be biochemically different, that this biochemical change may be detected by the loss of some antigens ABO(H) and the temporary expression and loss of others (T antigen). These surface changes may be paralleled by an aggressive biologic potential to invade.

As yet no final recommendations can be made for a specific patient based on ABO(H) antigens alone. It has been noted that particular care must be made in interpreting the results with type O patients because of the delicate nature of the O(H) antigen-antibody reaction. False negatives may be reported because of the inability of the laboratory to detect the presence of this antigen.[6, 9]

Cytogenetic studies of transitional cell cancer have not revealed a specific chromosomal change. The presence of marker chromosomes does appear to endow papillary tumors with a propensity for recurrence or invasiveness more than those tumors without such markers. Sandberg[22] reported that only one of 18 cancers without markers recurred whereas 11 of the 32 papillary cancers with markers recurred and became invasive.

Surgery

It has been demonstrated that with total extirpation of bladder mucosa, normal bladder mucosa regenerates in a week. The theory of mucosal denudation is that when all abnormal mucosa is removed, new, normal, mucosa will return. Long-term follow-up (4 years) shows that these patients had a recurrence rate of 60% and a tendency to recur at a higher grade.[7] This therapy is not believed to be effective.

Braken et al.,[2] reporting in 1981, reviewed 109 patients who underwent radical cystectomy without lymphadenopathy for superficial transitional cell cancer. Surgical indication was that the bulk and extent of the tumor could not be controlled with the combination of endoscopic surgery and intravesical chemotherapy. Average endoscopic procedures precystectomy was 2, and only 10% had 10 or more procedures. Most patients are recognized early as having fulminating disease. Five-year survival was 76% which was identical for age-matched controls. Of the 56 irradiated (5000 rads), 36% had all tumor eradicated and only 3% had local recurrence as compared to 9.45% in the nonirradiated group. Uretheral cancer was present in 9% of the patients. There was a 2.75% operative complications. Eight-four percent returned to their presurgery life style.

The role of surgery in superficial bladder tumors is both diagnostic and therapeutic. The surgeon initially attempts to control the tumor endoscopically. Cystectomy, unfortunately, is a common ultimate recommendation when the prognostic indicators suggest imminent invasion. Present investigations center around the use of markers as aides in indicating the timing of individual cystectomies.

Radiation

Van Der Werf-Messing, as reported by Matsumoto et al.,[13] showed that the 5-year survival rate for T_1 and T_2 bladder cancer after external supravoltage was 50 and 45%, respectively. Suprapubic radium implantation gave 90 and 65% 5-year survival rate, respectively, for T_1 and T_2, with recurrence rates of 12 and 20%, respectively. In 1980, Matsumoto *et al.*[13] reported on a one-shot high dose electron irradiation as a radical means of treatment of superficial bladder cancer (66 patients). The total dose was 2500–3000 rads between 15–20 days postoperatively. The 1-, 3-, and 5-year survival rates were 100 and 96.3%, respectively to T_a and T_1 lesions. Recurrence rate of solitary tumors was 5.7% and multiple tumors 23.1% for an overall recurrence rate of 10%. Five patients ultimately had cystectomies. One patient had a contracted bladder necessitating an ileal diversion. No other significant complications were noted.

INTRACAVITARY RADIATION

External radiation is not believed to be effective in low grade superficial tumors. Intracavitary radiation, with a dose of 4000 rads, has been reported as an alternative approach to superficial bladder tumors particularly in those patients who, failing intravesical chemotherapy, are not considered candidates for radical surgery.[8] This procedure is not commonly available. The method described is to fix a radium capsule in a 30-cc Foley retaining balloon catheter so that it would be at the center of the balloon. The Foley is left in for drainage. The technique allows a tissue dose of 1000 rads in 24 hours to the surface of the bladder. It is not used in conjunction with fulguration. Forty percent of the patients had moderate to severe radiation cystitis. The results showed 50% nonrecurrence or improvement in stage A, grade I and grade II patients.

Other Therapies

CRYOTHERAPY

Cryotherapy has been used in both prostate and bladder cancer. The European reports of this procedure, by use of a probe, seem to limit it to elderly, potentially risky, patients for a short procedure time of 4–5 minutes and a moderate hospital stay (less than 1 week). Some larger tumors were resected postcryotherapy.

Lack of American experience with the technique probably accounts for some of the complications reported. Theoretically, the simplicity, speed, lack of blood loss, and possible preservation of the prostate may allow this procedure to be considered in the future. At the present, the paucity of the data makes it impossible to compare it to conventional therapy.

HYPERTHERMIA

Reports on hyperthermia suggest that it is hazardous and should not be used as an alternative to cystectomy even in poor risk patients as the transitional cell carcinoma seems to be more resistant to the effects of the heat than the surrounding normal tissues.

HYDROSTATIC PRESSURE

Hydrostatic pressure therapy is an ischemic necrosis of tumor nests by pressure. The method is by instilling isotonic saline with antibiotics in patients under epidural anesthesia and producing a pressure between the systolic and diastolic blood pressure. This pressure is maintained from 3–5 hours. It is believed that some of the benefit of this therapy is mediated through the immune system.

ARGON LASER

Preliminary work has been performed using argon laser on superficial bladder tumors. Argon laser energy is absorbed by hemoglobin pigment and therefore erthematous lesions of the bladder may be treated selectively. Work thus far suggests that the necrosis extends to the lamina propria but not the muscularis. Bleeding is reported to be negligible. Long-term follow-up, and therefore the applicability of this treatment, is not yet established.

REFERENCES

1. Abrams, H., Choa, R. G., Gaches, C. G., Ashken, M. H., and Green, N. A. Controlled trial of single dose intravesical adriamycin in superficial bladder tumors. *Br. J. Urol.* *53:*585–587, 1981.
1a. Blumenreich, M. S., Needles, B., Yagoda, A., Sogani, P., Grabstald, H., and Whitmore, W. F. Jr. Cis platinum for supraficial bladder tumors. *Cancer 50:*853–865, 1982.
2. Braken, R. B., McDonald, M. W., and Johnson, D. E. Cystectomy for superficial bladder cancer. *Urology 18:*459–463, 1981.
3. Brosman, S. A. Experience with baccillus Calmerte-Guérin in patients with superficial bladder carcinoma. *J. Urol. 128:*27–20, 1982.
4. Byar, D., and Blackard, C. Comparison of placebo, pyridoxine and topical thiotepa in preventing recurrence of stage 1 bladder cancer. *Urology 10:*556–561, 1977.
5. Catalona, W. J. Practical utility of specific red cell adherence test in bladder cancer. *Urology 18:*113–117, 1981.
6. Emmott, R. C., Jadvadpour, N., Bergman, S. M., and Soares, T. Correlation of the cell surface antigens with stage and grade in cancer of the bladder. *J. Urol. 121:*37–39, 1979.
7. Hansen, R. I., Nerstrom, B., Djurhuus, J. C., and Lund, F. Late results from mucosal denudation for urinary bladder papillomatosis. *Acta Chir. Scand. 472:*73–76, 1976.
8. Hewitt, C. B., Babiszewski, J. F., and Antunez, A. R. Update on intra-cavitary radiation in the treatment of bladder tumors. *J. Urol. 126:*323–25, 1981.
9. Javadpour, N. Principles and management of urologic cancer. Williams & Wilkins. Baltimore, 1979.
9a. Jones, H. C., and Swinney, J. Thio-TEPA in the treatment of tumors of the bladder. *Lancet 2:*615–618, 1961.
10. Lamm, D. L., Thor, D. E., Stogdill, V. D., and Radwin, H. M. Bladder cancer immunotherapy. *J. Urol. 128:*931–935, 1982.
11. Lutzeyer, W., Rubben, H., and Dahm, H. Prognostic parameters in superficial bladder cancer, an analysis of 315 cases. *J. Urol. 127:*250–252, 1982.
12. Mautry, E. Benign and malignant tumors of the urinary bladder. Medical Examination Publishing Co., Yonkers, NY, 1971.
13. Matsumoto, K., Kakizoe, T., Mikuriya, S., Tanaka, T., Kondo, I., and Umegaki, Y. Clinical evaluation of intraoperative radiotherapy for carcinoma of the urinary bladder. *Cancer 47:*509–513, 1981.
14. McCarthy, J. P., Gravell, G. J., and LeBlanc, G. A. Transitional cell carcinoma of bladder in patients under thirty years of age. *Urology 13:*487–489, 1979.
15. Melicow, M. The role of urine in a patient with a bladder neoplasm. *J. Urol. 127:*660–663, 1982.
16. Mishina, T., Oda, K., Murata, S., Ooe, H., Mori, Y., and Takanashi, T. Mitamycin C bladder installment therapy for bladder tumors. *J. Urol. 114:*217–219, 1975.
17. Morales, A. Eidinger, D., and Bruce, A. W. Intracavitary bacillus Calmette-Guréin in the treatment of superficial bladder tumors. *J. Urol. 116:*180–183, 1976.

18. National Bladder Cancer Collaborative Group A. The role of intravesical thiotepa in the management of superficial bladder cancer. *Cancer Res. 37:*2916–2917, 1977.
19. Nocks, B. N., Nieh, P. T., and Prout, G. R. A longitudinal study of patients with superficial bladder carcinoma successfully treated with weekly intravesical thiotepa. *J. Urol. 122:*27–29, 1979.
20. Perry, S. B. Thorhallsson, P., and Hallgrimsson, J. Tumors in Iceland. *Acta Pathol. Microbiol. Scand. (A) 90:*175–183, 1982.
21. Robinson, M. R. G., Shetty, M. B., Richards, B., Bastable, J., Glashan, R. W., and Smith, P. H. Intravesical Epodyl in the management of bladder tumors: combined experience of the Yorkshire urological cancer research group. *J. Urol. 118:*972–973, 1977.
22. Sandberg, A. A. Chromosome markers and progression in bladder cancer. *Cancer Res. 37:*2950–2956, 1971.
22a.Schiegel, J. U., Pipkin, G. E., Nishimura, R., and Shultz, G. N. The role of ascorbic acid in the prevention of bladder tumor formation. *J. Urol. 103:*155–159, 1970.
23. Schulman, C. C., Robinson, M., Denis, L., Smith, P., Viggiano, G., dePauw, M., DaLesio, O., and Sylvester, R. Prophylactic chemotherapy of superficial transitional cell bladder carcinoma an EORTC randomized trial comparing thiotepa, an epipodophyllotoxin (VM26) and TUR alone. *Eur. Urol. 8:*207–212, 1982.
24. Shapiro, A., Kadmon, D., Catalona, W. J., and Ratliff, T. L. Immunotherapy of superficial bladder cancer. *J. Urol. 128:*891–894, 1982.
25. Soloway, M. S., Murphy, W., Rao, M. K., and Cox, C. Serial multiple-site biopsies in patients with bladder cancer. *J. Urol. 120:*57–59, 1978.

11

Cystectomy: Surgical Therapy of Deep Infiltrative Bladder Cancer

Howard M. Radwin, M.D.

Surgery for invasive transitional cell carcinoma of the bladder is performed primarily as an attempt to completely remove a lesion with life threatening potential. In the United States today, complete cystectomy is more commonly recommended than irradiation or partial cystectomy not only because of apparently superior survival rates, but also because of the threat of subsequent new lesions which may develop in the urothelium, which lesser techniques do nothing to prevent. Indeed, they may add to the difficulty in dealing with subsequent tumors with more complete surgery and chemotherapy. Thus, awareness of field change with epithelial atypia and carcinoma *in situ* potentially leading to the appearance of new invasive tumors is the major deterrent to partial cystectomy even when generous surgical margins are attainable.[1-5]

Recognition of the seriousness of this problem accounts for the general acceptance of the need for random biopsies at the time of the original transurethral excisional biopsy of the presenting lesion. The high positive yield attests to the validity of this concern. If adjuncts become available which are capable of controlling this progression, more limited tumor resection may become more prevalent. At this time, with few exceptions, it is advisable to perform complete cystectomy in the face of invasive disease. Radical cystectomy implies concomitant pelvic node dissection with the cystectomy. Its major justification is the reported significant incidence of 5-year survival in patients with a few proximate nodes found at surgery.[6, 7]

Survival rates with T_3 disease have improved in recent decades from approximately 20–50% following cystectomy with or without irradiation. Unfortunately, we appear to be approaching the maximum benefit achievable with purely regional therapy. This is indicated by the finding that two thirds of the failures in this group subsequently present with distant rather than local tumor spread. Caution is warranted in interpreting data because of the current lack of precision in staging. If more than a third of invasive lesions are understaged preoperatively, as verified by examination of the operative specimen, and a further group can be assumed to have micrometastases which are not revealed until even later, marked improvements in survival statistics can be achieved simply by more accurate staging. This would be accomplished by eliminating operative candidates as the result of better preoperative assessment of the stage of disease. This represents a major hazard in the use of historic controls to evaluate current management.[8, 9]

Nonseminomatous germ cell tumors of the testis serve as an example of real improvement in treatment of a urological neoplasm. If the reasons for this are analyzed it may be seen that much of this success is due to the ability to combine cytoreductive surgery with effective chemotherapy for metastases and to employ tumor markers to accurately judge the status of the disease. Neither of these last two factors are available in the management of bladder cancer today. The quest for tumor markers is being actively pursued with some encouraging results but effective chemotherapy remains elusive. Both chemotherapeutic and immunotherapeutic agents are being studied in this regard. The development of adjuncts, markers and methods to prevent malignancy from arising in susceptible urothelium will help to define the role of surgery in the control of vesical neoplasia, including invasive stages of the disease.

The radical cystectomy represents a challenge to the urological surgeon regardless of his skill and experience. Although a particular case may present technical problems to tax his ingenuity and skill, the major difficulty is the need to perform a procedure with many different components with consistent care and attention to detail.[10–12] A cystectomy performed well in 90% of its aspects can result in disaster. The preparation of the stoma, the ureteroileal anastomosis, the bowel anastomosis, hemostasis, the separation of the bladder and urethra from the rectum are all potential sources of danger if attention flags with fatigue. The question of speed should be regarded as an issue not so much requiring extreme nimbleness but of knowing what to do next, accomplishing and maintaining good exposure, and maintaining a pace for the entire operating team. As with most surgery much of this can be facilitated by preoperative planning in which various eventualities are considered and responses chosen in anticipation of their need. Some of this planning should be accomplished with the assistance of the patient. This is particularly true of such questions as whether to proceed with cystectomy if positive nodes are found and whether to perform palliative urinary diversion.

At the onset of the relationship between the urologist and the patient who is a candidate for definitive therapy, it should be made clear that the treatment decisions will be made jointly. It should be understood that it will be necessary to evaluate both the status of the tumor and the appropriateness of any therapy in relationship to the overall condition of the patient. The possibility of cystectomy is usually entertained when a transurethral biopsy demonstrates the presence of a lesion invading the muscle. However, it also may be considered in a variety of other circumstances including high grade tumor in the lamina propia, multiple lesions, carcinoma *in situ* refractory to other modalities, and intractable symptoms. In some of these circumstances studies such as the determination of the presence of cell surface antigens to suggest the virulence of the tumor may be of clinical use, but can not be expected, alone, to provide the final decision. Intravenous urography should demonstrate the extent of any upper urinary tract obstruction and roentgenographic evaluation of the chest may be used to rule out pulmonary metastases. The CT scan, although disappointing in its inability to provide precise information concerning lymphatic spread in the pelvis unless there is gross adenopathy, nevertheless may provide some information to the surgeon. It also permits visualization of the liver. This is supplemented by liver function studies to indicate possible hepatic metastases. Isotopic liver scanning has not been as helpful as had been hoped. While the evaluation of the neoplasm is proceeding, the patient's general health is evaluated to determine if he is a potential candidate for surgery. This includes thorough cardiovascular and pulmonary studies and, in the patient with a history suggestive of cardiac disease, the performance of a stress test. Certain patients who appear to be chronically ill and particularly those suffering significant weight loss will need a nutritional evaluation. If indicated, preoperative nutritional supplementation should be instituted. This is far more effective than is an attempt to deliver additional nutrients postoperatively during a period of obligatory catabolism.

A full liquid diet is given 48–72 hours prior to surgery and a 24-hour antibacterial bowel prep is administered. In addition, during the few days immediately preceding the operation, the patient is introduced to the enterostomal therapist and is made familiar with the circumstances of living with a urinary diversion. Since the patient is often more concerned with this aspect of the upcoming event than with the cystectomy itself, reassurance and support during this period is important. Selection of the stoma site is not complicated but should be performed prior to the operative day. It is not possible to do this satisfactorily with the patient in the supine position, particularly if there is any obesity. The position for the ostomy is best selected with the patient in the sitting position so that in addition to avoidance of obvious scars, any panniculus which is present does not interfere with bag placement. In the obese patient this often necessitates localization in a position which would appear surprisingly high while the patient is recumbent. Care should be taken to avoid proximity to the iliac spine as well as the umbilicus. A contralateral paramedian operative incision will also aid in allowing a smooth bed for the applicance. There can be some merit to having the patient wear an ostomy bag for a few days prior to surgery to familiarize himself with it.[13]

PLAN OF OPERATION

The patient is placed on the operating table in a low lithotomy position (Fig 11.1). This permits the second assistant to stand between the patient's legs where he not only can be of greater assistance in retraction

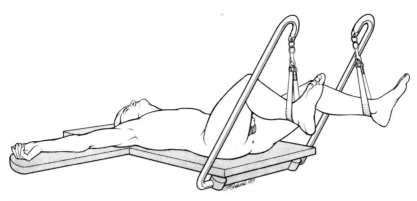

Figure 11.1. The patient is placed in a low lithotomy position permitting an assistant to be positioned between his legs. Hanging straps support the ankles and are padded (not shown).

but in those cases in which, because of previous radiotherapy, scarring, or other factors, there is anticipated difficulty in separating the prostate from the rectum, he can insert a finger into the rectum to assist the operating surgeon. The low lithotomy position is chosen over having the patient flat with his legs spread because the former choice permits some hip rotation which relieves strain on that joint. Care should be taken to avoid more lithotomy than necessary so as to prevent flexing of the pelvis with consequent deepening of its recesses. The slight elevation of the legs can improve venous drainage. Hanging stirrups should be used, instead of supports under the knees. A Foley catheter is placed in the bladder which is then slightly distended with approximately 200 ml of an antibacterial solution. Prior to making the operative incision, the abdominal wall is prepared for the stoma. A circle 2.5 cm in diameter is incised at the previously selected stoma site. This incision is carried directly through the skin and subcutaneous tissue to the abdominal wall fascia. Care should be taken that the surgical assistants in their effort to help do not distort the opening so as to cause it to deviate from a straight line. A circle of fascia of the same circumference is then cut in continuity and the muscle may be either excised with this or simply be subject to a cruciate incision. The plug of tissue which has been carried to, but not through, the peritoneum is now removed and a gauze sponge is left in the site. What has been created is a perfectly straight channel for the conduit in a manner far superior to that which can be done at the end of the operation with the abdominal wall open and an attempt made to realign the layers of the abdominal wall. If an inoperable lesion is subsequently discovered, closure of the stoma site presents a minor inconvenience.

A left paramedian incision is made which angles to the midline at its termination at the level of the pubis (Fig. 11.2). This choice permits adequate room for retention sutures which will not interfere with bag placement. At its most inferior portion the incision returns to the midline where the dissection of the prostatic urethra will occur. The rectus muscles are separated and the peritoneal cavity is entered. The first step in this phase of the operation consists of a general exploration

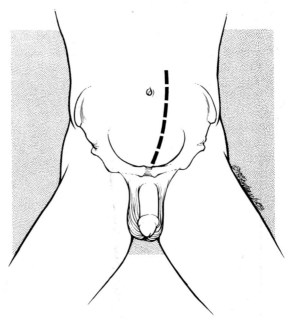

Figure 11.2. A left paramedian incision is made so as to provide adequate clearance for the ostomy appliance. The incision returns to the midline at its inferior aspect. The stoma site is not shown to emphasize that it must be individualized.

of the abdominal cavity with particular emphasis on examination of the liver for metastases. The periaortic region is palpated for adenopathy and any suspicious nodes are biopsied. The bifurcation of the aorta is exposed and a deliberate biopsy is made of nodal tissue in this area and sent for frozen section. Palpation of the pelvis is then performed and again suspicious nodes are biopsied if they are obvious at this point in the dissection.

Following the general exploratory phase of the surgery, the next procedure is the performance of the ileal conduit urinary diversion. This is done prior to the cystectomy for two reasons. First, in the event of a problem which may arise during the most traumatic portion of the operation, which is the cystectomy, urinary diversion has already been accomplished and the procedure may be terminated expeditiously. Second, the most meticulous and critical suturing is at the ureteroileal anastomosis and this is best performed when the operating team is fresh. A variety of specific techniques for constructing the ileal conduit are available but will not be described in detail here. The ureters are isolated and care is paid to bringing the left ureter retrocolic to the midline in a gentle arc so as to avoid kinking it on arterial structures emerging from the aorta. Frozen sections are taken of the distal end of the proximal ureter after division to ascertain the absence of carcinoma *in situ*. The ureteroileal anastomosis may be facilitated by inserting a sponge forceps through the distal conduit opening and permitting it to serve as an "embroidery frame" when placed directly under the small ileotomy which will receive each ureter (Fig. 11.3). This permits visualization of all layers of the intestinal wall so that precise placement of fine absorb-

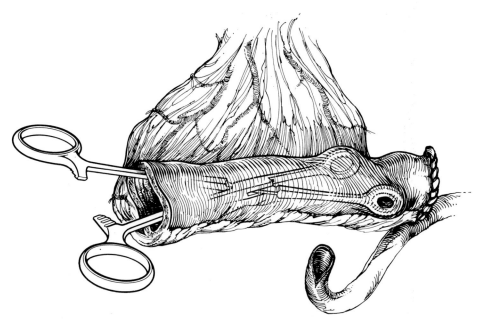

Figure 11.3. A ring forceps in the conduit aids in exposure of all layers of the ileotomy. Separate ileotomies are made for each ureter.

able sutures may then be done with accuracy. The proximal end of the ileal conduit is sutured to the sacral promontory but the distal end is not fixed at this time. If the conduit were to be secured both proximally and distally there is danger that during the subsequent node dissection and cystectomy the ureteroileal anastomosis may be disrupted by inadvertent traction. Ileoileostomy may be done with staples or sutures. This author's preference is for a two-layer open anastomosis.

Pelvic lymphadenectomy is performed next (Fig. 11.4). The purpose of including this step is not only the generally accepted 10–15% survival rate in patients with D_1 lesions, but also advantages which ensue in the performance of the cystectomy. Control of the vasculature of the bladder is accomplished during the lymphadenectomy procedure with direct exposure of the vesical arteries. This probably results in less blood loss than is seen with more random clamping and tying of tissue between the iliac vessels and the bladder itself. In addition, the lateral margins of the soft tissue dissection tend to be wider if a lymphadenectomy has been performed since the iliac vessels themselves serve as a lateral margin and perivesical tissue medial to them is removed. This may well assist in more complete surgical treatment of the patient with a c lesion. The lymphadenectomy itself begins at the bifurcation of the aorta and includes all nodal tissue along the common, external, and internal iliac arteries. The lateral margin of dissection is the genitofemoral nerve. Adipose and lymphatic tissue between these vascular structures also are removed and the obturator nerve is exposed. Dissection of potential nodal tissue in proximity to this nerve is accomplished so that it appears to stretch bare across the lateral wall of the pelvis. Dissection is extended to the inguinal ligament and Cloquet's node is removed. During the

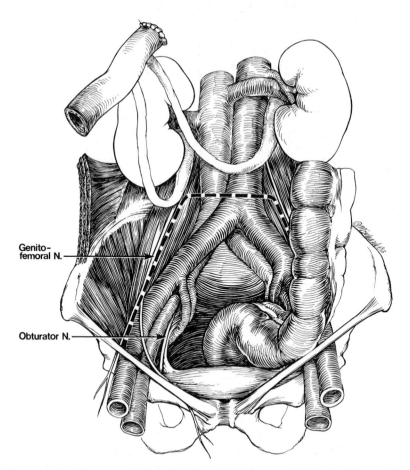

Genito-femoral N.

Obturator N.

Figure 11.4. The area of the pelvic lymphadenectomy is shown. The genito-femoral and obturator nerves mark the superficial and deep lateral margins of the dissection.

course of the dissection the vesical arteries are ligated, although branches from the superior hemorrhoidal artery will still be intact.

Removal of the bladder itself is begun by making two parallel incisions in the parietal peritoneum lateral to the dome of the bladder extending posteriorly to the peritoneal reflection (Fig. 11.5). These are then joined in the midline leaving a large section of peritoneum on the back of the bladder so that it will be included in the operative specimen. The posterior incision in the parietal peritoneum provides the entry for the subsequent separation of the base of the bladder and prostate from the rectum. As much as possible of this portion of the procedure is performed by sharp dissection but much of it will still require blunt dissection. In those circumstances in which tissue planes are not clear because of scarring or previous irradiation, it may be helpful for an assistant to insert a finger in the rectum to guide the surgeon. When this posterior dissection has been accomplished the puboprostatic ligaments are divided and the venous structures in Santorini's plexus are secured with suture ligatures (Fig. 11.6). If this is done prior to attempts at blunt dissection of the adiposal and fibrinous tissue overlying the prostate,

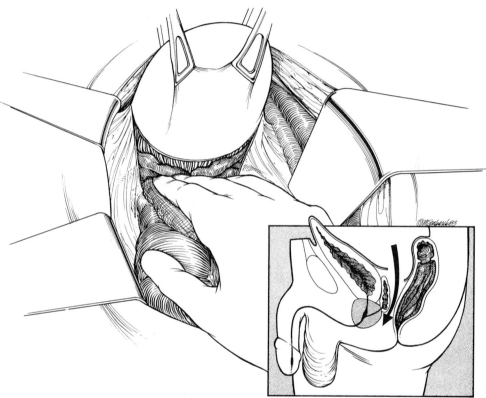

Figure 11.5. The parietal peritoneum is left on the posterior bladder wall. Separation of the bladder base, seminal vesicles and prostate from the rectum is begun through the posterior aspect of the peritoneal incision.

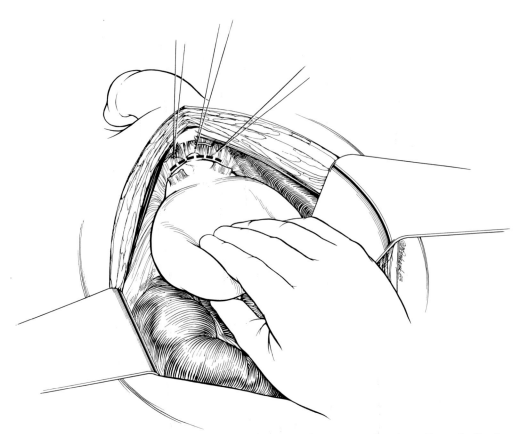

Figure 11.6. Transection of the membranous urethra is performed after hemostasis has been secured and the puboprostatic ligaments ligated.

blood loss can be reduced. Following this, the lateral borders of the prostate are freed with careful attention to hemostasis. If a urethrectomy is not to be performed, the urethra is severed at the urogenital diaphragm. If a urethrectomy is intended, this is accomplished with the lower urinary tract in continuity by means of a perineal incision which can be made by the surgeon stationed at the foot of the table. When the urethra has been freed from below, it can be removed in continuity with the bladder specimen through the abdomen. At this point intravenous indigo carmine is given and the ureteroileal anastomoses are carefully inspected for any leakage. The ileal conduit then may be brought through the abdominal wall and secured.[14] The need for drainage of the pelvis is controversial and is the choice of the surgeon. In the event of some persistent ooze from the undersurface of the pubis, a Foley catheter may be inserted through the urethra, the balloon inflated, and the catheter placed on traction. If a urethrectomy has been performed the catheter may be introduced through the perineum. In the female, the uterus and anterior vaginal wall are also removed. The abdominal wall itself is closed in layers and supplemental retention sutures are placed.

If a lesion can be excised with adequate margins it is difficult to escape the obvious question of doing a local resection, which in this case would imply a partial cystectomy.[15-17] Clearly the patient would prefer a procedure which did not involve urinary diversion. This is particularly tempting in the case of solitary lesions. Moreover in the elderly or poor risk patient the advantages of a more limited operation together with less hazardous recovery leave the burden of proof on those suggesting anything more extensive. Tumor in a diverticulum represents a related problem. These are commonly treated by diverticulectomy which, in essence, is a partial cystectomy. Diverticula do present special considerations, however, in that with the exception of urachal lesions, most vesical diverticula are actually pseudodiverticula. This is because a true diverticulum contains all layers of the wall of the organ, whereas in the bladder pseudoverticulum there is no muscle layer. Nevertheless, partial cystectomy is only performed today in most centers for specific indications. This is not usually due to problems with surgical margins but rather because of fear of the possibility of the development of other invasive lesions in the future. The recognition of the existence of "field change" in the urothelium suggesting the likelihood of a predisposition to further tumors is the overriding consideration. The question of surgical margins arises most commonly in lesions involving the trigone, where it may be impossible to circumscribe the tumor with enough normal tissue for confidence in the excision. For this reason some urologists would consider any lesion close enough to the trigone to require ureteral reimplantation as unacceptable for partial cystectomy. Because of these considerations the initial transurethral resection of the tumor should be accompanied by random biopsies of normal appearing urothelium proximate to the lesion as well as at randomly selected remote sites. The presence of epithelial atypia or carcinoma *in situ* in these biopsies would preclude further consideration of partial cystectomy.

From the above it is apparent that the most critical decision to be made does not involve details of technique but rather the judicious selection of patients for whom partial cystectomy is appropriate. With invasive lesions they remain the exception and not the norm. The operation is performed with the patient in a supine position. It is done through either a large Pfannenstiel or lower midline incision. A pelvic node dissection may be performed. The peritoneum is not separated from the bladder because any peritoneum overlying the lesion should be removed with the specimen. There should be an attempt to localize the involved area prior to opening the bladder. Stay sutures are used to circumscribe the lesion with at least a 2-cm margin. The bladder is entered outside of the area demarcated by the stay sutures and the interior is inspected. Whether the incision is then extended to the area of the stay sutures and then continued around them or whether a separate incision is used depends on the location of the tumor in the bladder. The stay sutures will be helpful in maintaining orientation by facilitating traction on the specimen. Following removal of the specimen, frozen sections are taken from the edges of the remaining bladder to ascertain that the margins are free of disease. A suprapubic tube is inserted and the bladder is closed in layers. The perivesical space is drained and the abdominal wall is reapproximated.

REFERENCES

1. Bowles, W. T., and Cordonnier, J. J. Total cystectomy for carcinoma of the bladder. *J. Urol., 90:*731, 1963.
2. Whitmore, W. F., Jr., and Marshall, V. F. Radical surgery for carcinoma of the urinary bladder. *Cancer 9:*596, 1956.
3. Cordonnier, J. J. Cystectomy for carcinoma of the bladder. *J. Urol. 99:*172, 1968.
4. Prout, G. R. Bladder cancer. *Urol. Clin. North Am. 3:*149, 1976.
5. Prout, G. R. Bladder cancer. *J. Urol. 128:*284, 1982.
6. Dretler, S. R., Ragsdale, B. D., and Leadbetter, W. F. The value of pelvic lymphadenectomy in the surgical treatment of bladder cancer. *Trans. Am. Assoc. Genitourin. Surg. 64:*1972.
7. Skinner, D. G., Tift, J. P., and Kaufman, J. J. High dose, short course preoperative radiation therapy and immediate single stage radical cystectomy with pelvic node dissection in the management of bladder cancer. *J. Urol. 127:*671, 1982.
8. Radwin, H. M. Radiotherapy and bladder cancer: a critical review. *J. Urol. 124:*43, 1980.
9. Mathur, V. K., Krahn, H. P., and Ramsey, E. W. Total cystectomy for bladder cancer. *J. Urol. 125:*784, 1981.
10. Skinner, D. G., Crawford, E. D., and Kaufman, J. J. Complications of radical cystectomy for carcinoma of the bladder. *J. Urol. 123:*640, 1980.
11. Drago, J. R., and Rohner, T. J., Jr. Bladder cancer: results of radical cystectomy for invasive and superficial tumors. *J. Urol. 130:*460, 1983.
12. Reiner, W. G., and Walsh, P. C. An anatomical approach to the surgical management of the dorsal vein and Santorini's plexus during radical retropubic surgery. *J. Urol. 121:*198, 1979.
13. Smith, R. B. Small bowel urinary conduit diversion. *Urol. Update Series*, Vol. *2:*7, 1979.
14. Bloom, D. A., Lieskovsky, G., Rainwater, G., and Skinner, D. G. Turnbull loop stoma. *J. Urol. 129:*715, 1983.
15. Brannan, W., Ochsner, M. G., Fuselier, H. A., and Landry, G. R. Partial cystectomy in the treatment of transitional cell carcinoma of the bladder. *J. Urol. 119:*213, 1978.
16. Novick, A. C., and Stewart, B. H. Partial cystectomy in the treatment of primary and secondary carcinoma of the bladder. *J. Urol. 116:*570, 1976.
17. Resnick, M. I., and O'Connor, V. J., Jr. Segmental resection for carcinoma of the bladder: review of 102 patients. *J. Urol. 109:*1007, 1973.

12

Role of Radiotherapy in the Treatment of Bladder Cancer

Sameer Rafla, M.D., Ph.D.
Ezzat Youssef, M.D.

In order to better evaluate the role of radiation in the treatment of bladder cancer, certain biological factors must be addressed.

RESPONSE OF NORMAL URINARY BLADDER TO RADIATION

The effect of irradiation on the normal bladder was primarily noted during the course of treatment of lesions of pelvic organs (*e.g.* uterine cervix) as the bladder is usually included in the irradiated volume. While the effect on a normal bladder is expected to be somewhat different from tumorous bladder, certain basic findings are common in both situations. Among the various integuments which form the envelope of this hollow viscus, the mucus membrane is most prone to acute radiation effect, especially during the early changes. The muscular wall does not display substantial early changes even after high doses of radiation of the order of 70 grays (7000 rads). Late changes occurring as part of the process of healing, starting as early as 3 months or so after the end of a treatment course, are rather different since substantial changes can be seen in the muscular wall and blood vessels including fibrosis, vascular narrowing and occlusion of small lumen vessels. Areas of the membrane which received the brunt of radiation damage will show evidence of pallor and atrophy to which telangectasia is added later on, several months after treatment. The three bladder "sphincters"—ureteric and urethal—are influenced both by the early changes affecting the mucous membrane causing reflex spasm following the incidence of mucous membrane congestion or mucositis and the late fibrotic atrophic changes resulting in the loss of sphincteric action of ureteric orifices with reflux. These may occur in the case of urethral incontinence, especially in the female. The clinical findings that manifest all these changes are also classified into acute and chronic phases.

ACUTE PHASE

Mild radiation mucositis occurs after delivering 40 grays in 4 weeks causing frequency due to bladder irritability. Edema and occasionally submucosal petichae are seen during this phase.

With increased dose up to 70 grays in 7–8 weeks, intense urinary frequency and even incontinence may occur. Microscopical inflammation of the mucous membrane and submucosa, engorged capillaries, round cell infiltration and edema are seen. This reaction lasts for about 3 weeks and subsides with rest, urinary antiseptics and bladder muscle relaxants.

CHRONIC PHASE

Usually manifests within 1–4 years after completion of therapy. Patient may present with persistent frequency (contracted bladder) and occasionally hematuria. With excessive damage, fistula may occur.

On cystoscopic examination the blood vessels are dilated and tortuous. Ulceration may be seen.

Secondary infection may be superimposed and in long-standing cases may lead to ascending pyelonephritis. Urine diversion may be needed in extreme cases.

In bladder with carcinoma, radiation tolerance is lower than in a normal bladder due to impaired vascularity, previous surgeries (*e.g.* transurethral resection (TUR), and fulgeration) and excessive organ trauma which predisposes to infection. Not only are radiation effects more accentuated but the process of repair is usually sluggish and often incomplete.

EFFECT OF BIOLOGICAL MODIFIERS

The use of biological modifiers to enhance neoplastic radiation damage (sensitizers) or supplement normal tissues protection (protectors) has been actively investigated over the last few years.

Radiosensitizers

Several agents were used to increase tumor sensitivity to radiation and maximize tumor cell kill, misonidazole and hyperbaric oxygen are the two widely tested.

The effect of the addition of misonidazole is to increase cellular and radiation effect which influences both tumor tissue and bladder mucous membrane,[3] resulting in more intense acute reaction which tends to eventually heal completely. No increased chronic effect is noted in the cases studied so far, but since most cases were rather late with limited survival, this aspect of possible enhanced radiation damage is not yet fully clear.

The clinical gain from the use of misonidazole is far from established yet. Studies by Abratt *et al.*,[1] and Awwad,[3] claimed a salutary effect and better regression rate (73% *versus* 43% in historical control) but studies by the Radiation Therapy Oncology Group have not confirmed this.

Further randomized studies are in progress to evaluate the role of radiosensitizers in the management of bladder tumors.

Hyperbaric Oxygen

The technique of treatment of bladder cancer patients by radiation under hyperbaric oxygen claims its roots from the biological fact that tumors irradiated under full oxygenation respond much more readily to radiation as compared to those treated under hypoxic conditions.[23] Tumor hypoxia especially noted in huge necrotic lesions is widely accepted as an important factor denoting and explaining their poor radiosensitivity. By increasing the oxygen pressure (up to 3 atmospheric) under which patients are treated, blood oxygen content is increased and hypoxia is reduced thus promoting more tumor radiosensitivity.

While the above biological facts are not disputed, clinical results did not follow in tandem.

Cade et al.[13] showed in a randomized collaborative study of 24 patients that hyperbaric oxygen associated with radiation therapy as a primary method of treatment did not improve survival over a period of 5 years. Cases were evenly distributed among different stages (T_1 and T_2, 113 cases; T_3 and T_4, 128 cases). Plenk,[32] on the other hand claimed that patients treated by hyperbaric oxygen have an improved survival rate at 36 months: 43% versus 11% in a group of 27 patients randomly treated. However, this difference all but disappeared after 48 months of follow-up.

Certain technical difficulties have hampered the widespread use and a more complete evaluation of this modality, however.

Hyperthermia

It has been known for over a 100 years that heat treatment destroys cancer cells.[16] Ogura et al.[30] demonstrated the cytotoxic effect of heat on transitional cell carcinoma in vitro. This was applied successfully to transplanted transitional cell carcinoma in rats.[30] Survival was improved by the addition of radiation therapy to hyperthermia. Newsam et al.[29] were able to demonstrate the beneficial effect of treating patients suffering from intractable malignant hematuria with hyperthermia applied after radiotherapy (2-hour intervals) at a temperature of 45 °C. Seven out of eleven patients responded for periods of 2–6 months.

Chemotherapy

The biological effect of chemotherapy on mucous membrane lesions and the enhancing of radiation effect seen during the treatment of pelvic tumors in children lead to the concept of considering several chemotherapeutic agents such as cyclophosphamide (Cytoxan), actiniomycin, doxorubicin (Adriamycin), bleomycin and cis-platinum DDP as modifiers of radiation biological effect. All these agents seem to intensify the acute radiation effect, initiate it at lower doses and reinduce it even after the heating of the primary reaction (recall phenomenon). The utilization of this enhancement for the purpose of therapeutic gain has been tested in few studies. Recently, Shipley et al.[39] reported on a trial of the National Bladder Cancer Collaborative Group A where the addition of DDP (70 mgm/Xmn^2 every 3 weeks for 8 courses) to a course of radical external irradiation (about 6500 in 7 weeks to bladder volume) have resulted in a complete response rate of 83% in a group of 23 patients suffering from invasive bladder cancer (T_2, T_3, T_4) with an actuarial 2-year survival of 53%. This improved radiation response rate seems to have been achieved without a significant increase in evidence of acute radiation damage. While this pilot study signifies the validity of the concept of biological effect enhancement, the extent of therapeutic gain remains to be more fully investigated and verified.

Upon the suggestions of Adams[2] and others[25] that hyperthermia, chemotherapy and radiation interact favorably to modify radiation response and increase tumor cell kill, few trials were launched to test this hypothesis. Kubota,[25] in a pilot study, compared the results in patients treated by a combination of hyperthermia (42–43 °C for 1 hour), and radiotherapy (35–40 grays/about 6 weeks) and intravesical bleomycin with those treated by radiotherapy alone or radiotherapy and bleomycin. Radiation response was intensified both by hyperthermia and bleomycin but the therapeutic benefit was short-lived (median of 28 months) and never reached level of statistical significance.

FACTORS WHICH AFFECT THE RESULT OF RADIATION THERAPY

For a logical evolution of a policy for the treatment of bladder cancer, clear understanding of the impact of certain prognosticators on results of treatment is paramount.

Clinical Staging

Clinical staging seems to be the main factor that determines eventual prognosis (Table 12.1).

While it is recognized that clinical staging is less accurate than the surgical one[5, 6, 14, 35] not all patients undergo open surgery aimed at adequate staging, a fact that leaves clinical staging as the only alternative. We believe that the accuracy of clinical staging is directly proportional to the meticulous care taken by the urologist to achieve this end. Bimanual examination under satisfactory anesthesia, deep adequate biopsies and CT scans are but a few of the steps that are necessary.

Nevertheless, certain inherent limitations continue to weaken the impact of clinical staging such as determination of nodal status, especially that even recent generations of CT scanners can only identify nodes larger than 2 cm. Moreover clinical staging does not take into consideration data relevant to tumor grading and gross tumor characteristics (size and number).

The suggestion advanced by Goffinet[22] of performing staging exploratory laparotomy with femoral and periaortic nodal sampling in the deeply invasive tumors to improve the accuracy of staging prior to definitive therapy may prove to be a better alternative.

Table 12.1
Results of Treatment by Clinical Staging

Author	Year	A	B	B$_2$	C	Remarks
		%	%	%	%	
Milner	1954	70	57			Transurethral resection
Nichols	1956	81				Transurethral resection
Cox	1968	47	8			Transurethral resection
O'Flynn, et al.	1975	62	59			Transurethral resection
Jewett, et al.	1964	58	58			Segmental resection
Cox	1968	43	73	20		Segmental resection
Long	1972	80	67	43		Segmental resection
Resnick	1973	75	57	55		Segmental resection
Utz	1973		68	47		Segmental resection
Evans	1975		69	43		Segmental resection
Bramman	1978		79	80		Segmental resection
Cummings	1978	100	79	80		Segmental resection
Pomerance	1972	77	27	15		Simple cystectomy
Cordonnier	1974		46	52		Simple cystectomy
Crigler	1966	0	57	44	35	Radiotherapy 5-yr survival
Caldwell et al.	1967	60	48	25	15	Radiotherapy 5-yr survival
Werf-Messing et al.		64	34	10		Radiotherapy 5-yr survival
	(T$_1$)	(T$_2$)	(T$_3$)			
	1972	45	35	27		Radiotherapy central
Pederson et al.	(T$_1$)	(T$_2$)	(T$_3$)			Source 5-yr survival
	1972	75	60	56		Disappearance rate
Walbom-Jorgensen[41]	(T$_1$)	(T$_2$)	(T$_3$)			Radiotherapy

However, despite all the problems that beset the accuracy of clinical staging, it remains the best prognostic parameter, as can be seen in Table 12.1 which summarizes the experience in several large published series.

Grading

Although some early authors[10] denied the effect of tumor grade on survival, it is now widely accepted that it affects the prognosis.

Pomerance[33] studied the relationship between the pathological features of bladder carcinomas in cystectomy specimen and the subsequent clinical course. He found strong correlation between the depth of invasion, tumor grading and lymphatic invasion.

Collins et al.[17] showed that survival is strongly related to the tumor grade. Among tumors of the same invasive characteristic (or clinical stage) the 5-year survival in 362 patients with a T_1, G_1 tumor was 92% versus 68% in 24 patients with T_1, G_2 tumors. A similar differential was noted between the T_2, G_1 tumors and the T_2, G_2 tumors (69 and 50%, respectively).

Cell Type and Pattern of Growth

Transitional carcinomas form about 95% of bladder carcinoma cases, followed by squamous cell carcinoma which comprise about 4%[38] and adenocarcinoma in about 1%. This is a fortuitous arrangement since transitional cell carcinoma cases have a better prognosis as compared to adenocarcinoma where prognosis is the worst. The 5-year disease-free survival of patient with squamous cell carcinoma amounted only to 17% in a group of 52 patients reported recently by Prempree.[34]

Sarcomas including leimyosarcoma and rhabdomyosarcomas are highly malignant with a poor salvage rate (<10%).[21,47]

The impact of *the pattern of growth, number of lesions and their site* is somewhat contentious. It is claimed that papillary lesions have a better prognosis than sessile or ulcerating lesions.[8] This better prognosis is partially explained by the fact that sessile and ulcerating lesions display a deeper and wider extent of invasion as compared to papillary ones, in addition to the predominance of advanced grade tumors. Whether papillary tumors display better radiation response as compared to sessile and ulcerative ones for the same grade and depth of invasion is not settled yet.

Age

Age plays an important role. The older the patient, the higher the chances of having systemic and arteriosclerotic diseases which adversely affect the blood supply to the bladder and the malignant lesion, thus reducing response to radiotherapy. Bloom et al.,[11] in a randomized study for T_3 bladder cancer, found better results in younger patients (<60 years of age) especially when an aggressive combination of surgery and radiotherapy was used. Patients older than 60 displayed inferior results when treated with the same aggressive combination and seemed to do better when treated with radiation alone.

Tumor Size

Scant data exists in the literature for adequate evaluation of this factor. Conceptually, a larger tumor would be less responsive to radiation than a smaller one, by virtue of several factors including a larger number of hypoxic cells, and generally a more substantial tumor burden. Bloom[11] and others[8] were able to demonstrate in a randomized trial that patients with tumors smaller than 5 cm fare better than those with larger tumors when both populations were treated by radical radiotherapy. The 5-year survival for both groups was 33 and 18%, respectively.

On the other hand, patients treated with combined preoperative radiotherapy and surgery showed no such differential. More studies are needed to confirm these findings since it has a clear impact on the choice of treatment strategy.

Transurethral Resection of Bladder Tumors (TURB)

The role of TURB as a prognosticator in bladder cancer subsequently treated by radiation is unclear since the presence of many variables cloud conclusions drawn from various studies. The fact that repeated transurethral resections lead to a fibrotic contracted bladder with a compromised blood supply and a substantial burden of hypoxic cells is established.[8] Recently Keys et al.[24] demonstrated the deleterious impact of transurethral resection of prostatic lesions on the results of treatment by radiation, with the 10-year survival after TURB being 0% *versus* 50% after needle biopsy. A similar finding was noted in a group of 310 cases of bladder cancer treated in our department[36] and followed-up for varying periods up to 14 years (mean, 7 years).

RESULTS OF TREATMENT ACCORDING TO MODALITY OF RADIATION USED

The modality of radiation used in the treatment of bladder cancer plays a definitive role in the outcome. For a proper evaluation of the role of surgery with its different techniques other chapters of this work should be consulted.

Curative radiotherapy is delivered by many differing techniques or modalities; intracavitary insertion, interstitial implant of radioactive sources, external radiation therapy or a combination of external and interstitial irradiation. The role of a combined approach by radiation and surgery will also be discussed.

Intracavitary Insertion

Two techniques were utilized towards this end: an intracavitary radioactive central source, or distension of the bladder by radioactive material.

The basic concept of this technique is that sources of irradiation with varying depths of penetration, when inserted into the bladder, would treat the whole of the bladder mucosa. The extravesical tissues and, to a lesser extent, the bladder wall would receive only a minimal amount of radiation.

The methods used vary from a central source to the instillation of radioactive solutions. ^{60}Co or radium is the central source usually employed, contained in a balloon. While theoretically such a central source may irradiate the bladder mucosa homogenously, any variation in the geometry caused by the tumor would result in a gross distortion of the dose. Generally, the bladder wall is more intensely irradiated with this method. The resultant radiation damage limits the use of this method. The ideal indication is that of multiple small tumors which have not penetrated beyond the submucosa. Pedersen *et al.*[31] reported on the treatment of 145 patients with a central radium source (using a so-called modified Walter Reed technique) in two sessions of 120 hours each, delivering a dose of approximately 35 grays (at the balloon surface) in each session. The total dose to tumor cells lying 10–12 mm deep (or away from the balloon) is about 35 grays. While the results seem encouraging, only 8% (10 of 121) of patients treated were alive and well after 5 years without any surgical interference. However, a further 40 patients (33%) were alive after salvage surgery.

Intracavitary solutions are either ^{60}Co (not used because of hazards of spillage combined with a long half-life) or colloidal yttrium,[19] but it tends to settle on bladder base when mixed with urine or colloidal gold.[18, 41] Radioactive sodium in the form of NaCl and radioactive bromine in the form of ammonium were used by Wallace[42] by inserting them under pressure into a modified Miller-Abbott tube. Colloidal gold, on the other hand, was instilled directly into the bladder as it is not absorbed through the bladder mucosa. As radioactivity would surround a papillary lesion from all directions, it is presumed that the dose to these lesions is several times that to the normal smooth mucosa. Dickson[18] treated patients with two instillations, 8 weeks apart, delivering 3000 rets to the bladder mucosa in each session which lasts 2–3 hours. Again, the ideal indication is where several mucosal papillary lesions exist and are considered to be too extensive for diathermy.

Wallace[42] reported on 41 patients treated with colloid ^{198}Au with 25 surviving 5 years (61%) and 16 surviving for 10 years (39%). However cystectomy was carried out as salvage in 12 patients, 6 because of severe hemorrhages. Metastases occurred in 20% of the patients and tumor recurrences were found even after the urothelium was completely destroyed by irradiation (may be attributable to errors in staging). Only five patients survived without evidence of recurrence (12%).

Complications of intracavitary instillations are unfortunately very high with 30% of the patients suffering from severe bleeding and 15% suffering from markedly contracted bladder. The incidence of contracted bladder was higher with radioactive bromine.

Interstitial Implant

This can be permanent using either gold grains ^{198}Au or ^{525}I or a removable implant using either radium needles, or radioactive tantalum wire,[49] or ^{192}Ir.[12] It is ideal for lesions not exceeding 5 cm in diameter and penetrating to a depth not exceeding the superficial muscle. The implant is performed through suprapubic cystostomy. Lesions situated in almost any region of the bladder wall are accessible, although those situated in the dome and the trigone need particular attention and good expertise. An assessment of this technique is rather difficult because of paucity of results published.

Werf-Messing[44–46] reported on the use of radium needles implanted submucosally in a single plane or a two-plane configuration, depending on the depth of the lesion. For more penetrating lesions interstitial irradiation was supplemented by external irradiation to bladder, paravesical regions and the scar. Results indicate that superficial lesions (T_1) responded very favorably with long-term relapse-free survival of 85% *versus* 18% for TUR only where the majority of patients needed further therapy. A boost by external irradiation is necessary for more invasive lesions (T_2 and T_3) to prevent scar recurrence. The 5-year results with and without the boost for T_2 lesions were 55 and 40%, respectively.[44] The scar recurrence rate was reduced to half by the addition of the boost.[44] Bloom,[10] in an earlier publication, using gold grain implants, demonstrated superior results in well differentiated mucosal lesions (70% 5-year survivals) as well as satisfactory outcome when the tumor has extended to muscle (49% 3-year survivals). However, in the poorly differentiated lesions, the control rate was shown to be noticeably less.

It seems that for the control of a well differentiated T_1 or T_2 lesions an interstitial implant is a highly satisfactory modality provided the lesions are within 5 cm in diameter. Supplement by external irradiation seems to be indicated in the more extensive or deeply invasive lesions (T_3).

Werf-Messing et al.[44-46] reported on a small group of patients with limited T_3 tumors (>5 cm) who were treated with a modest dose radium implant (about 35 grays) sandwiched between two courses of external irradiation (10 grays and 30 grays) with encouraging results (57% 3-year actuarial survival). However, cases suitable for such approach are rather limited.

External Radiation Therapy

This is the most widely used modality in the application of radiation therapy to bladder cancer. An essential step in delivery of safe and effective external irradiation is careful treatment planning to avoid overirradiation of the rectum.

Computed tomography (CT) scan became an important tool in detecting the extent of the disease of bladder cancer as well as in planning the treatment.

The standard method for planning the treatment is a localizing cystogram performed by instilling radiopaque dye in the bladder, followed by injection of air (20–40 cc). Films are taken in arteroposterior and lateral views as well as CT cuts (where available). A contour of the patient at the center of the field is taken, and the target volume is transferred to the contour. A treatment plan is produced to deliver an optimal dose to the target volume and avoid irradiating the surrounding structures as much as possible, mainly the rectum and bowels.

The inability of the localizing cystogram to detect the extent of tumorous extravesical spread and other details of pelvic structures indicates the advantages of a high resolution CT scan.

Rothwell[37] compared the target volumes of radical radiotherapy treatment plans in 60 patients done through both the conventional localization cystogram and CT scan. He found that the cystogram failed to delineate extravesical spread of the tumor in 30% of cases. Also the CT scan is more accurate in obtaining the contour of the patient enabling a treatment plan to be done directly and according to the real measurements of the patient, increasing substantially the degree of accuracy— especially since some authors[4,36] claimed that discrepancies between target volumes determined by localized cystograms alone and those determined by both methods amounted to 85% of cases reported.

Treatment beams used must always be of the high quality type, accelerator beams of the magnitude of 4–12 Mev or X or ^{60}Co beam with an 80-cm source skin distance (SSD).

Treatment fields depend on the target volume size and the total dose to be delivered.

In the preoperative course, parallel opposed fields or four-field box technique are applied to deliver 40–50 grays (4000–5000 rads) with the conventional fractionation (2 grays or 200 rads/fraction).

When early stages are treated with radical radiation therapy, the treatment volume should be limited to the bladder alone since incidence of lymph node metastases is relatively low. Field arrangements may be a configuration or 360° rotation, which is used more advantageously in patients with a balanced globular contour.

In advanced stages (T_2 or T_3) the bladder and the regional pelvic lymph nodes are included in the target volume by using a three- or four-field plan.[36] A dose of 40–50 grays (4000–5000 rads) in about 5 weeks is delivered to this volume which is followed by a boost to the bladder (and perivesical region), 20–25 grays (2000–2500 rads) in 2 or $2\frac{1}{2}$ weeks.

Dose/Time/Fractionation: Most authors seem to agree that a tumor (or volume) dose of 60–65 grays (6000–6500 rads) in 6 weeks in about 24–30 fractions is well tolerated with optimum results. Higher doses of 65 grays in about 5 weeks (2.5 grays, daily fractions) and 65 grays in 4 weeks (3 grays, daily fractions) were reported by Finney[20] with increasing incidence of rectal complications (8, 39 and 67%, respectively). However, the author[20] also claimed that 3-year survivals were better with higher biological doses (25, 31 and 75%, respectively). Nevertheless such findings were not substantiated by others and must be viewed as experimental.

EVALUATION OF THE ROLE OF EXTERNAL IRRADIATION

A critical *evaluation of the role of external irradiation* in the treatment of bladder cancer is essentially an evaluation of the role of radiotherapy as a modality since most cases reported are treated by external irradiation. Moreover a multivariate analysis of results published is necessary to take into account the effect of the many prognosticators mentioned earlier. Since clinical stage and histological grade seem to be the most commonly used factors for categorization of results we propose to discuss the role of external irradiation accordingly.

T_1 Lesions

Table 12.2 summarizes the results of treatment of patients suffering from T_1 lesions as published by various authors. It is clear that an average 5-year survival of 55%[15] using external irradiation (^{60}Co or accelerator beam) in the well differentiated group is not as favorable as the survival claimed after interstitial implant. On the other hand, results in the poorly differentiated group of cases (G_2 and G_3) are rather different with external irradiation achieving a certain degree of superiority above interstitial implant, 65 *versus* 55%. Such comparison can be persuasive in determining the place of external irradiation in T_1 lesions where it seems to be preferred in the poorly differentiated tumors. Patients who are not good surgical risks or who suffer from large or multiple lesions are better candidates for external irradiation.

T$_2$ Lesions

Table 12.3 summarizes results of treatment of T$_2$ lesions as reported by various authors according to the modality of radiation used and grade of tumors. For solitary lesions less than 5 cm interstitial implant along with external irradiation boost seem to give control results of 50–60%,[11, 14, 43] with the better results in well differentiated tumors.

For larger or multiple lesions radical external irradiation seems to be the method of choice with a control rate of 40–50%, with high grade tumors performing worst.

T$_3$ Lesions

Table 12.4 summarizes the results of treatment of these deeply invasive tumors by external irradiation. It is obvious that results of treatment using radical external irradiation alone is far from satisfactory, averaging about 20%, which is very similar to results after cystectomy alone.[22, 42, 49] However when salvage cystectomy is used systematically the control rate is substantially improved. Bloom[11] reported on a small group of

Table 12.2
Results of Treatment of T$_1$ (Radiotherapy)

Author	Year	Five-year Results	Remarks
		% (No. of Cases)	
Frank	1970	45 (12)	
Finney	1971	24 (29)	
Morrison	1960	44	3-Year results for T$_1$ and T$_2$
Bloom	1960	70	Interstitial implant
Ellis	1963	16	
Crigler	1966	32	Stage 0, T$_1$, T$_2$ included; treated by external irradiation
Buschke	1967	44	T$_1$ and T$_2$ included
Sell	1967	40 (22)	Intracavity radiation
Pedersen et al.	1972	56 (51)	Intracavity radiation
Werf-Messing	1965	64 (23)	Interstitial radiation

Table 12.3
Results of Treatment of T$_2$ (Radiotherapy)

Author	Year	Five-year Results	Remarks
		% (No. of Cases)	
Frank	1970	51 (53)	
Finney	1971	23 (77)	
Bloom	1960	40	Interstitial implant
Ellis	1963	9	Cases included T$_2$ and T$_3$
Sell	1967	29 (7)	Intracavity radiation.
Pedersen et al.	1972	36 (24)	Intracavity radiation.
Caldwell et al.	1967	43 (68)	T$_1$ and T$_2$ radical cystectomy
		50 (38)	T$_1$ and T$_2$ external radiation
Werf-Messing	1965	34 (82)	Interstitial radiation

Table 12.4
Results of Treatment of T_3 (Radiotherapy)

Author	Year	Five-year Results	Remarks
		% (*No. of Cases*)	
Frank	1970	22 (55)	
Finney	1971	33	
Morrison	1960	26	3-Year results of T_3 and T_4
Crigler	1966	28	External radiation
Buschke	1967	14	
Sell	1967	11 (9)	Intracavity radiation
Pedersen *et al.*	1972	20 (20)	Intracavity radiation
Whitmore *et al.*	1968		
Caldwell *et al.*	1967	31 (77)	Extensive radiations: 3½-year result
		20 (45)	Radical radiotherapy
Jergensen	1972	28 (43)	Radical radiotherapy
Miller and Johnson	1973	20 (109)	Radical radiotherapy
Edsmyr	1975	29 (125)	Radical radiotherapy
Goffinet *et al.*	1975	28 (218)	Radical radiotherapy
Wallace and Bloom	1976	21 (91)	Radical radiotherapy

patients treated by radical radiotherapy (65 grays in 7 weeks) followed by salvage cystectomy with 60% 5-year disease-free survival. However, morbidity and mortality of such combinations is rather high, amounting to almost 11% mortality rate especially among the older group of patients. Morbidity including delayed healing, wound disruption and infection may also occur at substantial levels. Other authors who reported on the results of such aggressive combination failed to show such high survival figures. Batata et al.[7] reported 40%, 5-year survival and Smith et al.[40] reported 37%. On the other hand the incidence of complications continued to be pronounced occurring in one-third of patients in Smith's study.

A less aggressive approach utilizing external irradiation given in modest doses (20 grays in 1 week or 45 grays in 41/2–5 weeks) followed by cystectomy seems to be gaining more acceptance. Table 12.5 summarizes results of treatment as reported in recent literature.

Preoperative radiation therapy aims at shrinking the tumor and downstaging (or reducing the depth of infiltration) the lesion, thus improving prognosis. Reduction of dissemination of neoplastic cells during surgery both locally (minimizing local recurrence) and systemically as well as the sterilization of minimal tumor in the lymph nodes are other objectives.

Whitmore et al.[48] compared two programs, of 40 grays in 4 weeks to the true pelvis, followed 6 weeks later by radical cystectomy (group 1), and 20 grays in 1 week followed by similar surgery within 1 week in a mixed (stage) group of patients (group 2). He claimed that the advantages of the integrated therapy was apparent mainly in the deeply infiltrating lesions (T_3). Moreover, the determinate 5-year survival without evidence of recurrence was almost the same in both groups of combinations (43 and 42%, respectively). However, stage reduction occurred in 40% of

Table 12.5
Result of Treatment of Combined Radiation Therapy (Modest Dose) and Surgery in T_3 Tumors

Author	Year	Five-year Survival	Remarks
Whitmore *et al.*	1977	34 and 40	After 4000 rads and 2000 rads preop
Werf-Messing	1979	45	4000 rads preop
Hall	1981	60 and 30	4000–4500 rads preop Depending on downstaging
Bloom *et al.*	1982	38	4000 rads preop
Miller	1973	53	5000 rads preop controlled trial
Boileau "M. D. Anderson"	1980	50	5000 rads preop
Prout	1976	36	4500 rads preop

cases in the first group as compared to 27% in the second one. The surgical morbidity amounted to 13% in group 1 compared to 9% in group 2 but there was no difference in incidence of serious complications. A further analysis of both groups[9] revealed a better survival for those who received preoperative irradiation to the whole pelvis, as compared to those where only the true pelvis was treated, with a lower incidence of local recurrence in the former group which was reduced from 28% after cystectomy alone to 14–16% with true pelvic irradiation and 8% with whole pelvis irradiation.

The conclusion that the impact of the two differing doses of preoperative radiation (40 grays and 20 grays) on survival is the same is disputed by some[28] but it seems that all agree about the superiority of the larger dose given to an adequate volume for control of local recurrence and affecting tumor downstaging.

Werf-Messing *et al.*[44] reported that downstaging occurred in 68% of 141 patients with stage T_3 Nx Mo who were treated with preoperative 40 grays (in two gray fractions over a period of 4 weeks), followed by simple cystectomy.

The superiority of the combined approach over external irradiation alone or cystectomy alone was confirmed in two randomized trials, one by Miller[27] and the other by Bloom *et al.*[11] The dose of preoperative radiation used varied somewhat among both series (50 grays and 40 grays, respectively) which seems to have affected the results marginally (46 and 33%, respectively). Survivals after radical radiotherapy alone in both series was very similar, 22 and 21%, respectively. It is to be noted that both groups of patients received very similar total dose levels (70 grays and 65 grays, respectively in about 7 weeks).

Tumor downstaging or complete disappearance, which has been reported consistently and seems to be dose-dependent, has a salutory effect both on survival and incidence of lymph node metastasis. Bloom[11] reported the 5-year survival in patients who showed downstaging to be 68% *versus* 27% when no such effect was noted. Similarly, lymph node metastases occurred in 5 and 34%, respectively.

THE SANDWICH COMBINATION

A recent approach to combined external irradiation and surgery in T_3 cases was introduced recently and piloted by the Radiation Therapy Oncology Group in a small group of patients with encouraging results. Patients received 5 grays in a single fraction, followed on the same day or day after with cystectomy (with or without pelvic node dissection). Patients with high grade B_1 tumors or B_2–C tumors were treated to the whole pelvis by external irradiation to a dose of 45 grays in 5 weeks.

The 3-year actuarial survival in 39 patients was rather outstanding, reaching 85–90% in B cases and 78% in C cases. This promising approach seems to have the potential of breaking new ground and further confirmatory studies are needed.

T_4 Lesions

These are treated mainly palliatively with external radiation therapy to prevent bleeding or pain (see below).

The 5-year survival in this group of patients is dismal, amounting to less than 10% even after radical course of radiation therapy.

Postoperative Radiotherapy

Most radiotherapists favor preoperative radiation especially since the results are rewarding.

There are few studies regarding postoperative irradiation. Miller[27] reported a 34% pelvic recurrence rate with postoperative therapy.

Postoperative irradiation is delivered in high risk patients and for control of local or regional failure.

Postoperative radiation therapy is considered important for a known residual disease, invasion of adjacent organ or involvement of pelvic nodes. Five-year survival may be improved marginally but the complication rate is high, especially after a radical cystectomy.

SUMMARY

It is clear from the above discussion of the role of various modalities of radiation in the treatment of different stages of bladder cancer that several alternatives exist. Our recommended approach towards this problem is seen in Table 12.6.

Place of Irradiation in Palliative Therapy

Palliation still plays a major role in management of bladder cancer since over one-third of the patients seen are beyond cure by present day therapy. Moreover symptomatic bladder cancer is very distressing and palliation is important for improving quality of life. The most important symptom where radiation is highly effective is hematuria, with frequency and dysuria closely behind.

Hematuria is very amenable to radiotherapy which exercises a rather rapid styptic effect which reaches its zenith by the 3rd or 4th week of treatment[26] when the tumor dose is about 30 grays (3000 rads). Short

Table 12.6
Recommended Radiation Therapy for Bladder Carcinoma

Modality	T_1	T_2	T_3	T_4
Interstitial implant	×[a]	×[a]		
External radiotherapy	×[b]	×[b]	×[c]	×[f]
Combined interstitial plus external radiotherapy		×[d]		
Combined radiotherapy plus surgery			×	×[e]

[a] In multiple or large lesions (<5 cm) external irradiation to bladder region is recommended. A booster dose of external irradiation to anterior abdominal wall is recommended to avoid scar recurrence.
[b] Recommended for multiple lesions.
[c] Recommended either when surgery is refused or not applicable. On occasions, radical external irradiation, with salvage surgery in case of failure, is recommended for young patients with well differentiated tumors.
[d] Recommended in larger lesions but still within 5 cm when tumor is poorly differentiated.
[e] Recommended in T_4 only if tumor is mobile and limited to pelvis with no nodal disease outside pelvis.
[f] Largely palliative.

courses of palliative radiation have been tried and recommended by some with effect. However, when the dose delivered is biologically less than 40–45 grays (4000–4500 rads) in about 41/2 weeks, hematuria is likely to recur in about 4–6 months—then a rather disturbing occurrence since patients are generally more feeble and the tumor is less responsive to treatment.

Dysuria and frequency are interrelated in their incidence and etiology which may not always be exclusively neoplastic. Infection, repeated prior TURB and trigone involvement are often present. Moreover radiation does contribute to incidence of dysuria and frequency in the early weeks by augmenting the congestive irritative reaction displayed by vesical mucous membrane. The treatment of frequency and dysuria must therefore be a multipronged attack consisting of proper antibiotics—as determined by sensitivity tests—given for adequately long periods coupled with plain muscle relaxants and pain killers. Response to treatment is generally partial and slow but improvements should be detected by 3rd or 4th week following the end of radiation therapy. Nocturnal frequency can be disturbing especially to male patients and it is wise to restrict intake of fluids and caffeine-containing drinks (*e.g.* tea or coffee) early in the evening to help reduce sleep interruption episodes. The dose recommended to obtain enough tumor regression to improve neoplastic-induced dysuria is in the range of 50 grays (5000 rads) in about 5 weeks.

Suprapubic pain or back pain are rarely present in the case of intravesical tumors but extensive bladder lesions involving prostate or posterior paravesical pelvic structures may cause local pain which can be relieved by radiation treatment of the neoplastic process. However, pain relief is slow and necessitates a rather high tumor dose of about 50 grays (5000 rads) in 5 weeks since such relief is related to an adequate degree of tumor regression. The rate of relief is generally related to tumor regression reaching its zenith during the 7th week and, on occasions, may be delayed even further. Pain killers must also be used freely in order to break the pain cycle and it is noted that patients who respond favorably to radiation display a gradually subsiding need of analgesics.

Management of Complications of Radiation Therapy

The bladder and colo-rectum are the organs that bear the brunt of radiation effect during a course of therapy. Such effect is maximal after a course of radical external irradiation delivered to the whole pelvis which may be exaggerated further by preexisting conditions such as infection (cystitis, colitis) or trauma (multiple TURB or open surgery). Older men form the population that is most vulnerable. Dose fractions larger than 2 grays (200 rads) are often more injurious.

ACUTE

Cystitis: Cystitis (or bladder irritation) occurs usually around the 3rd week of treatment. However, bladder mucosa is often infected and irritated with disease as well as prior trauma, with patients often displaying symptoms of cystitis (frequency, dysuria) when referred. The frequency and intensity of symptoms demonstrated by Walbom-Jorgensen[41] where 24% of 429 patients treated by radical external irradiation suffered from cystitis but only 1% had their treatment interrupted because of severity of symptoms. Management of cystitis depends mainly on combat of infection (antibiotics, long-acting sulfa drugs and change of urinary pH) in addition to antispasmodics (to relax bladder muscle) such as propantheline bromide (Pro-Banthine) and analgesics such as aspirin, Percodan or meperidine (Demerol). Mild antiseptics such as phenazopyridine (Pyridium) may sometimes prove valuable.

Rectal Reactions: These vary from simple loose bowels to severe diarrhea and tenesmus leading to eventual dehydration. While mild diarrhea may be expected during the last 2 weeks of treatment, earlier severe reactions may be predisposed to by preexisting diseases such as diverticulitis, colitis or uremia. Certain treatment factors such as large volumes irradiated and large fractions, especially if one field only is treated each session, will also predispose to pronounced reactions. A plan of treatment where the brunt of a radical dose is applied to the rectum, such as the use of two opposing fields, must be shunned if such complications are to be avoided. Walbom-Jorgensen[41] showed that while about half the patients suffered from simple diarrhea, only about 5% had their treatment interrupted because of severity of symptoms. In our series of 310 patients treatment was interrupted because of diarrhea in 10 patients (3%).

Simple diarrhea can be combated by dietary restrictions (fresh fruit, vegetables and fruit juices) in addition to Kaopectate and Lomotil tablets. Mixtures of chalk and morphine are also effective. Predisposing factors should be corrected.

Uremia: This complication is particularly threatening where the disease has involved ureteric openings. Early mucous membrane edema which occurs in the first few weeks of treatment may tip the balance in a borderline case leading to increasing levels of blood urea. The radiotherapist should proceed with the treatment carefully (and perhaps slowly) in such cases with frequent estimates of blood urea. High levels of blood urea (above 40 mg/100 ml) and createnine may be an indication for temporary suspension of treatment in addition to proper hydration of the patient and other supportive measures necessary to avoid open uremia.

Anemia: Anemia is rarely encountered and then only when large volumes, including both pelvic bones, are used. Unexplained early or profound anemia should alert the physician to other etiologies such as uremia or second malignancy.

General constitutional disturbances including nausea, anorexia and weight loss are unusual symptoms except in advanced disease. An unexplained occurrence warrants detailed investigations for possible other causative factors.

CHRONIC

Bladder: 1. Hemorrhagic cystitis due to telangectasis may occur after several months from end of treatment, usually after 1 year. Caldwell *et al.*[15] reported an incidence of 15% in 104 patients. This is a most troublesome and often serious complications. Antibiotics, bladder wash and cystoscopy (to ascertain cause of bleeding) are usual conservative measures. The employment of compression balloons in addition to diluted solutions of silver nitrate for bladder wash may succeed in combating the bleeding. Sometimes the only treatment is cystectomy.

Bleeding may be caused by recurrent neoplasm, in which case repeat palliative radiotherapy may be considered if there is a margin of tolerance.

2. Contracture of the bladder leads to marked frequency. In the absence of tumor this complication is often self-correcting. Rarely, urinary diversion and ileal loop bladder may be necessary.

3. Vesicovaginal (or vesicorectal) fistula: This is a very rare complication and is invariably due to recurrence of disease with involvement of the vesicovaginal septum.

Rectum: 1. Rectal stricture rarely leads to lasting symptoms since the stricture is usually of the pliable type and usually not enough to cause intestinal obstruction. Such a complication may indicate high level of rectal irradiation which should be avoided by proper planning.

2. Colonic complications: The incidence of such complications is rather rare and usually mild. Serious complications such as gut perforation are even more rare, Walbom-Jorgensen[41] reported such occurrence in about 1% of cases studied (5/429).

Bones: Bone necrosis and pathological fractures of the femur are exceedingly rare especially if careful planning and proper beams were carried out.

REFERENCES

1. Abratt, R. P., *et al.* Radical irradiation and misonidazole in the treatment of T_2 grade 3 and T_3 bladder cancer. *Int. J. Radiat. Oncol. Biol. Phys. May* 9:629–632, 1983.

2. Adams, G. E., *et al.* Structure-activity relationships in the development of hypoxic cell radiatosensitizers. *Int. J. Radiat. Biol. 35:*151–160, 1979.
3. Awwad, H. K., *et al.* Misonidazole in the preoperative and radical radiotherapy of bladder cancer. *Cancer Clin. Trials 3:*275–280, 1980.
4. Badcock, P. C. *Int. J. Radiat. Oncol. Biol. Phys. 9:*905–911, 1983.
5. Baker, R. The accuracy of clinical *vs.* surgical staging. *JAMA 206:*1770–1773, 1968.
6. Baker, R. Pitfalls of clinical *versus* microscopic staging of cancer of the bladder in relationship to potential curability. *Am. Surg. May:* 269–275, 1970.
7. Batata, M. A., *et al.* Patterns of recurrence in bladder cancer treated by irradiation and/or cystectomy. *Int. J. Radiat. Oncol. Biol. Phys. 6:*155–159, 1980.
8. Batata, M. A., *et al.* Factors of prognostic and therapeutic significance in patients with bladder cancer. *Int. J. Radiat. Oncol. Biol. Phys. 7:*575–579, 1981.
9. Batata, M. A., *et al.* Preoperative whole pelvis *versus* true pelvis irradiation and/or cystectomy for bladder cancer. *Int. J. Radiat. Oncol. Biol. Phys. 7:*1349–1355, 1981.
10. Bloom, H. J. G. Treatment by interstitial irradiation using tantelum 182 wire. *Br. J. Radiol. 33:*471, 1950.
11. Bloom, H. J. G., *et al.* Treatment of T$_3$ bladder cancer: controlled trial of preoperative radiotherapy and radical cystectomy *versus* radical radiotherapy. *Br. J. Urol. 54:*136–151, 1982.
12. Botto, H., *et al.* Treatment of malignant bladder tumors. *Urology 16:*467–469, 1980.
13. Cade, I. S., *et al.* Hyperbaric oxygen and radiotherapy: a Medical Research Council trial in carcinoma of the bladder. *Br. J. Radiol. 51:*876–878, 1978.
14. Caldwell, W. L. Radiotherapy: definitive, integrated and palliative therapy. *Urol. Clin. North Am. 3:*129–148, 1975.
15. Caldwell, W. L., *et al.* Efficacy of linear accelerator X-ray therapy in cancer of the bladder. *Engl. J. Urol. 97:*294–300, 1967.
16. Cockett, A. T. K., *et al.* Enhancement of regional bladder megavoltage irradiation in bladder cancer using local bladder hyperthermia. *J. Urol. 97:*1034, 1967.
17. Collins, W. E., *et al.* Management of primary bladder cancer by a multidisciplinary team. *Can. J. Surg. 22:*431–434, 1979.
18. Dickson, K-J. *et al.* Treatment of papillomas of the bladder with radioactive colloidal gold. *AJR 83:*116–122, 1960.
19. Durant, K. R., *et al.* Treatment of multiple superficial papillary tumor of the bladder by intracavitary yttrium −90. *J. Urol. 13:*480, 1975.
20. Finney, R. The treatment of carcinoma of the bladder by external irradiation. A clinical trial II. *Clin. Radiol. 22:*225–293, 1971.
21. Flint, L. O., *et al.* Myosarcoma of the urinary bladder: preliminary report of a favorable case. *Lakey Clin. Bull. 6:*181, 1949.
22. Goffinet, D. R., *et al.* Bladder cancer: results of radiation therapy in 384 patients. *Radiology 117:*149–143, 1975.
23. Hall, E. J. *Radiobiology for the Radiologist.* Harper & Row, New York, 1982.
24. Keys, H. M. *et al.* The negative impact of transurethral resection of long-term survival. *Int. Radiat. Oncol. Biol. Phys. 9:(Supp.1):*103, 1983.
25. Kubota, Y. Hyperthermia therapy of the bladder cancer. *Nippon Hinyokika Gakkai Zasshi 6:*742–751, 1981.
26. Kurohara, S. S., *et al.* Analysis in depth of bladder cancer treated by supervoltage therapy. *AJR 95:*458–67, 65.
27. Miller, L. T$_3$ Bladder cancer. *Cancer, April Suppl:* 1875–1878, 1980.
28. Mohiuddin, M., *et al.* Preoperative radiotherapy for bladder cancer. *Urology 17:*515–520, 1981.
29. Newsam, J. E., *et al.* Hyperthermic perfusion of the distended urinary bladder in the management of recurrent transitional cell Ca. *Br. J. Urol. 54:*64, 1982.
30. Ogura, K., *et al.* Hyperthermia in experimental bladder tumors. *Eur. Urol. 7:*100–104, 1981.
31. Pedersen, M., *et al.* Intracavitary radium treatment of malignant tumors of the urinary bladder. *Acta Radiol. Thera.* (Stockh.) *11:*369–385, 1972.
32. Plenk, H. P. Preliminary results of a randomized study of cancer of the urinary bladder and review of the oxygen experience. *AJR 114:*1152–1157, 1972.
33. Pomerance, A. Pathology and prognosis following total cystectomy for carcinoma of

bladder. *Br. J. Urol. 44*:451–458, 1972.

34. Prempree, Th. Radiation management of squamous cell carcinoma of the bladder. *Int. J. Rad. Oncol. Biol. Phys. 9*:(Suppl)72, 1983.
35. Prout, G., *et al.* Preoperative irradiation as an adjuvant in the surgical management of invasive bladder carcinoma. *J. Urol. 105*:223–231, 1977.
36. Rafla, S., *et al.* in *"Introduction to Radiotherapy,"* Mosby, St. Louis, 1974.
37. Rothwell, R. I. Radiation treatment planning for bladder cancer: A comparison of cystogram localization with computed tomography. *Clin. Radiol. 34*:103–111, 1983.
38. Rotman, M., *et al.* Carcinoma of the urinary bladder. The Radiological Society of North America Meeting, Chicago, 1979.
39. Shipley, W. U., *et al.* 4000 Rad preoperative irradiation followed by prompt radical cystectomy for invasive bladder carcinoma; a prospective study of patient tolerance and pathologic downstaging. *J. Urol. 127*:48–51, 1982.
40. Smith, J. A., *et al.* Salvage cystectomy for bladder cancer after failure of definitive irradiation. *J. Urol. 125*:643–645, 1981.
41. Walbom-Jorgensen, S. W. Treatment of bladder carcinoma with 6 mev linear accelerator. *Scand. J. Urol. Nephrol. 6*:(Suppl.) 15–113, 1972.
42. Wallace, D. M. Intracavitary radiation for multiple noninfiltrating bladder tumors. *Br. J. Urol. 43*:177–180, 1971.
43. Wassif, S. B., *et al.* Treatment of bladder cancer at the Rotterdam Radiotherapy Institute. *Urol. Res. 6*:241–247, 1978.
44. Werf-Messing, *et al. Therapeutic Radiology. New Directions on Therapy.* Medical Examination Publishing Co., New York, 1983.
45. Werf-Messing, *et al.* T$_3$ NxMo carcinoma of the urinary bladder treated by the combination of radium implant and external irradiation. A preliminary report. *Int. J. Radiat. Oncol. Biol. Phys. 6*:1723–1725, 1980.
46. Werf-Messing, *et al.* Carcinoma of the urinary bladder category T$_3$ NxMo, treated by the combination of radium implant and external irradiation: second report. *Int. J. Radiat. Oncol. Phys. 9*:177–180, 1983.
47. Whelock, M. C. Sarcoma of urinary bladder. *J. Urol. 48*:628, 1942.
48. Whitmore, W. F., *et al.* A comparative study of two preoperative radiation regimens with cystectomy for bladder cancer. *Cancer 40*:1077–1086, 1977.
49. Winston, *et al. Urol. Res. 6*:249–251, 1978.

13

Integrated Irradiation and Cystectomy for Bladder Cancer

Jerome P. Richie, M.D.
Ralph R. Weichselbaum, M.D.

The ideal method of therapy, or combination of therapy, for patients with invasive carcinoma of the urinary bladder has yet to be defined. Prior to the 1970s, opposing schools of thought existed concerning the appropriate therapy for high grade invasive carcinoma of the bladder. One school advocated that such patients should be treated by definitive radiation therapy in the range of 6000–7000 rads delivered by conventional fractionation over a 6–8 week time span with possible salvage cystectomy in those patients who failed radiation. The other school believed that appropriate therapy consisted of simple or radical cystectomy with some type of urinary diversion without any radiation therapy. Proponents of definitive radiation therapy were quick to cite excessive morbidity and mortality associated with anterior exenteration, along with impotency and the necessity for urinary diversion, requiring adaptation to a different life-style. Proponents of surgical extirpation alone pointed out the significant complications and hazards of high dose radiation therapy, the significant failure rate with radiation therapy alone, and the inability of radiation therapy to prevent subsequent recurrence elsewhere in the bladder. With either radiation therapy or radical cystectomy as a single modality of therapy, one undeniable fact was obvious—failure of therapy due either to local tumor recurrence or distant metastases was noted in a high percentage of patients. The five-year survival rate for invasive bladder cancer with either modality was consistently between 15 and 30%.

Miller,[1] in 1971, reported on the results of definitive radiation therapy in 529 patients treated at the M.D. Anderson Hospital. A mortality rate directly attributable to radiation was reported in 5%, and a 15% major complication rate was reported with respect to bladder, rectal or small bowel injuries. Other factors that were thought to contribute to the failure of radiation therapy included portal size inadequate to encompass the entire tumor, undetected metastases prior to initiation of radiation therapy, the inability of radiation therapy to prevent subsequent recurrence in the bladder mucosa, and ineffectiveness of radiation therapy to sterilize the hypoxic relatively radioresistant cells in the center of large bulky tumors with necrosis or anoxia.

Radical exenterative surgery also had potential mortality and morbidity. Whitmore and Marshall,[2] in 1956, reported significant postoperative complications of urinary or enterocutaneous fistula, small bowel obstruction, and major wound infections in approximately 30% of patients. As with radiation therapy, there are certain factors inherent in failure of surgical therapy. The extent of operation may be insufficient to remove all local tumor, undetected metastases might be present prior to surgery, local tumor spill may lead to pelvic recurrence, and tumor manipulation at the time of cystectomy may increase the possibility of dissemination of tumor cells.

The failure rate of either radiation therapy or radical cystectomy as a single definitive modality of therapy, and the possibility that combination of the two modalities of therapy could improve survival rates by eliminating some of the inherent disadvantages of each, led to trials of combinations of radiation therapy and cystectomy. Prior to consideration of the results of some of these trials, the theoretical and experimental manifestations of radiation therapy and its combination with extirpative surgery will be considered briefly.

RADIATION THERAPY: THEORETICAL CONSIDERATIONS

The effects of radiation therapy, either direct or indirect, are random in nature. The major biological effect of radiation concerns interaction with DNA. A cell that sustains enough damage to the DNA content may lose its reproductive integrity and thus face cell death when or after it attempts cell division. A cell that has sustained radiation-induced lethality may given rise to several daughter cells that ultimately will die when they face cell division. Thus, cells with a long doubling time may appear morphologically viable for extended periods of time prior to attempted cell division and subsequent death.

When cells are treated with irradiation, lethal damage can occur or the damage may be modified so that cell death need not occur. This modification of damage is referred to as repair and can be divided into potentially lethal damage repair and sublethal damage repair. When damage sufficient to prevent reproduction has been sustained, the cell has been sterilized and will no longer be clonogenic (lethal damage). Sublethal damage represents injury to the cell that can be repaired prior to the next dose of therapy. An enhancement in survival that occurs when a dose of radiation is divided as compared to a single dose has been interpreted as the repair of sublethal damage in survivors of the first dose. Sublethal damage can be accumulated and accounts for the initial shoulder seen in cell survival curves after treatment with radiation. Potentially lethal damage is damage which, if unmodified, will lead to cell death. However, if the postirradiation conditions are modified to allow repair, cells which would have died ordinarily can be salvaged. Those postirradiation conditions that suppress cell division are most likely to promote repair of potentially lethal damage.[3] Sublethal and potentially lethal damage repair may be important in relating cell culture studies in human tumors to the clinical response *in vivo*.

Bladder cancer cells may have a variable response to radiation therapy, depending upon the innate responsiveness of the tumor cell and the conditions under which radiation therapy is applied. Radiosensitivity (D_0), the innate sensitivity of cells to radiation, is the inverse of the slope of the radiation survival curve. Radioresponsiveness is a term defining the clinical appearance of tumor regression promptly following moderate doses of radiation therapy. Radioresponsiveness does not necessarily indicate that the tumor will be controlled permanently, since radioresponsiveness is a function of the radiosensitivity of the cell itself and also a function of the active cell kinetics (cell kill and cell loss factor) of the tumor. Since most cells do not die until they face mitosis, rapidly proliferating tumors will regress more rapidly than slowly proliferating tumors. Tumors with a high growth fraction and a high cell loss may show moderate regression without moderate cell kill. Conversely, slowly growing tumors may be controlled at a high frequency but regress slowly. Radiocurability means that the normal tissue relationships of the tumor are such that a potentially curative dose of radiation can be delivered without excessive damage to the normal tissue.

The theoretical rationale for radiation therapy in the treatment of invasive bladder cancer has been based on the assumption that bladder cancer cells are radiosensitive and that the environment of these radiosensitive cells is conducive to the therapeutic effects of radiation. Experiments by Powers and Palmer[4] have shown that normal and tumor cells derived from transitional epithelium are radiosensitive both *in vivo* and *in vitro*. In addition to inherent radiosensitivity to radiation, the environment of cells at the time of radiation may have a great deal to do with the radioresponsiveness. Factors such as blood supply and the degree of oxygenation have been postulated to be as important as the inherent cellular radiosensitivity in determining the beneficial effects of radiation therapy in the treatment of a particular type of neoplasm. The oxygen enhancement ratio, the ratio of dose required for equivalent cell killing in the absence as compared to the presence of oxygen, varies from about 2.5–3.5. This means that for a given survival level, 3 times as much radiation is required under hypoxic conditions than under normal oxygenated conditions.[5]

One final consideration with radiation therapy is the fractionation or size and number of radiation treatment increments. Fractionation of radiation therapy dose dates back to the early part of this century when it was observed that fractionation allowed more effective tumor cure without excessive complications to normal tissue. Thus, the total dose, the dose delivered per fraction and the time between fractions seem to be important for both tumor control and damage of normal tissue. The ratio of tumor damage to normal tissue damage is defined as the therapeutic ratio. The patient tolerance of radiation also depends upon the volume irradiated, the amount and type of dose-limiting normal tissue, the age of the patient, and the quality of the radiation (*i.e.* orthovoltage or supervoltage). All of this must be taken into account in planning for radiation therapy.

In addition to the above-mentioned factors, several other important principles of radiation therapy have emerged. A relatively small dose of 500–1000 rads may inactivate a substantial portion of the total cell population. A large dose of 6000–7000 rads is necessary in order to ensure enough cell kill to provide a high probability of cure.[6] Since radiation therapy kills by first order kinetics, the proportion of cells inactivated with each incremental dose of radiation appears to remain unchanged. Therefore, additional doses of radiation, which inactivate the same proportion of cells, actually affect a progressively smaller total number of cells.[7]

The dose required to eradicate small tumor foci has been shown to be proportional to tumor size. Suit[8] found that spherical tumor nodules of 10^5 fully oxygenated cells (0.57 mm in diameter) required 2400 rads for eradication, 10^3 (0.12 mm in diameter) needed 1600 rads, and 10^2 cells (0.06 mm in diameter) needed 1240 rads.

Although these principles have ramifications for definitive radiation therapy they also have important ramifications for radiation therapy as an adjunct to surgery. The factors thought to account for early failures in cancer treatment by operation alone—microscopic tumor extension, tumor spill, or dissemination during manipulation—would lend themselves well to the adjunctive use of radiation therapy and thereby, hopefully, improve the effectiveness of overall local therapy.

Certain experimental studies would lend credence to the effectiveness of radiation therapy as an adjunct to surgery. Hoye and Smith[9] found that tumor take was diminished by 90% by the use of subcurative preoperative radiation therapy. In animal experiments using five different transplantable tumors, the growth of tumor disseminated intravascularly, intramuscularly, or into an axillary wound was decreased by more than 90% using radiation doses as small as 715 rads. Perez,[10] in 1970, reviewed the literature and attempted to define the optimal dose of radiation, optimal timing of operation, and optimal fractionation of the dose for a variety of experimental studies in animal tumor systems.

Inch and McCredie,[7] utilizing the C3H mammary tumor in mice, needed 6000 rads to effect a 90% cure rate. However, with doses of 2000 rads preoperatively compared to surgery alone, recurrence rates at 3 months postoperation were 61% with surgery alone and 42% with irradiation and surgery when excision was done 6 days after the irradiation. There was no significant difference, however, when excision was done 1 day or 12 days postirradiation. They also showed that local tumor recurrence was reduced from 45 to 10% by the addition of 2000 rads 24 hours prior to removal of a murine carcinosarcoma.

All of the above mentioned studies tend to support the thesis that small doses of preoperative irradiation can favorably influence the survival rate with certain tumors.

RADIATION THERAPY: CLINICAL EFFECTS IN BLADDER CANCER

In consideration of the hypothetical role of radiation therapy as an adjunct to bladder cancer, several important ramifications must be evaluated in a clinical setting. First, are transitional cell tumors of the urinary tract radiosensitive tumors? If the tumor cells are in fact radiosensitive, does the addition of radiation therapy prevent local pelvic recurrence? Does preoperative radiation therapy damage cells so that they are incapable of implantation as distant metastases and thereby decrease the incidence of distant disease during tumor manipulation? Does radiation therapy in an adjunctive setting increase the overall long-term survival rate? Each of these aspects is important but the last mentioned aspect, that of long-term survival, is of the utmost importance.

Radiosensitivity of Transitional Cell Carcinoma

Several observations have suggested innate radiosensitivity of transitional cell carcinoma to the effects of radiation therapy. Preoperative radiation therapy has produced a marked diminution in the implantation in the subcutaneous tissue of cancer cells after partial cystectomy.[11] Additionally, preoperative radiation therapy has been shown to decrease tumor stage (downstaging), sometimes even to the absence of tumor in the resected specimen.[12, 13]

Van der Werf-Messing[11] has clearly shown that low doses of preoperative radiation therapy, as small as 1000–1500 rads, can eliminate local wound recurrence in the cystotomy incision in patients receiving interstitial radiation therapy.[11] She showed that wound implants, documented in 7 of 29 patients with stage T_3 bladder cancer without preoperative radiation therapy, were reduced to 3 of 53 (5.7%) in patients who received 1500 rads preoperatively and 0 of 34 in patients who received 1050 rads preoperatively. The most important benefit was seen in patients with stage B_2 or C (T_3) bladder cancer, whereas patients with B_1 (T_2) bladder cancer had very few wound implants with or without preoperative radiation therapy.

Downstaging of bladder cancer by radiation would be another important indication of radioresponsiveness. Van der Werf-Messing[14] described a series of 59 patients with clinical stage B_2 or C (T_3) bladder cancer in which $2/3$ were downstaged after 4000 rads of external beam irradiation. In a more recent series, van der Werf-Messing[12] analyzed 42 patients who were found to have absence of tumor in the surgical specimen after completion of 4000 rads of preoperative radiation therapy. Of these patients, 25 (60%) had documented cancer in the muscle in the initial biopsy specimen, suggesting a marked radiation therapy response in $2/3$ of this series of patients.

Prout and associates,[13] with the National Bladder Cooperative Study, reported that preoperative radiation therapy of 4000–4500 rads would lead to tumor downstaging in 50% of patients and that 30% of patients were found to have no tumor in the cystectomy specimen. In their subsequent series, approximately 8–10% of patients were found to have no tumor in the cystectomy specimen, presumably on the basis of the transurethral biopsy alone. Therefore, the difference, approximately 25%, would appear to have been radiosensitive and radioresponsive with downstaging to P_0 after radiation therapy.

Although these observations do suggest a major impact on tumor growth by radiation therapy, the implications of the significance of presumed tumor downstaging have been questioned. Downstaging has been noted more frequently with papillary tumors rather than those with a solid appearance.[15] Papillary tumors, however, tend to invade muscle on a more superficial basis than do those of a solid configuration.[16] Papillary tumors on giant histologic sections are found to invade in a finger-like fashion rather than on a broad front of cells.[16] Papillary-type tumors also tend to involve the bladder vasculature and lymphatics less frequently than do solid tumors. Taken together, these features could suggest that papillary lesions might be more amenable to total resection by simple transurethral methods.

Control of Regional Disease and Local Recurrence by Radiation Therapy

One potential area of major benefit for adjunctive radiation therapy has been in the control of regional nodal involvement and prevention of local tumor recurrence. Van der Werf-Messing[12] has reported that downstaging of tumors carried a lower incidence of regional nodal involvement (8%) as compared to patients who were not downstaged after radiation therapy (37%). Bloom and associates,[17] in a large controlled series of preoperative radiation therapy and cystectomy *versus* radical radiotherapy for deeply invasive bladder cancer, reported that only 5.5% of patients who were downstaged after radiation therapy were noted to have metastases to the regional lymph nodes as compared to 34% of patients who did not experience downstaging.[17] These findings have been interpreted to suggest a radiosensitivity of the regional pelvic lymph nodes that correlates with the radiosensitivity of the primary tumor.

Radiosensitivity and radioresponsiveness as documented by downstaging should also correlate with a decreased incidence of pelvic tumor recurrence. This fact was observed by Whitmore,[18] who reported a decrease in clinical pelvic recurrence from 37% of patients with T_3 tumors who had undergone cystectomy alone to 20% of patients after 4000 rds, and 18% after 2000 rads of preoperative irradiation. Furthermore, in those patients who experienced downstaging of their primary tumor, pelvic recurrence was only 6% after 4000 rads and 4% after 2000 rads. Wallace and Bloom[19] reported that in patients who had received 4000 rads of preoperative radiotherapy, the incidence of pelvic lymph node metastases was 23% and when the cystectomy specimen showed no evidence of tumor, regional lymph node involvement was present in only 8%. This stands in marked contrast to the 40–50% expected regional lymph node involvement in their series.

Control of Distant Disease by Radiation Therapy

The question as to whether radiation therapy can affect dissemination of viable cells during surgical manipulation has not been answered effectively. Approximately 50% of patients who present with clinical stage B bladder cancer will subsequently die of distant metastases.

Whether these distant metastases represent preexisting unrecognized implantation or whether the metastases occur as a result of surgical manipulation cannot be answered at the present time. The occurrence of metastases is a complex problem representing a cascade of events from lymphatic permeation, to survival in the blood stream, to implantation at a distant site. The recognition of cancer cells appearing in the blood stream following surgical manipulation has been recognized following radical mastectomy and other major operative procedures. An unanswered question is how viable these manipulated cells are and how likely they are to subsequently implant and cause metastases. In experimental models, undifferentiated tumors were found to be most likely to shed cells directly into lymphatics and blood vessels and that more anaplastic tumors were found to favor cellular detachment.[20, 21] Importantly, the phenomena of tissue invasiveness and subsequent metastases may occur in the course of a tumor, possibly even before the local malignancy has been recognized.[22]

Thus, in bladder cancer, metastases may take place at an early phase of development of the tumor, especially with the solid, more anaplastic, cancers. If this were the case, then radiation therapy in the prevention of distant metastases would be expected to have a minimal effect.

Effect of Radiation Therapy on Long-Term Survival

The most important documentation of the effectiveness of radiation therapy as an adjunct in patients with bladder cancer rests on whether or not it enhances survival. Much of the experience recorded in the literature has been in the form of retrospective or phase II studies which, unfortunately, do not include a control arm. Although most reports have suggested that radiation therapy does enhance long-term survival, these conclusions have been based upon comparisons with historical groups or groups receiving radiation therapy alone compared to radiation and cystectomy together. For the most part, studies that have attempted to compare cystectomy alone with preoperative radiation plus cystectomy in a randomized fashion have been flawed by patient selection, inadequate staging, and large numbers of patient exclusions.[23] Radwin[23] has suggested that improvements in survival attributed to radiation therapy may have reflected factors other than radiation therapy, such as reduced operative mortality in more series, earlier recognition and institution of treatment, and better selection for particular types of treatment.

Despite the potential criticisms of these studies, a review of them may provide some insights into the rationale for integrated preoperative radiation therapy and cystectomy. In 1973, Miller and Johnson[24] reported a prospective randomized study that compared definitive radiation therapy to combined radiation therapy and radical cystectomy without lymph node dissection. With the integrated radiation therapy plus cystectomy, these authors reported a 53% 5-year survival rate for patients with stage B_2 or C bladder cancer. The therapeutic program was well tolerated. The local recurrence rate was reduced by one-third with the addition of radiation therapy and cystectomy and the 5-year survival for stage B_2 and C bladder cancer was tripled. Thus, there seems little argument that radiation therapy combined with surgery was superior to radiation therapy alone.

During the 1960s, Whitmore and others began to combine radiation therapy with surgery. In a pilot series of 30 patients treated with 4000 rads of preoperative radiation therapy followed by radical cystectomy, Whitmore[25] reported a 37% 5-year survival rate for stage B_2 or C tumors compared to a 17% 5-year survival rate for a group of patients treated by cystectomy alone. This series has been expanded by sequential treatment groups—137 patients treated by surgery alone from 1949–1959, 119 patients treated by 4000 rads of preoperative radiation therapy followed by radical cystectomy from 1959–1966, and 86 patients treated by 2000 rads of preoperative radiation therapy from 1966–1971.[26] A detailed analysis of their data reveals that the overall impact of preoperative radiation therapy on the results of cystectomy was negligible. However, in patients with T_3 tumors subjected to cystectomy, planned preoperative irradiation improved the survival rate from 16–46%. The favorable effects of preoperative irradiation therapy were largely restricted to those patients in whom tumors were downstaged and most specifically to those that were found to have no tumor within the bladder specimen. Long-term high dose (4000 rads) irradiation was not found to be superior to short-course low dose (2000 rads) irradiation. The pelvic recurrence rate in their series was 10% and treatment failures were largely attributable to metastatic systemic disease. In general, the radiation therapy given was well tolerated and there were no adverse effects from the use of preoperative irradiation except for minor delay in wound healing and mild radiation enteritis. Although these studies were sequential and not with randomized concordant control, the dramatic decrease in pelvic recurrence and the overall increase in survival for tumors that were downstaged does suggest a role of radiation therapy as an adjunct to radical cystectomy.

In 1964, the National Cooperative Bladder Cancer Group began to evaluate preoperative radiation therapy and cystectomy compared with radical cystectomy alone. Preliminary results suggested that preoperative irradiation therapy did not improve overall survival; however, later analysis revealed that the 5-year survival rate for irradiated patients who had no tumor in the cystectomy specimen was 44% as opposed to 25% for patients who were not irradiated and who did have tumor remaining in the bladder.[27] Furthermore, following transurethral resection of the bladder tumor alone, 10% had no residual tumor as compared with 35% who had no residual tumor after receiving radiation therapy in addition to transurethral resection of the bladder. The subgroup of patients who appeared to have been helped by preoperative irradiation therapy were predominantly those with papillary carcinomas as opposed to solid tumors—stage reduction to P_0 (no residual tumor) occurred in 42% of the papillary tumors compared with 30% of the solid tumors. In those patients who received preoperative radiation therapy, fewer pulmonary metastases were noted as the first evidence of treatment failure than in those patients who had undergone cystectomy alone. This may have a bearing in such a way that cells disseminated by operative manipulation are less capable of implantation.

In an elegant study by Bloom and associates,[17] a controlled clinical trial of preoperative radiation therapy and radical cystectomy was compared to treatment with radical radiation therapy alone or with salvage cystectomy. Four thousand rads of preoperative radiation therapy plus cystectomy *versus* 6000 rads of definitive radiation therapy for stage T_3 or B_2/C tumors was explored in a multicenter prospective randomized trial involving 189 patients. The 5-year survival rate for integrated treatment was 44% compared to 31% with radiation therapy alone, with or without salvage cystectomy. Patients who were downstaged had a significant survival advantage over those patients whose tumors remained deeply infiltrating, 64% *versus* 27%. Those patients who experienced complete response to definitive radiation therapy, with no evidence of tumor on repeat cystoscopy, had a 49% 5-year survival compared to 25% with a partial response and 10% with no response. Most importantly, in patients who responded to radiation therapy, the survival rate was superior in the integrated radiation therapy and cystectomy group *vis-a-vis* those patients who experienced a response to radiation therapy, 64% *versus* 41% 5-year survival. Equally importantly, in those patients who did not experience tumor downstaging, the 5-year survival was superior for integrated irradiation therapy compared to definitive irradiation and salvage cystectomy, 27% *versus* 14%. These results indicate that the survival is superior for tumors that have been downstaged but that, overall, radiation therapy plus surgery was superior to radiation therapy alone in each subgroup. Although radiotherapy followed by salvage cystectomy is clearly inferior to planned integrated therapy in terms of survival, some patients who cannot accept the sequellae of cystectomy may opt for purportedly less morbid treatment.[28]

Evidence from these studies supports the contention that radiation therapy given in a preoperative adjuvant fashion has a profound effect on the primary invasive bladder cancer and that it can be safely combined with radical surgery. It can improve the survival rate in patients with deeply invasive tumors, particularly those whose tumors are downstaged by radiation. It is worthwhile to recall, however, that not all patients benefitted from preoperative radiation therapy.

CONCLUSIONS

Although controversial, there is evidence to support the combination of preoperative radiation therapy followed by cystectomy as an integrated form of therapy that can improve survival. Although evidence has been presented that some of the improved survival can be related to surgical technique and management, there does remain a subset of patients who do respond to radiation therapy with tumor downstaging and this subset clearly benefits from preoperative radiation therapy. The idea of avoiding a cystectomy in patients whose bladder tumors disappear after radiation therapy is attractive but dangerous, as demonstrated by Sagerman et al.[29] and Engel et al.[30] Sagerman et al.[29] describe two patients who had negative biopsies after 3000 rads of external beam radiation therapy and then received an additional 3000 rads; both were noted to have recurrences in less than a year. Engels' group[30] described

12 patients with partial cystectomy after apparent disappearance of tumor; 6 subsequently suffered recurrences.

Clearly, although all patients do not benefit from radiation therapy preoperatively, a group of patients with radiosensitive and radioresponsive tumors does exist. There has been great interest in identifying this subset of patients whose tumors will disappear after radiation therapy, as opposed to those who will not. If this group could be distinguished, therapy could be administered to those patients who would benefit, while the patients who would not be expected to benefit would be spared preoperative irradiation therapy. Slack and Prout[31] have described the heterogeneity of invasive bladder cancer, looking specifically at downstaging and its association with lymphatic permeation and tumor appearance. They reported that patients with solid tumors and lymphatic permeation tended to have persistent tumor in the cystectomy specimen, experiencing a 20% 5-year survival rate. Patients with papillary tumors and no lymphatic permeation most often experienced tumor downstaging to P_0 and a 5-year survival rate of approximately 80%. Their conclusion was that preoperative radiation therapy not be indicated in patients with solid tumors and lymphatic permeation.

The M. D. Anderson group has reviewed 159 patients who had undergone preoperative radiation therapy and radical cystectomy.[32] They concluded that precystectomy evaluation of stage, grade, appearance, or lymphatic permeation did not allow prediction of downstaging or disappearance of the tumor. However, this group found that both downstaging and the absence of muscle invasion were associated with significantly higher 5-year survival rates and disease-free intervals.

All the above studies point out the need to identify predictive factors in patients with bladder tumors, and thus allow more tailored therapy. We have investigated the effects of ionizing radiation on human bladder cell lines as an *in vitro* study of radiobiology.[33] We have shown that a reasonable degree of consistency can be demonstrated for the radiobiologic characteristics of human transitional cell lines maintained *in vitro*. If this technique can be utilized for the evaluation of bladder tumors *ex vivo* following limited biopsy, then perhaps a more rational selection of radiation therapy as a preoperative adjunct can be made. As in many other tumor systems at the current time, our inability to recognize distinctions in the heterogeneity of the tumor and its implications for behavior have hampered our therapeutic efforts. The search must continue to further define parameters that will allow prediction of the best results of integrated therapy, be it adjunctive radiation therapy, adjunctive chemotherapy, or some newer forms of therapy as yet unrecognized.

REFERENCES

1. Miller, L. S. Clinical evaluation and therapy for urinary bladder: radiotherapy. In *Diagnosis and Management of Cancer: Specific Sites*, p. 283. Year Book Medical Publishers, Chicago, 1971.
2. Whitmore, W. F., Jr., and Marshall, V. F. Radical surgery for carcinoma of the urinary bladder. *Cancer 9:*596, 1956.
3. Richie, J. P., Weichselbaum, R. R., and Little, J. B. Importance of repair of potentially lethal damage in assays of cytotoxic agents. *Surgery 92:*380, 1982.
4. Powers, W. E., and Palmer, L. A. Biologic basis of preoperative radiation treatment. *AJR 102:*176, 1968.

5. Belli, J. A., Discus, G. J., and Bonte, F. J. Radiation response of mammalian tumor cells. 1. Repair of sublethal damage *in vivo. J. Nat. Cancer Inst. 38:*673, 1967.

6. Powers, W. E., and Tolmach, L. J. A multicomponent x-ray survival curve for mouse lymphosarcoma cells irradiated *in vivo. Nature 197:*710, 1963.

7. Inch, W. R., and McCredie, J. A. Effect of a small dose of x-radiation on local recurrence of tumors in rats and mice. *Cancer 16:*595, 1963.

8. Suit, H. D. *Textbook of Radiotherapy,* p. 91. Lea & Febiger, Philadelphia, 1966.

9. Hoye, R. C., and Smith, R. R. The effectiveness of small amounts of preoperative irradiation in preventing the growth of tumor cells disseminated at surgery. An experimental study. *Cancer 14:*284, 1961.

10. Perez, C. A. Preoperative irradiation in the treatment of cancer. Experimental observation and clinical implications. *Front. Radiat. Ther. Oncol. 5:*1, 1970.

11. van der Werf-Messing, B. Carcinoma of the bladder treated by suprapubic radium implants. The value of additional external irradiation. *Eur. J. Cancer 5:*277, 1969.

12. van der Werf-messing, B. Preoperative irradiation followed by cystectomy to treat carcinoma of the urinary bladder category T_3 Nx, 0-4MO. *Int. J. Radiat. Oncol. Biol. Phys. 5:*395, 1979.

13. Prout, G. R., Jr., Slack, N. H., and Bross, I. D. J. Irradiation and 5-fluorourcil as adjuvants in the management of invasive bladder carcinoma. A cooperative group report after 4 years. *J. Urol 104:*116, 1970.

14. van der Werf-Messing, B. Carcinoma of the bladder treated by preoperative irradiation followed by cystectomy. *Cancer 32:*1084, 1973.

15. Slack, N. H., Bross, I. D., and Prout, G. R., Jr. Five-year follow-up results of a collaborative study of therapies for carcinoma of the bladder. *J. Surg. Oncol. 9:*393, 1977.

16. Soto, E. A., Friedell, G. H., and Tiltman, A. J. Bladder cancer as seen in giant histologic sections. *Cancer 39:*447, 1977.

17. Bloom, H. J. G., Hendry, W. F., Wallace, D. M., and Skeet, R. G. Treatment of T_3 bladder cancer: controlled trial of preoperative radiotherapy and radical cystectomy *versus* radical radiotherapy. Second report and review (for the Clinical Trials Group, Institute of Urology). *Br. J. Urol. 54:*136, 1982.

18. Whitmore, W. F., Jr. Management of bladder cancer. *Curr. Prob. Cancer 4:*1, 1979.

19. Wallace, D. M., and Bloom, H. J. G. The management of deeply infiltrating (T_3) bladder carcinoma: controlled trial of radical radiotherapy *versus* preoperative radiotherapy and radical cystectomy (first report). *Br. J. Urol. 48:*587–594, 1976.

20. Weiss, L. Cell detachment and metastasis. In *Cancer Metastasis, Approaches to the Mechanism, Prevention and Treatment,* p. 25, edited by P. G. Stansly and H. Sato. Tokyo University Press, Tokyo, 1977.

21. Golinger, R. C., Gregorio, R. M., and Fisher, E. R. Tumor cells in venous blood draining mammary carcinomas. *Arch. Surg. 112:*707, 1977.

22. Fisher, B., Slack, N., Katrych, D., and Wolmark, N. Ten-year follow-up results of patients with carcinoma of the breast in a cooperative clinical trial evaluating surgical adjuvant chemotherapy. *Surg. Gynecol. Obstet. 140:*528, 1975.

23. Radwin, H. M. Radiotherapy and bladder cancer: a critical review. *J. Urol. 124:*43, 1980.

24. Miller, L. S., and Johnson, D. E. Proceedings: megavoltage irradiation for bladder cancer: alone, postoperative, or preoperative. *Proc. Natl. Cancer Conf 7:*771, 1973.

25. Whitmore, W. F., Jr. The treatment of bladder tumors. *Surg. Clin. North Am. 49:*349, 1969.

26. Whitmore, W. F. Integrated irradiation and cystectomy for bladder cancer. *Br. J. Urol. 52:*1, 1980.

27. Prout, G. R., Jr. The surgical management of bladder carcinoma. *Urol. Clin. North. Am. 3:*149, 1976.

28. McNeil, B. J., Weichselbaum, R. R., and Paucker, S. Speech and survival: trade-offs between quality and quantity of life in laryngeal cancer. *N. Engl. J. Med. 305:*982–987, 1981.

29. Sagerman, R. H., Veenema, R. J., Guttmann, R., *et al.* Preoperative irradiation for carcinoma of the bladder. *AJR 102:*577, 1980.

30. Engle, R. M., Urtasum, R. C., Jewett, J. H., and Lott, S. J. Treatment of infiltrating

188   BLADDER CANCER

bladder cancer by cobalt 60 radiation: recurrence of tumor in bladder after initial disappearance. *J. Urol. 101:*859, 1969.

31. Slack, N. H., and Prout, G. R., Jr. The heterogeneity of invasive bladder carcinoma and different responses to treatment. *J. Urol. 123:*644, 1980.

32. Boileau, M. A., Johnson, D. E., Chan, R. C., and Gonzales, M. O. Bladder carcinoma: results with preoperative radiation therapy and radical cystectomy. *Urology 16:*569, 1980.

33. Richie, J. P., Weichselbaum, R. R., Dahlberg, W., and Little, J. B. Effects of ionizing radiation on human bladder cell lines: an *in vitro* radiobiologic study. *Surg. Forum, 34:*674–675, 1983.

14

Chemotherapy of Bladder Cancer

Michele Pavone-Macaluso, M.D.
Maria Tripi, M.D.
Carlo Pavone, M.D.
Giovan Battista Ingargiola, M.D.

Since the advent of chemotherapy in the oncological armamentarium after World War II it has been hoped that this new weapon would be of great help in addition to the conventional methods of treatment of bladder cancer. We have been interested in this topic for the last 20 years and our early experimental and preliminary clinical results and considerations have appeared in the current urological literature.[1,2] Our further experience was mainly obtained through multicenter cooperation in Europe within the activities of the European Organization for Research on Treatment of Cancer (EORTC) urological group.[3]

As pointed out by Smith,[4] who acted for many years as a leader of this group, the management of tumors of the bladder still leaves much to be desired. Those which are superficial can usually be controlled by transurethral resection but tend to recur. Even in the best hands radical radiotherapy, cystectomy and combination of radiotherapy and surgery cannot offer 5-year survivals in excess of 40% for patients with category T_3 lesions. Few patients with category T_4 bladder cancer survive longer than a year. These figures have shown very little improvement over the last decades. The members of the EORTC urological group believed, therefore, that the time had come to evaluate alternative treatments with special reference to the use of cytotoxic chemotherapy.

Patients with bladder tumors fall naturally into three groups, those with T_1 lesions for whom intravesical chemotherapy may be helpful, those with T_2 and T_3 lesions in whom adjuvant chemotherapy (in addition to either radical surgery or radiotherapy, or both) may be life-saving, and those with T_4 cancer or metastatic disease in whom chemotherapy may produce some remission.

Rather than trying to produce a complete review of the entire literature which would be an enormous task, we prefer to concentrate our efforts on providing an updated review of the European experience, with special emphasis on the work of the EORTC urological group. For more extensive reviews of the whole area of chemotherapy of bladder the reader is referred to some recent surveys, articles and books, related to this field.[5-10]

CHEMOTHERAPY OF ADVANCED BLADDER CANCER

When Carter and Wasserman[11] reviewed the status of systemic chemotherapy of bladder cancer from the current literature existing in 1975, it appeared that only three agents had been adequately evaluated. Namely, mitomycin C, 5-fluorouracil (5-FU) and doxorubicin (Adriamycin) had been reported to produce remission rates of 25, 30 and 35%, respectively. Further experience with doxorubicin showed a remission rate of 11%, with a median remission duration of 3 months.[12] Doxorubicin-based combinations failed to show a longer duration of remissions.

Combinations of doxorubicin with cyclophosphamide or Teniposide (VM-26) were not superior to doxorubicin alone. The EORTC urological group[13] reported that the combination of doxorubicin and 5-FU was well tolerated, with a remission rate of 40%, but could not provide any demonstration of the superiority of the combination over the single constituents. It was suggested, however, that doxorubicin was likely to be the more active of the agents employed, since no patient who responded relapsed while on the doxorubicin treatment, but many did so after the maximum dose of doxorubicin (550 mg/m^2) had been given and the patients were kept on maintenance with 5-FU alone. Cyclophosphamide had shown activity in relatively old studies[14] but was not adequately tested with modern criteria thereafter.

Conversely, another old drug, methotrexate, has been widely employed in recent years[15] and found to be among the most effective agents. Median remission duration is 6 months and remission rate varies between 53% in the series from the Royal Marsden Hospital and 28% in that from the Memorial Sloan Kettering Cancer Center. It should be noted, however, that the remission rate was 42% when methotrexate was administered in previously untreated patients.

Cisplatin is now considered to be the most active single agent in the treatment of advanced bladder cancer.[16] Remission rate in nonpretreated patients is 40–50% and median remission duration is 6 months. The overall response rate, adding together 120 patients from various series, is 35%. Cisplatin-based combinations (cisplatin and cyclophosphamide or doxorubicin or both, or cisplatin and 5-FU), again display a median remission duration of 6 months and response rates ranging from 40–57% in well documented series.

There is no evidence, however, that cisplatin combinations improve the clinical results, while it appears that the addition of side-effects from multiple drugs may represent an increased burden of toxicity for the patient.

If we take into consideration the most extensively employed agents, the results can be summarized as shown in Table 14.1.

Table 14.1
Response Rates in Advanced Bladder Cancer From Chemotherapy with Three Widely Used Agents

Drug	Response rates (from the current literature)	
	Pretreated Patients	Non Pretreated Patients
	%	%
Cisplatin	35	45
Methotrexate	30	40
Doxorubicin	15	25

The EORTC urological group, after the first phase II trials mentioned above,[12,13] has implemented further studies with the objective of evaluating the combination of cisplatin with other drugs and to discover new active agents. A strict selection of patients was adopted, accepting only transitional cell carcinoma, and excluding epidermoid carcinoma or other rare histotypes. Only patients with measurable primary or metastatic disease were entered. Those having only vaguely "evaluable" lesions were not eligible.

It was also requested that patients with poor performance status, reduced renal function or congestive heart failure be excluded from the studies.

Three consecutive studies (30771, 30802 and 30821) were aimed at finding successful cisplatin combinations. Studies of new drugs initiated so far include vincristine (30797) and mitoxantrone (30823). A short report of published studies and preliminary information about on-going studies will be given here in some detail. The most important data are summarized in Table 14.2.

EORTC Study 30771

The objective of this study was to establish the actual response rate of the combination of cisplatin, doxorubicin and cyclophosphamide, administered intravenously at the dose of 40, 40 and 400 mg/m^2, respectively, every 3 weeks. This combination, known as CISCA or CAP, had been submitted to preliminary evaluation in other institutions with an initial report of a 90% response rate in a rather limited number of patients.[17] In the report from EORTC Urological Group[18], 52 patients were registered, 5 were ineligible and 5 were unevaluable. Of the 42 patients evaluable for response, 5 (11.9%) had a complete and 12 (28.6%) had a partial response with an overall objective response rate of 40.5%. The toxicity was not negligible, since all patients presented alopecia and suffered from nausea and vomiting. Severe nephrotoxicity was observed in 3 of 52 (6%) patients evaluable for toxicity. Bone marrow depression, when present, was rather mild. The conclusion was that the CAP combination did not seem to yield better results than would be expected from cisplatin alone.

EORTC Study 30802

The rationale for this combination was that preliminary experience from the same group[12] had shown some activity of Teniposide (VM-

Table 14.2
EORTC Urological Group: Trials of Systemic Chemotherapy for Advanced Bladder Cancer

Trial No.	Coordinator	Drug (s)	Number of Evaluable Patients	Response Rate	In Reference
				%	
1	M. Pavone-Macaluso	Doxorubicin	18	11.1	12
		VM-26	30	16.6	
		Bleomycin	33	15.1	
2	M. Robinson and P. H. Smith	Doxorubicin +5-FU	52	40.0	13
30771	J. H. Mulder	Cisplatin + Doxorubicin + Cyclophosphamide	44	34.0	18
30797	B. Richards	Vincristine	26	19.2	20
30802	G. Stoter	Cisplatin + VM-26	41	51.0	19

26), with an overall response rate of 17% (2 complete and 3 partial remissions in 30 extensively pretreated patients) and that synergism exists between cisplatin and epipodophyllotoxins.

This regimen was given with the following modalities: cisplatin, 70 mg/m^2 I.V. on day 1; and VM-26 100 mg/m^2, I.V. on days 1 and 2. Such a course was repeated every 3 weeks and the patients were considered evaluable for response after a minimum of two courses. The rules for patient selection were similar to those outlined for the previous study. Of 57 patients registered, 8 were ineligible, 8 unevaluable and 41 were evaluable for response. It should be noted that 44% had sustained previous radiotherapy and 15% had had intravesical instillations with chemotherapeutic agents, but no patient had received prior systemic chemotherapy. Of the 41 evaluable patients, 4 (10%) had a complete and 17 (41%) a partial remission, leading to an overall 51% objective response rate. No change was seen in 11 (27%), there was progression in 7 (17%) and early death from malignancy in 2 (5%) patients. Prior radiotherapy did not seem to affect the results. The side effects were quite marked in some patients. Nausea and vomiting led to cessation of the treatment in six patients, and myelotoxicity required dose reduction in seven. The lowest leukocyte count was 1400/mm^3 and the nadir of platelets was 85,000. Questionable renal toxicity could be seen in only one patient. Again, the median response duration was of 6 months and the results were not significantly better than those that could be expected from cisplatin alone in patients not pretreated with systemic chemo-therapy.[19]

EORTC Study 30821

As shown in Table 14.1, it is presently believed that cisplatin and methotrexate are the two most active drugs in the treatment of bladder cancer. It was hoped, therefore, that their combination could be effec-tive, but there was also considerable concern about its safety, since both drugs, especially cisplatin, are potentially nephrotoxic. Methotrexate is excreted to a large extent by the kidneys and it was feared that if renal function is impaired by cisplatin, methotrexate retention would result with a secondary increase in its toxicity.

A pilot phase I study showed, however, that if cisplatin is administered at the dose of 70 mg/m^2 I.V. on day 1 and methotrexate at the dose of 40 mg/m^2 I.V. on days 8 and 15, and such a cycle is repeated every 3 weeks, this regimen is well tolerated and only simple precautions are needed. The study is still in progress and no final results are available, but preliminary analyses from this and similar studies have shown a very encouraging trend, insofar as the complete response rate approaches 25%, *i.e.* is much higher than that obtainable with either drug used alone.[19] If confirmed, these results might form the basis for a successful chemotherapy program to be employed in the adjuvant situation.

EORTC Study 30797

Vincristine is not a new drug, but had never been given an adequate trial in bladder cancer treatment. The EORTC urological group started this as a second choice study for patients who were not eligible to be entered in one of the cisplatin combination trials, especially in view of the fact that vincristine is neither myelotoxic nor nephrotoxic. A schedule of 1 mg/m^2 I.V. weekly for 8 weeks and every 2 weeks thereafter was adopted. Of 43 registered patients, 6 were ineligible, 6 not evaluable and 31 were fully evaluable for response of whom 1 showed a complete remission (3%), 2 a partial remission (6%), with an overall response rate of 10%. Side effects, especially from neurotoxicity, were quite severe and response duration ranged between 2 and 7 months. The conclusion is that vincristine has very little, if any, role to play in the treatment of bladder cancer.[20]

EORTC Study 30823

Mitoxantrone is a new anthracycline derivative, with less cardiotoxicity than doxorubicin in the experimental animals. The study is still on-going and no results are yet available.

Comments

In spite of carefully planned studies from the EORTC urological group, other cooperative forces and large specialized institutions, no significant progress has been made in the field of systemic chemotherapy of advanced bladder cancer.

In spite of a couple of anecdotal cases of long-lasting responses, it can be held that anticancer chemotherapy is still unable to achieve a complete cure of this disease. Its maximum success can be envisaged, therefore, in the prolongation of survival, rarely exceeding a year, in a responding patient in whom objective reduction of tumor mass brings about a symptomatic improvement, such as palliation of pain caused by tissue infiltration or compression due to cancer. If this is kept in mind, the only ethical justification for chemotherapy in this field consists of the likehood of achieving a better quality of life in patients with distressing symptoms, and of the possibility of finding better drugs or drug combinations for future patients. It is imperative, under this regard, that the patients should be treated within the frame of well designed clinical trials, whose results can be adequately and correctly analyzed and interpreted.

It can also be concluded that, if quality of life is our main concern at the present time, attention to side effects from any given treatment should outweigh slight differences in reported response rates.

Until the superiority of combination chemotherapy over the administration of single agents can definitively be proved, much care should be taken to avoid the indiscriminate use of highly toxic cocktails of drugs.

ADJUVANT CHEMOTHERAPY OF INVASIVE BLADDER CANCER

Adjuvant chemotherapy is very appealing to every urologist who is not satisfied with the results of either cystectomy or radical irradiation or both in the treatment of deeply infiltrating bladder cancer.

Adjuvant chemotherapy has become an established way of treatment following surgery of breast cancer, but unfortunately its results have been quite disappointing in other fields of clinical oncology and in almost all other forms of solid tumors. The prerequisites for a successful adjuvant chemotherapy to be used in conjunction (before, during or after) other forms of more effective treatment can be summarized as follows:

1. A regimen of chemotherapy should be available that is capable of completely destroying all residual cells that can escape removal by surgery or destruction by irradiation. This should include prevention of both local recurrences and distant metastases from occult deposits not detectable clinically (so called micrometastases).
2. Such an adjuvant treatment is unlikely to be successful if it is unable to induce a high rate of complete remissions (10–20%) and of overall regressions (50–60%) in the metastatic situation.
3. Adjuvant treatment will unnecessarily be given to patients who will recover even in its absence and therefore must not be exceedingly toxic or potentially lethal.
4. Adjuvant treatment is not be advised if a high rate of complete remissions and permanent cures can be obtained with chemotherapy, should distant metastases appear in the future. In this case, salvage chemotherapy rather than adjuvant chemotherapy is preferable.
5. Routine adjuvant chemotherapy is not recommended until controlled clinical trials have demonstrated a significant increase in survival, a prolongation of free time to progression and lack of severe toxicity.

With regard to bladder cancer it can be stated that, until the encouraging results of the methotrexate-cisplatin combination can be confirmed, none of these prerequisites has been fulfilled. In particular, only a few reports have been published, but they refer to uncontrolled studies, where the value of adjuvant treatment was suggested but never demonstrated. A few well planned randomized clinical trials (chemotherapy *versus* lack of treatment after cystectomy) have been started but, unfortunately, most of them have been stopped and other ones proceed at a rather slow pace, so that their results are not yet available. It should be noted that the tolerance has been, in general, rather poor, especially when dealing with patients who have undergone a lot of traumatic aggressions such as a cystectomy, a lymphadenectomy and a urinary diversion, with or without preoperative irradiation.

Tolerance appears to be especially poor for cisplatin or its combinations, leading to severe nausea and vomiting, which may jeopardize the already unstable nutritional balance of these patients, so that continuation of the treatment is often refused after the first dose. Methotrexate alone is better tolerated and it has been possible for a British study to proceed for some years.[21] Its final results are expected with the greatest interest. Finally, chemotherapy can be used in conjunction with radiotherapy. Although the addition of doxorubicin and 5-fluorouracil after radiation failed to improve the results of radiation alone in a British study, there are some encouraging results from the use of cisplatin together with radiotherapy.[22,23] A wider experience and a longer follow-up will be requested before this can be considered superior to standard irradiation and be adopted as an accepted form of treatment.

LOCO-REGIONAL CHEMOTHERAPY

Intra-arterial chemotherapy is virtually impossible without escape of the drugs into the systemic circulation. Its use has been restricted to only few centers. Encouraging results were recently reported in Europe and in Japan, using intra-arterial infusions of doxorubicin.

Intravesical chemotherapy, already mentioned previously, can be administered for therapy or for prophylaxis. A therapeutic topical treatment can be performed with the aim of obtaining the regression of already established lesions, such as multiple or diffuse superficial neoplastic growths that cannot be removed completely by endoscopy or other methods of conservative surgery, and for carcinoma *in situ* (primary or secondary to concomitant or subsequent exophytic or infiltrating growth).

Intravesical chemotherapy with anticancer drugs is over 20 years old, since the first reports on the topical use of thiotepa. Intravesical instillations are now an accepted treatment for the therapy of superficial papillary tumors that are too extensive to be removed with the resectoscope. In such conditions a complete disappearance of all visible lesions can often be obtained following the use of various drugs, but also a partial response can be of value, insofar as it can enable the surgeon to perform a complete transurethral resection (TUR) of all remaining tumors. Topical chemotherapy has been employed with variable success in the treatment of flat carcinoma *in situ*.

Intravesical instillations can also be employed in the prophylaxis of new tumor formation after TUR of T_a or T_1 transitional cell carcinoma. Detailed reviews of intravesical chemotherapy have been published elsewhere in recent years.[7,9]

Many drugs have been employed for this purpose and, according to our experience and to current literature, they can be divided in various groups, as shown in Table 14.3. Topical immunotherapy with bacillus Calmette-Guérin (BCG) has been reported to be helpful.

The EORTC urological group has implemented four randomized trials in order to compare different drugs among themselves and with lack of postoperative treatment. The most significant data are reported in Table 14.4.

Table 14.3
Treatments Having Been Employed for Chemotherapy, Immunotherapy or Chemoprophylaxis of Papillary Bladder Tumors

Group 1
  Active—Relatively few side effects
    Doxorubicin (Adriamycin)
    Etoglucide (Epodyl)
    Mitomycin C
    BCG
Group 2
  Active—Possibility of systemic toxicity
    Cisplatin (anaphylaxis)
    Thiotepa (myelotoxicity)
Group 3
  Moderately active
    Teniposide (VM-26)
Group 4
  Reported to be active but insufficiently tested
    Daunorubicin
    Mechloretamine
    Peptichemio
Group 5
  Little activity
    Bleomycin
    Cyclophosphamide
    5-fluorouracil (5-FU)
    Methotrexate
Group 6
  Not yet tested
    Etoposide (VP-16)
    Vinca alkaloids
    Actinomycin C
    Various drug combinations

Table 14.4
EORTC Urological Group: Trials of Chemoprophylaxis after TUR for Superficial Bladder Tumors

Trial No.	Coordinator	Drug	Route of Administration	Number of Evaluable Patients	Recurrence Rate	In Reference
30751	C. Schulman	Thiotepa	Intravesical	105	5.4	24
	M. Staquet	Teniposide	Intravesical	99	6.6	25
		None		104	8.9	
30781	M. Robinson	Pyridoxine	Oral			
		Placebo	Oral	On-going		27
30782	L. Denis	Thiotepa	Intravesical			
		Doxorubicin	Intravesical	On-going		26
		Cisplatin	Intravesical			
30790	K. H. Kurth	Doxorubicin	Intravesical	73	2.91	
		Epodyl	Intravesical			27
		None		47	9.17	

Trial 30751

The main points of interest, which have derived from this study have been published in two different papers[24, 25] the first dealing chiefly with the results, the other with the value of the prognostic factors. The design of the study was as follows: there was a preliminary stratification in two groups: primary and recurrent tumors. After urethrocystoscopy and bimanual palpation under anesthesia the papillary tumors were resected by TUR. After histological confirmation of lack of muscular infiltration, but irrespective of the grade (therefore all G_1, G_2 and G_3 were included), the patients were randomized into three groups: thiethylenethiophosphoramide (thiotepa) 30 mg in 50 ml normal saline; Teniposide (VM-26) 50 mg in 50 ml; and lack of treatment. The drugs were retained in the bladder for 1 hour. The first instillation was started only 1 month after TUR. The next instillations were then repeated at weekly intervals for a month and then at monthly intervals for a year, up to a total number of 15 instillations. Blood counts were performed before each instillation. Cystoscopies were repeated every 3 months for the first year. If a recurrence was found, it was resected and considered a true recurrence only after histological confirmation. The drug was not changed, but a weekly regimen was again instituted for the next 4 weeks. After 370 patients were admitted, a trial was closed to entry, but the patients are still being followed-up.

Neither thiotepa nor Teniposide reduced the number of patients showing recurrences as compared to patients receiving no treatment. However, the effects of the treatment can be shown by adopting a parameter which is defined as "recurrence rate," which takes into consideration the total number of recurrent tumors cumulatively discovered in all control cystoscopies per patient per month. To avoid the use of decimals this is multiplied by 100, so that the definition of recurrence rate in this and in the further studies reads "number of recurrent tumors per 100 patients/months." By the use of this formula it was shown that thiotepa was statistically better than no treatment.

Neither a marked bone marrow depression nor a severe chemical cystitis was produced by either thiotepa (30 mg) or Teniposide instillations.

Relevant prognostic factors were identified (or confirmed). Recurrent *versus* primary, multiple *versus* single and high grade *versus* low grade tumors showed a higher recurrence rate. However, the most important single prognostic factor leading to high recurrence rate was the number of recurrent tumors at the presentation followed by those discovered in the year preceding the entry of the patients in the study. This high risk group benefitted the most from intravesical treatment especially with thiotepa.

Free time until first recurrence was not greatly modified by the treatment, although a trend in favor of thiotepa can be suggested, especially in high risk groups. Otherwise the results of instillation were more or less the same, both in primary and in recurrent urotheliomas.

Trial 30781

Study 30781 was aimed to compare oral pyridoxine to a placebo and to correlate recurrence rate with the changes in the urinary excretion of tryptophan metabolites, which are supposed to be endogenous carcinogenic agents, and to be reduced by the oral administration of pyridoxine.

The need for a central laboratory performing the tryptophane metabolites determinations has restricted this study to investigators in Yorkshire. The study has been closed to entry, but no preliminary results have been given either for this or for the next study.

Trial 30782

The design of study 30782 is similar to that of 30751. The main differences consist in the fact that there is no control group. Two new drugs are tested, namely doxorubicin (Adriamycin) and cisplatin, and the dosage of thiotepa has been increased to 50 mg. All drugs are used at the dose of 50 mg in 50 ml. Only patients with recurrent tumors are eligible. The interval between TUR and the first instillation is shortened.

Two subgroups will be analyzed retrospectively, those starting treatment within 2–3 days from TUR and those approaching the maximum allowable interval of 2 weeks.

The incidence of chemical cystitis appeared to be somewhat high in trial 30782, in which it was reported in 12% of patients given doxorubicin. Only in 3% was it severe enough to warrant discontinuation of the treatment. Chemical cystitis was also present in 14% of patients given cisplatin, but was never reported after thiotepa.

The systemic side-effects of local chemotherapy are even more interesting. Thiotepa, 50 mg, produced systemic side-effects in 10% of patients, under the form of leucopenia or, more often, of thrombocytopenia. The latter was quite severe in one patient (23,000 platelets/mm^3) requiring the treatment to be discontinued. This was not unexpected, although most toxicity data reported in the literature resulted from higher doses of thiotepa.

More interesting was, instead, the finding that cisplatin instillations were followed by rather severe systemic side-effects in 14% of the patients. The toxic effect was under the form of anaphylactoid shock, sometimes preceded by a rash, which required interruption in treatment in all patients and was considered life-threatening in some of them. It appeared as a late phenomenon, occurring in the last months of treatment and was described independently by participants from different institutions.[26]

This observation would suggest that, unless cisplatin shows itself to be therapeutically more active than the other drugs, its use should not be encouraged as a topical agent for protracted use. The efficacy results of study 30782 are therefore awaited with the greatest interest.

Trial 30790

This trial, which is running parallel to the previous one, presents the following features: a different geographical distribution (mainly from the Netherlands and Germany); entry permitted not only to recurrent but also to primary patients; randomization into three groups, one of which involves a control group receiving no treatment. The two other groups receive instillations of either doxorubicin 50 mg, or etoglucide

(Epodyl), 1.3 g in 100 ml. The control group has been recently dropped out, after the first analysis of the preliminary results. In study 30790 the only complaint was chemical cystitis which occurred in 4% of patients in both treatment groups (doxorubicin or etoglucide).

Some preliminary results are available for study 30790, since an interim analysis showed that lack of treatment was significantly worse than treatment with either doxorubicin or etoglucide, with a p value less than 0.001. No significant difference between the two drugs was apparent but the difference between recurrence rate in treated patients (2.91) and those not receiving treatment after TUR (9.17) was so great that the study Coordinator, Dr. Kurth, in agreement with the Data Center, decided to stop the randomization of patients in the no-treatment arm.

Comments

The EORTC studies have shown that various drugs, such as thiotepa, doxorubicin and etoglucide, can effectively reduce recurrence rate. Teniposide (VM-26) and cisplatin appear to be less active or more toxic. Not all treated patients, however, respond to this form of treatment and there are local and systemic side-effects that vary according to the drug employed. The need for a local chemotherapy appears at least in conditions in which a high risk of multiple recurrence can be anticipated and in this context it was found, using multivariate statistical techniques, that the number of tumors at presentation was the most important factor, followed, in order of importance, by the recurrence rate at entry and the size of the primary tumor.

It can be concluded, that any further trial designed to improve the tolerance and the efficacy of intravesical chemotherapy should take into consideration not only a comparison of different drugs, but also the choice of various modalities of treatment.

SUMMARY

Systemic chemotherapy of inoperable or metastatic bladder cancer can produce palliation and transient regression in some patients but does not lead to a really permanent cure. Adjuvant chemotherapy after radical surgery or irradiation is still experimental and cannot be recommended in general practice.

Local chemotherapy is more rewarding, as complete disappearance of diffuse superficial papillary bladder tumors can be obtained by different drugs in a variable number of patients.

Topical chemotherapy has also been widely adopted as a prophylaxis measure to prevent recurrences after TUR of superficial urotheliomas. The preliminary results of the randomized trials conducted by the EORTC urological group are of special interest in this regard.

REFERENCES

1. Burt, F. B., Pavone-Macaluso, M., Horns, J. W., and Kaufman, J. J. Heterotransplantation of bladder cancer in the hamster cheek pouch: *in vivo* testing of cancer chemotherapeutic agents. *J. Urol. 95:*51, 1966.

2. Pavone-Macaluso, M. Chemotherapeutic agents in the treatment of bladder tumors. In *Verhandlungsberichte der deutschen Gesellschaft für Urologie*, p. 186. Springer Verlag, Heidelberg, 1969.

3. Pavone-Macaluso, M. Il gruppo cooperativo urologico dell'EORTC. Struttura, scopi, ricerche, risultati. In *The Tumors of Genito-Urinary Apparatus*. p. 19, edited by M. Pavone-Macaluso. COFESE, Palermo, 1976.

4. Smith, P. H. Chemotherapy of bladder cancer. In *The Tumors of Genito-Urinary Apparatus*, p. 24, edited by M. Pavone-Macaluso. COFESE, Palermo, 1976.

5. Jacobi, G. H. Chemotherapy for urinary bladder cancer: developments, trends and future perspectives. In *Clinical Bladder Cancer*, p. 93, edited by L. Denis, P. H. Smith and M. Pavone-Macaluso. Plenum Press, New York, 1982.

6. Schulman, C. C. Intravesical chemotherapy for superficial bladder tumors. In *Clinical Bladder Cancer*, p. 101, edited by L. Denis, P. H. Smith, and M. Pavone-Macaluso. Plenum Press, New York, 1982.

7. Pavone-Macaluso, M., and Ingargiola, G. B. Local chemotherapy in bladder cancer treatment. *Oncology 37:*71, 1980.

8. Pavone-Macaluso, M., Smith, P. H., and Edsmyr, E. *Bladder Tumors and other Topics in Urological Oncology*. Plenum Press, New York, 1980.

9. Hallwachs O., and Altwein, J. E. (eds) *Intravesikale Chemotherapie und transurethrale Verfahren zur Behandlung und Rezidivprophylaxe*. Steinkopff Verlag, Darmstadt, 1982.

10. Yagoda, A. Progress in the chemotherapeutic treatment of advanced bladder cancer. In *Clinical Bladder Cancer*, p. 113, edited by L. Denis, P. H. Smith, and M. Pavone-Macaluso. Plenum Press, New York, 1982.

11. Carter, S. K., and Wasserman, T. H. The chemotherapy of urologic cancer. *Cancer 36:*729, 1975.

12. Pavone-Macaluso, M., and EORTC genito-urinary tract cooperative group A V. Single drug chemotherapy of bladder cancer with adriamycin, VM-26 or bleomycin. *Eur. Urol. 2:*138, 1976.

13. EORTC urological group B. The treatment of advanced carcinoma of the bladder with a combination of adriamycin and 5-fluorouracil. *Eur. Urol. 3:*276, 1977.

14. Fox, M. The effect of cyclophosphamide on some urinary tract tumor. *Br. J. Urol. 37:*399, 1965.

15. Hall, R. R., Bloom, H. J. G., Freeman, J. E., Nawrocki, A., and Wallace, D. M. Methotrexate treatment of advanced bladder cancer. *Br. J. Urol. 46:*431, 1974.

16. Yagoda, A. Future implications of phase 2 chemotherapy trials in ninety-five patients with measurable advanced bladder cancer. *Cancer Res. 37:*2775, 1977.

17. Sternberg, J. J., Bracken, R. B., Handel, P. B., and Johnson, D. E. Combination chemotherapy (CISCA) for advanced urinary tract carcinoma; a preliminary report. *JAMA 238:*2282, 1977.

18. Mulder, J. H., Fossa, S. D., De Pauw, M., and Van Oosterom, A. T. Cyclophosphamide, adriamycin and cisplatin combination chemotherapy in advanced bladder carcinoma: an EORTC phase II study. *Eur. J. Cancer Clin. Oncol. 18:*111, 1982.

19. Stoter, G., Van Oosterom, A. T., Mulder, J. H., De Pauw, M., and Fossa, S. D. Combination chemotherapy with cisplatin and VM-26 in advanced transitional cell carcinoma of the bladder. *Eur. J. Cancer Clin. Oncol.* 1984, (In press).

20. Richards, B., Newling, D., Fossa, F., Bastable, J. R. G., Denis, L., Jones, W. B., De Pauw, M., and members of the EORTC genito-urinary tract cancer cooperative group. Vincristine in advanced bladder cancer: a European Organization for Research on Treatment of Cancer (EORTC) phase II study. *Cancer Treat. Rep. 67:*575, 1983.

21. Williams, G. Methotrexate adjuvant study in carcinoma of the bladder: an interim report. *Proceedings of the 13th International Congress of Chemotherapy*, p. 118. Vienna, 1983.

22. Richards B. Adjuvant chemotherapy following primary irradiation in T_3 bladder cancer. In *Bladder Tumors and Other Topics in Urological Oncology*, p. 395, edited by M. Pavone-Macaluso, P. H. Smith, and F. Edsmyr. Plenum Press, New York, 1980.

23. Soloway, M. S., Ikard, M., Scheinberg, M., and Evans, J. Concurrent radiation and cisplatin in the treatment of advanced bladder cancer: preliminary report. *J. Urol. 128:*1031, 1982.

CHEMOTHERAPY OF BLADDER CANCER 201

24. Schulman, C. C., Robinson, M., Denis, L., Viggiano, G., De Pauw, M., Dalesio, O., Sylvester, R., and members of the EORTC genito-urinary tract cancer cooperative group. Prophylactic chemotherapy of superficial transitional cell bladder carcinoma: an EORTC randomized trial comparing thiotepa, an epipodophyllotoxin (VM-26) and TUR alone. *Eur. Urol. 8:*207, 1982.
25. Dalesio, O., Schulman, C.C., Sylvester, R., De Pauw, M., Robinson, M., Denis, L., Smith, P. H., Viggiano, C., and members of the EORTC genito-urinary cancer cooperative group. Prognostic factors in superficial bladder tumors: a study of the EORTC genito-urinary tract cooperative group. *J. Urol. 129:*730, 1983.
26. Denis, L. Anaphylactic reaction to repeated intravesical instillation with cisplatin. *Lancet 1:*1378, 1983.
27. Kurth, K. H., Schulman, C., Pavone-Macaluso, M., Robinson M., De Pauw, M. Sylvester, R., and members of the EORTC protocols for superficial bladder cancer. *Proceedings of the 13th International Congress of Chemotherapy,* Part 240, p. 12. Vienna, 1983.

15

Bilharzial Bladder and Carcinoma

Anwer Halim, Ph.D., F.R.C.S.
I. Hussain, M.B., F.R.C.S.

Urinary schistosomiasis is perhaps the most widely written about, and yet the least understood of diseases. It remains as serious an affliction today as it was some 50 years ago, and there is evidence that it is spreading still further afield.

The effects in man, of the worm *Schistosoma haematobium*, are as fascinating to study, as they are dreadful to witness. There is now a vast body of literature on all facets of these effects, and it continues to excite the interest of a widening array of scientific enthusiasts that include not only clinicians and pathologists but epidemiologists, immunologists, malacologists and ecologists.

In the past, we have perhaps suffered because of too insular an approach to the study of the disease—there was the disease in Egypt, that in the Mozambique, in East and South Africa, in Iraq, and in South Arabia. With the great mobility of populations today, bilharzia has become a worldwide problem, reflected perfectly by our personal experience of the disease, gained entirely in a nonendemic area.

EPIDEMIOLOGICAL IMPACT OF BILHARZIAL BLADDER CANCER

Geographical Distribution of Urinary Schistosomiasis

Schistosomiasis is one of the major health problems, affecting more than 200 million people.[1] In areas irrigated by the Nile and in regions watered by the Tigris and Euphrates, infection with *S. haematobium* is intense. It is in such areas that high prevalence of bladder cancer has been established.[2] Cancer in the bladder has been known to afflict man from ancient times, and there are records of the disease in inscriptions from the Mesopotamian Valley, Babylonia, the Pharaonic tombs, and in a papyrus dated circa 1600 B.C.[3]

Relationship to Mortality in Endemic Areas

The impact of the disease in areas of high endemicity is reflected by the study of 190 consecutive autopsies, by Smith and his associates,[4] performed at the Cairo University Hospitals, over a 4-month period (Table 15.1).

Urinary schistosomiasis was recorded in 61% of these autopsy cases, and was the direct, or indirect, cause of death in 17.2% of all 116 cases.

In those with severe schistosomiasis, the disease resulted in, or contributed to, death in 42.7% of cases.

Incidence of Bladder Cancer in Bilharzial Populations

The fact that the chronic bilharzial bladder is more frequently predisposed to the development of carcinoma is now established.

A causal relationship was first suggested by Fergusson[5] in 1911, and a look at the figures in Table 15.2 showing the incidence of bladder cancer in the 1950s is fairly suggestive of such an association. Makar[6] reported a rather high incidence of bladder cancer in Egypt. In a more recent study of cases seen at the Cairo Cancer Institute, El-Sebai et al.[7] recorded an incidence of 27.6% of all malignancies. It is certainly the commonest solid tumor occurring in adult males in Egypt.

The frequency with which malignant change occurs in a bilharzial bladder seems to vary from one endemic area to another, and appears to be influenced by a number of factors, all of which are not yet entirely defined. However, the clinical and laboratory data supports Hicks'[2] hypothesis that cancer is initiated by exposure to an environmental or locally produced chemical carcinogen being excreted in the urine, which reacts with the mucosal surface of the bladder to produce an irreversible and potentially carcinogenic change in the DNA of one or two of the urothelial cells (see Chapter 35).

RACIAL DIFFERENCES

Chapman[8] reported the frequency with which bladder cancer was seen in three racial groups in Durban, over a 5-year period (Fig. 15.1.).

Table 15.1
Relationship of Urinary Schistosomiasis to Mortality[a]

No schistosomiasis found	74 cases
Schistosomiasis detected	116 cases
10.4%	Direct or underlying cause of death
6.8%	Contributed to death
23.3%	Concomitant severe schistosomiasis
59.5%	Incidental schistosomiasis

[a] 190 consecutive autopsies in Cairo University by Smith *et al.* 1974.[4]

Table 15.2
Incidence of Bladder Cancer in 1950s

London (Harnet, 1942)	3% of all fatal cancer
Egypt (Makar, 1955)	40% of all malignancies

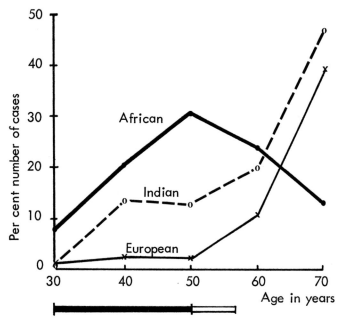

Figure 15.1. Racial differences in age distribution of bladder cancer in Durban, South Africa. (Reproduced by permission from Bhagwandeen, 1964 (quoted in Ref. 8).

Although the figure shows all bladder cancers, over 80% occurred in proven bilharzial bladders, an experience which is very similar to that in Egypt, and in other highly endemic areas such as Mozambique. The age incidence of the larger group of African patients was again similar to that reported in Egypt—the peak is in the 4th and 5th decades, and 70% of those with bilharzia were under the age of 50.

The surprising feature is that although there are many more Indians reporting with urinary bilharziasis in Durban, these were 4 times as many Africans who developed carcinoma in their bilharzial bladders. There are two possible explanations for this: (1) Either the Africans made light of their symptoms whenever infected and did not report for treatment, as all the Indians did; or (2) The African patient with bilharzia is more susceptible to the development of bladder cancer.

Three-quarters of the Indians with cancer in a bilharzial bladder were below the age of 40. The age-relatd frequency of cancer in Europeans was very similar to that in the United Kingdom.

PATHOGENETIC MECHANISMS

Life cycle of *Schistosoma haematobium*

The life cycle of *Schistosoma haematobium* has been described in many textbooks including the one published by one of the authors.[9] Suffice to say that the adult worm resides in the systemic veins of the pelvis, especially those of the urinary bladder. The female worm deposits its eggs in a bead-like row, often deep into the wall of the bladder. The eggs in the tissue of the bladder undergo development and a fully developed miracidium is formed in about 1 week. The urine containing the eggs is then shed in fresh water and the miracidia, after its release, penetrates the susceptible species of *Bulinus* snail. There is asexual reproduction in the snail and the cercariae penetrate human or animal skin, and subsequently proliferate and mature in the portal system of the infected host.

Changes Related to Tissue Egg Burden

In the study described earlier, Smith[4] attempted to correlate tissue egg burdens of *S. haematobium* with the severity of change in various regions of the urinary tract (Fig. 15.2.). The figures represent the mean number of eggs obtained after mincing and digesting tissue with potassium hydroxide, at various levels in the genitourinary tract. The bladder, lower ureters, and seminal vesicles, showed high tissue egg burdens, while the kidneys showed the least. (Inexplicably, the right lower ureter appeared more heavily burdened than the left.).

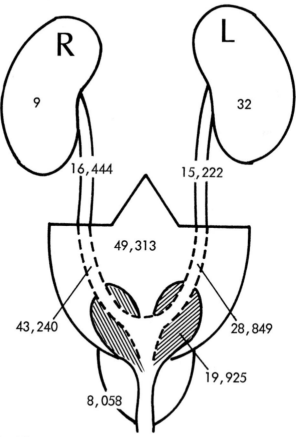

Figure 15.2. Tissue egg burden of *Schistosoma haematobium* in genitourinary organs. (Reproduced by permission from J. H. Smith *et al. American Journal of Tropical Medicine and Hygiene 23:*1053, 1974.)

There is a strong correlation between bladder egg burden and the histological severity of disease. Urothelial hyperplasia, metaplasia and dysplasia, are all associated with severe schistosomal infection. Metaplasia and dysplasia is especially marked in those cases that show evidence of superimposed bacterial infection of the lower tract.

Sites of Egg Concentration Related to Malignant Change

In the bladder, the coupled worms migrate as close to the submucosa as they can, and the eggs are discharged into the lamina propria, where they excite a severe granulomatous reaction. Eventually, there is erosion of the urothelial lining and the eggs are released into the urine. The severity of the granulomatous reaction will also depend upon the immunological response of the host to the lytic antigenic secretion of the eggs. There may be severe local tissue necrosis, characterized by infiltration with eosinophils—the Hoeppli phenomenon.

Not uncommonly, the local tissue response is severe enough to incite a hyperplastic response, so that the change known as polypoidal cystitis emerges. Nodules may grow into pedunculated growths, the site of preference being the bladder trigone, and usually the paraureteric regions.

The natural history of these early proliferative lesions may be somewhat gauged by series of clinical observations, performed in infected and treated patients, at various ages.

An interesting feature arising from this study[10] was that, in the bladder, schistosomal ova appear to concentrate in the submusoca, close to the epithelial lining, and there is a sparse scattering in the deeper muscle and perivesical tissues (Fig. 15.3). In the ureter, however, the concentration of ova is very largely in the outer muscle layer, and in the periureteric tissues. This is an important finding and may readily, and

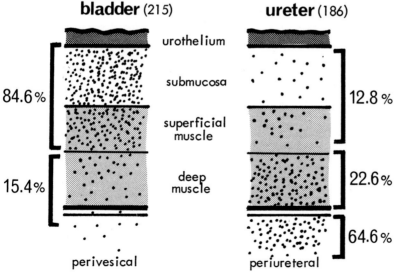

Figure 15.3. Sites of concentration of deposited bilharzial ova in bladder and ureter. (Reproduced by permision from M. M. Zahran *et al. Urology* 8:73–79, 1976.)

very simply, explain why it is that bilharzial change in the bladder manifests as serious epithelial lesions, with metaplasia and carcinoma—while, in the ureter, the change is mural and fibrotic, and affects mainly its functional capacity in the onward transport of urine. Carcinoma is known to be exceedingly rare in the bilharzial ureter.

PATHOLOGICAL FEATURES

Gross Pathological Features in the Bladder

A look at the complete spectrum of bilharzial lesions that present in the bladder shows that we have already discussed those active, or early, lesions that may present as tumors—namely, tubercles, and polypoid lesions (Table 15.3).

The fibrocalcific polyp is usually seen in the older, adult patient (and in bilharzia, this implies, over the age of 20). These are single, pedunculated, and the overlying musoca is yellowish and granular, suggesting old, inactive infection. Biopsy reveals an underlying healed granuloma, and there is usually calcification.

The "sandy patch" is so well-known—even to the most inexperienced endoscopist—and so difficult to capture on photography, as the granular appearance is made typical by light reflection.

Bilharzial ulcers may be seen in the active stage of infection, appearing as erosions, or they may be chronic and indurated, and may even show malignant change.

Other late proliferative lesions may be associated with urothelial metaplasia or dysplasia, and we will look at these in a little more detail, before going on to carcinoma.

Rounded downgrowths of hyperplastic urothelium may form nests of cells, first described by von Brunn, or they may become excavated, so as to appear as cystic spaces, in the change known as cystitis cystica.

The Spectrum of Histopathological Change

In a recent histopathological study of bilharzial tissue specimens obtained at surgery, Zahran and his associates[10] at Cairo University recorded the relative frequency of the urothelial changes in the bladder and ureter (Table 15.4).

Cystic changes were the most frequently encountered, and the ureter was almost as equally affected as the bladder. Involutionary epithelial

Table 15.3
Bladder Lesions in Bilharziasis

Pseudo tubercle	
Bilharzial polyp	Active granulomatous papillomatous or villous fibrocalcific
"Sandy patch"	
Ulcer	Active or chronic
Cystitis cystica or glandularis	
Squamous metaplasia or leukoplakia	
Carcinoma	

Table 15.4
Histopathologic Changes in Ureteral and Bladder Specimens Obtained at Endoscopy or Surgery[a]

Condition	Bladder (215 specimens)	Ureter (186 specimens)
	%	%
Cystica change	63.25	51.6
von Brunn nests	53.4	13.9
Glandularis change	48.8	6.45
Squamous metaplasia	15.3	0

[a] M. M. Zahran et al, 1976

hyperplasia, with the formation of von Brunn' nests in the lamina propria, is more frequent in the bladder—as also is glandular configuration. Squamous metaplasia appears to occur almost exclusively in the bladder, and is rarely seen in the ureter.

It would appear, therefore, that this epithelial hyperplastic response to bilharzial infection becomes less prominent with increasing age, and that this is not too significantly related to the occurrence or frequency of reinfestation.

It is possible that the fibrosis following the primary infection makes it somewhat difficult for subsequently infesting worms, and their ova, to gain superficial access to the bladder urothelium, thereby exciting the more severe tissue response in successively deeper layers. It is precisely such circumstances that is thought to induce the worms into migrating, through shunting venous channels, to the ureters—so as to satisfy the biological need to discharge ova as freely as possible.

A more likely explanation, however, is that there is the development of an increasing immunological host resistance, modifying tissue response following the primary infection, at successive reinfestation.

The major pathogenic agent is the egg containing the living miracidium. However, both the adult worm and the egg have been shown to secrete antigenic material that invoke a relatively specific sensitization, and experiments in animals have demonstrated a cell-mediated type of immunological response.

A dramatic increase in both total IgE and of specific IgE antibody, has also been shown to occur in human infections with *S. haematobium.*

It has, indeed, been suggested that the severe changes seen in some bilharzially infected patients, may be more closely related to some defect in cell-mediated immunity, rather than to intensity of the primary infection, or to other factors, such as bacterial infection and repeated reinfestation.

FREQUENCY OF CHANGES IN THE BLADDER AND URETER

A comprehensive study of 200 Egyptian men and boys with bilharzia, by Lehman and his associates,[11] has been reported. The majority of these patients (82.5%) were excreting live bilharzia ova and therefore had active disease. However, an uncertain proportion of this active disease was undoubtedly superimposed upon previous bilharzial changes, as reinfestation is a feature, especially common in Egyptian patients.

A notable finding is that the filling defects seen on urography, both in the bladder and ureter, tends to decrease with age. Around 42% have proliferative bladder changes before the age of 14, while only 6.7% show the same changes after the age of 20.

Lehman also noted "striking improvement" of these filling defects in serial urography in some patients, performed as early as 7 days after the completion of antischistosomal treatment.

Other investigators[12, 13] have reported similar findings, and it appears that the polypoidal cystitis, associated with active and early bilharzial infection, is benign, and often shows complete resolution, providing treatment is adequate. Resolution of these early proliferative changes is accompanied by breakdown of the bladder urothelial lining, the shedding of ova and, subsequently, healing by fibrosis, and a steady increase towards calcification.

METAPLASTIC CHANGES AND THEIR SIGNIFICANCE

Cystic changes, as earlier noted, occurs with almost equal frequency, in the ureter and the bladder, and there is little doubt that it is a benign lesion. Some observers have suggested that it may have premalignant significance, on account of its frequent co-existence in the malignant bilharzial bladder, but this must be incidental. Cystitis cystica is known to occur in other types of benign and chronically inflamed bladders.

Occasionally, the epithelial cells of the down-growing cysts show columnar metaplasia, appearing as glandular structures, very similar to those seen in the large bowel, and may even secrete mucus (Fig. 15.4). Although this change is also seen, rarely, with long-standing bacterial infections, cystitis glandularis has a natural history that is believed to lead to the subsequent development of adenocarcinoma.

Squamous metaplasia is associated with all forms of chronic cystitis, and is frequently seen in the chronically infected bilharzial bladder, and in those showing malignant change (Fig. 15.4). There is also believed to be an association with vitamin A deficiency, and this may be a predisposing factor in some poorly developed endemic communities.

Khafagy and his associates[14] noted that a little over half of these lesions are nonkeratinizing, the rest either showing surface keratosis or basal cell atypia.

When surface hyperkeratosis is excessive, the thickened epithelial patch becomes identifiable at cystoscopy as thick, whitish plaques in the condition recognized as leukoplakia. There is also, invariably, some degree of basal cell hyperplasia. In bilharzia, leukoplakia, which is without doubt a premalignant lesion, must be differentiated from calcific plaques in the bladder mucosa, and this is only possible by biopsy.

CARCINOMA IN THE BILHARZIAL BLADDER

The clinicopathological behavior of cancer occurring in a bilharzial bladder has been succinctly outlined by Ghoneim.[15]

The average age of incidence in males is 46.7 years and 46.3 in the female, with a male-to-female ratio of 4:1 (El Bolkainy, et al.)[16]

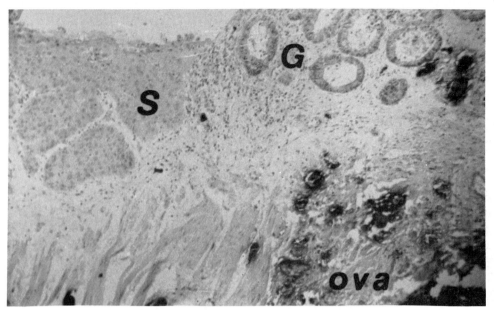

Figure 15.4. Microphotograph showing squamous (S) and glandular (G) metaplastic changes in the same bilharzial bladder lesion. Clusters of dead *S. haematobium* ova are evident in the deeper layers of the bladder wall muscle.

The main presenting symptom is cystitis accompanied with painful micturition. Hematuria, although common in the bilharzial bladder, may alter with malignant changes. In the above mentioned study,[16] 25% of cases seen were inoperable. This confirmed the findings of other investigators that these tumors present in an advanced stage. The main reason for this is overlapping of symptoms of simple bilharzial cystitis with malignant changes. The tumor is generally of the nodular, fungating type and occupies the fundus, posterior or lateral walls of the bladder. The trigone seems rarely involved. It may grow to a large size, may be necrotic in places, and there is usually a good deal of fibrosis and phosphatic encrustation.

In spite of their bulk, and the fact that they present late, it is fortunate that the incidence of regional node involvement is relatively low—varying from 15–17% in most surgical series. Autopsy series record the frequency of distant metastases to be less than 4%.

Numerous factors must play a role in suppressing the invasiveness of these tumors. These include the extensive preexisting bilharzial fibrosis that limits local spread, and the heightened immunological response in the host that is generated by the presence of the parasite and its eggs.

CLINICAL FEATURES AND EVALUATION

Clinical Presentation

The finding that males are more frequently disposed, not only to the development of bladder carcinoma, but also to bilharzial infection itself, has intrigued us all (Table 15.5).

Women are undoubtedly as frequently exposed to infestation, from

Table 15.5
Clinical Features of Carcinoma Occurring in a Bilharzial Bladder

Predominantly males	4:1 ratio
Mean patient age 46.5 years	30–50 age range
Symptoms of frequency, dysuria and haematuria	

childhood, as are men—and yet they appear to show a greater immunity towards the development of the more serious complications. Various workers have shown, experimentally, that progesterone and stilbestrol can suppress the sexual drive of the mating worms and, indeed, Wallace[17] found that a week of treatment with stilbestrol reduced egg load in the urine of two young, unmarried males with active bilharzial infection. This relationship of endogenous host hormones, with the reproducing worm, has not yet been fully investigated and may have a future practical application.

The average patient age incidence is at least 10–20 years younger than that in cancer occurring in nonbilharzial bladders.

The symptoms are really nonspecific, if they are seen in context with those occurring in a bilharzial population at large. Hematuria, in a bilharzial patient, does not bear the significance that it does, to patient and clinician alike, in nonendemic areas. Moreover, bleeding is almost always associated with painful micturition and symptoms of cystitis.

In effect, the patient only seeks help if the rather familiar bleeding becomes unduly troublesome, and the clinician, faced with the logistic difficulty of treating a large volume of patients, tends to consider cystoscopy in a few selected cases.

Certainly, all this would explain the finding, by El Bolkainy, *et al.*[16] that most bilharzial bladder cancers present in an advanced stage, and 25% may be considered inoperable at first presentation.

Diagnosis

Urine cytology is proving to be a useful tool in the early detection of such tumors. El Bolkainy, *et al.*[18] found seven carcinomas, when screening some 3000 subjects in the Mansoura region of Egypt. Four of these were early P_1 tumors and would certainly not have been picked up clinically until quite later.

A further development may arise in the screening of patients at risk of developing cancer in bilharzial bladders by the detection of nitrosamine carcinogens excreted in their urine. From animal experimental studies, Mariam Hicks[2] has postulated that nitrosamine compounds act as an initiating, predisposing factor for bladder cancer, which may then develop, years later, as a result of promotion by *S. haematobium*. These *N*-nitroso compounds are the products of the breakdown of ingested nitrates, to nitrites, by the action of bacteria infecting such tracts. Sources of dietary nitrates may be from drinking water supplies, or vegetables, particularly in those areas where agriculture is heavily dependent on the use of synthetic fertilizers. There is a current investigation into these urinary carcinogens in patients in the Qualieb area of Egypt by Hicks and her associates, and the results are awaited with interest (see Chapter 3).

Radiological Features

Calcification of the bladder is a feature in some 50% of patients with bilharzia and, when present, it usually shows a fairly contiguous line (Fig. 15.5A). It has been noted that such calcification appears to diminish with advancing age. The bilharzial calcification mentioned earlier may be disrupted, suggesting the presence of a tumor (Fig. 15.5B).

In certain endemic regions, calcification may rarely be a feature of bilharzial infection, and we have noted this in our patients from Oman. In spite of the apparent low intensity of infection in such regions, we have had at least three patients from Oman with carcinoma in bilharzial bladder. Almost all our Egyptian patients, however, seem to show calcification in some measure. The tumors are usually solid looking and broad based, and there is generally concomitant chronic bilharzial change in the upper tracts.

Intravenous urography and cystography are essential to the diagnosis of the bilharzial bladder carcinoma. The bladder may be contracted due to severe and prolonged infection. Cystography sometimes reveals filling defects of proliferative bladder lesion but are by no means diagnostic of malignancy (Fig. 15.6). Computerized tomographic scans are now being used by us to show the extent of the growth and its operability. Critical evaluation of the bladder lesion, however, requires endoscopic examination.

Cystoscopy and EUA

Endoscopy will confirm the presence of tumor and there is usually evidence of other bilharzial changes—the waxy, yellow, granular mucosa, sandy patches, and nodules.

The early submucosal lesion is manifested clinically as a hemorrhagic cystitis and, on endoscopy, the very typical bilharzial pseudotubercles are seen as seedlike, yellowish specks, surrounded by an area of inflammation. Larger, coalesced lesions are sometimes called bilharzial nodules.

Polyps may be encountered as single growths, adjacent to a ureteral orifice, usually red, and surrounded by angry mucosa, studded with bilharzial tubercles. Occasionally these may be multiple or clustered. Such granulomatous polyps are always benign and are the most frequent bilharzial growths seen in children and young adults. At times, these active growths may be seen to be fairly large, and villous or raspberry-like, so that they may be indistinguishable from vesical papillomata seen in the nonbilharzial bladder. Biopsy of these lesions, however, will always reveal the characteristic bilharzial granuloma at the base. Again, a rather characteristic feature is their invariable proximity to the ureteral orifices.

Although it is useful to stage these tumors, with the standard clinical method of bimanual pelvic palpation under anesthesia, assessment must take into account any existing perivesical fibrosis from the chronic bilharzial infection.

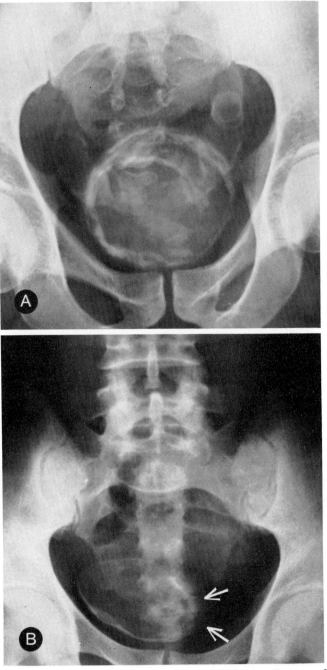

Figure 15.5. *A*, benign calcification in a bilharzial bladder. Detrusor function is often surprisingly well preserved, and the lines of calcification are relatively uninterrupted. *B*, erosion of calcification in the left wall of a bilharzial bladder, due to the development of malignancy.

Biopsy and Tumor Staging

There appears to be a tendency towards understaging the extent of the disease and, in a series of 135 radical cystectomies, Ghoneim[15] recorded a clinical error in staging of 37.2%. Over half the tumors in

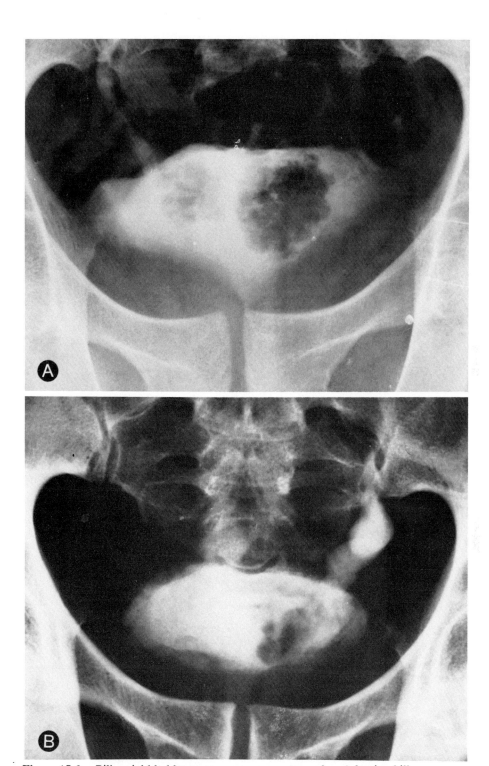

Figure 15.6. Bilharzial bladder tumors seen on cystography. *A*, benign bilharzial polypi appearing as "grapelike" clusters in each paraureteric region. The left upper tract is obstructed. These lesions successfully respond to endoscopic resection and chemotherapeutic treatment. *B*, carcinoma in a bilharzial bladder.

his series showed infiltration into deeper muscles, and 12.8% showed extravesical spread.

The histological features in around two-thirds of these tumors is that of squamous cell carcinoma, the majority being well differentiated and showing low malignancy (Fig. 15.7).

Most observers have recorded the occurrence of multicentric lesions in many of these tumors. Khafagy, et al.[14] in 1972 showed squamous metaplasia in 65%. Even in those few cases where the tumor appears predominantly of transitional-celled type, there may be areas of squamous cell metaplasia, or glandular change.

Tumors may show extensive squamous and glandular metaplasia, with huge nodular masses of calcified ova, and a relatively small area of carcinoma of transitional cell type. The pattern may be confusing, but the overall picture is one of low grade malignancy.

Carcinoma *in situ* is often associated with bilharzia. The bladder is generally noted to be inflamed, red, and bleeds easily with overdistension. There may also be areas of ulceration. Although the incidence of this change is not yet known, biopsy is essential for diagnosis.

MANAGEMENT

Endoscopic Resection

This method is limited to obtaining biopsy material for histopathological diagnosis and staging of the tumor. The generally advanced stage and the large bulk of the bilharzial bladder tumor makes it difficult to resect it urethrally. To date there are no reports in the literature about this procedure.

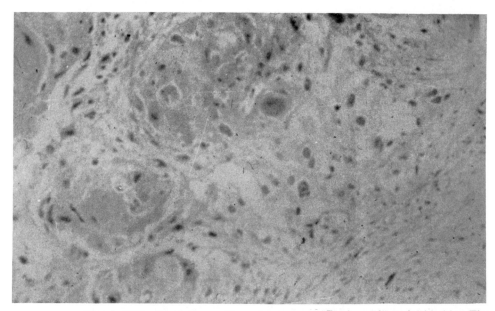

Figure 15.7. Squamous cell carcinoma occurring in a bilharzial bladder. The microscopic appearance is typical and there is differentiation into whorls of epithelial "pearls."

Segmental Resection

The low grade malignancy of these tumors, and their reluctance to spread far, together with the fact that they seldom involve the trigonal area of the bladder, has encouraged some surgeons to attempt local resection, with or without augmentation. Undoubtedly, this is an attractive surgical choice in areas where social taboos about urinary diversion exist. However, segmental resection of the bladder should be limited to small, solitary tumors not involving the trigone. In a series reported by Ghoneim,[15] only 10% of tumors were judged suitable for this procedure, and the 5-year survival was recorded at 26.5%.

Radical Cystectomy

Radical cystectomy with urinary diversion remains the most logical surgical approach. However, care should be taken to excise the bladder along with its perivesical fat, peritoneal covering, prostate, and seminal vesicles, together with lymph nodes from common, internal and external iliac groups. In the female, the radical cystectomy includes the bladder, urethra, uterus, and upper two-thirds of the vagina, with pelvic cellular tissue and the aforementioned lymph nodes.

The postoperative mortality ranges from 10–12.5% in various series. The chief causes of mortality are peritonitis and intestinal obstruction. The present 5-year survival rate ranges from 27–33%.

Urinary Diversions in Endemic Areas: Although the ileal loop is the preferred method of urinary diversion in the young patient, it poses problems in the developing world. Socioeconomic factors and climate not only entail difficulties in the care of the stoma, but the continuous supply of sophisticated and expensive appliances is beyond the reach of common farmhands and laborers. Equally, the care of the stoma becomes more difficult due to environmental stresses. Ureterocolic anastomosis also poses technical problems due to the thick, dilated ureter with intense periureteritis. The complications of ascending infection, pyelonephritis and metabolic acidosis are severe and lead to early and progressive renal failure.

The isolated rectum as a bladder substitute was first described by Mauclarie[19] in 1895. The method was reintroduced in Egypt in 1968 by Ghoneim and Safwat.[20]

The rectal bladder with terminal colostomy has been found to be a suitable method of urinary diversion in Egypt. The procedure described by Ghoneim[15] is technically simple and hence reduces morbidity. It separates the feces from the urinary stream, thus diminishing ascending infection. Biochemical disturbances are minimal as the absorbent surface area is limited. Terminal colostomy does not require as much care as an ileal loop diversion. The patient can be taught to regularly evacuate his bowel once or twice daily. It does away with expensive ileostomy apparatus. However, the method is not completely devoid of problems. Ascending pyelonephritis is a problem but Ghoneim has been able to reduce this by the use of submucosal tunnel. Nocturnal urinary leakage has also been reported by many surgeons, this too can be controlled by moderate doses of imipramine hydrochloride (Tofranil).

Radiotherapy

The beneficial effects of preoperative radiation followed by cystectomy have already been established with nonbilharzial cancers and significant improvement in survival rates have been demonstrated. Radiation inactivates smaller cell burden in the deeply infiltrating parts of the tumor, as well as microextensions into the perivesical cellular tissue or lymphatics. Such foci are expected to show a better response relative to the main tumor since they are better oxygenated and, although fewer, have a high cell birth rate.[21] A number of clinical trials are under way in Egypt using different combinations. Some of these trials are showing marginally better results in terms of disease-free survival, others in morbidity or mortality. The one conclusion that most authors have agreed on is that surgery alone, despite being radical, is inadequate to deal with the extent of the "local" pathology. Adjuvant radiotherapy directed to the pelvis improves the results of treatment, but external beam therapy, alone, for definitive control of bilharzial bladder tumors is disappointing. Not only does the coexisting bilharzial lesion interfere with local tissue tolerance, but the substantial population of hypoxic tumor cells increase radioresistance. Tissue tolerance can be improved 80% with the use of split course of radiotherapy. Awwad[21] carried out a clinical trial where a preoperative radiation (4000 rads) was given prior to cystectomy. Radiation was delivered in two dose-time schedules: conventional fractionation (200 rads/day) and hyper-fractionation (1000 rads/day, divided into 17 hourly fractions of 60 rads each). The latter regime is a stimulation of continuous low-dose irradiation and was used in an attempt at augmenting local tissue tolerance. The disease-free survival rate was reported as 53% for the irradiated group and 19% among controls. Results did not differ between the two groups. A similar trial using a lower dose of irradiation (2000 rads) delivered in five daily increments (400 rads each), through wide portals including the regional lymph nodes, is under way in Mansoura University (Egypt). The above regime has the theoretical advantage of being applicable on a large scale, since the required logistics are simple. However, the expected therapeutic value is compromised by the presence of a large proportion of hypoxic cells, the oxygenation of which could be improved with a more protracted fraction.[15]

Chemotherapy

Gad El-Mawla[22] in 1978 evaluated some of the chemotherapeutic agents at the Cancer Institute of Cairo University with unresectable T_4 lesions. With hexamethylmelamine, partial remission was reported in 10 out of 26 cases, with a median duration of 9 months. VM-26, methotrexate, bleomycin, and doxorubicin (Adriamycin) showed less favorable results. Our own results with doxorubicin have been disappointing. Trenimone and cisplatin are under trial at Cairo Cancer Institute.

PROGNOSIS WITH TREATMENT

The prognosis with radical cystectomy appears, however, to be somewhat better and, in a recent series, Ghoneim[15] and his associates have

Table 15.6
Radical Cystectomy for Bilharzial Cancer

Author	No. of Cases	5-Year Survival
		%
El-Sebai (1977)	1007	27.0
Ghoneim et al (1979)	138	32.6

recorded an overall 5-year survival of 32.6%. With adjuvant preoperative radiotherapy, the survival was reported to be increased to 53% (Table 15.6).

These results are encouraging, and indicate that they could be better, providing the tumors are diagnosed at a less advanced stage.

FUTURE PROSPECT

Research efforts are currently directed to explore the value of chemical hypoxic cell sensitizers for promotion of the radioresponsiveness of these tumors and the application of more optimized fractionation systems.

The screening of urine in rural populations at risk is currently being investigated by Mansoura University in Egypt. Contrary to beliefs, the technique is proving fairly accurate. The early detection of patients with bladder cancer will certainly improve the results of existing methods of treatment or allow for a less radical approach to the problem.

REFERENCES

1. Chatelain, C. *La Bilharziose Uro-genitale*, Masson, Paris, 1977.
2. Hicks, R. M. Urinary bilharziasis: carcinogenic implications. *Tropical Urology*, Chapt. 14. Churchill & Livingstone, London, 1984.
3. Breasted, J. H. *The Edwin Smith Surgical Papyrus*, pp. 367, 403. University of Chicago Press, Chicago, 1930.
4. Smith, J. H., Kamal, I. A., Elwi, A., von Lichtenberh, F. A quantitative postmortem analysis of urinary schistosomiasis in Egypt. I. Pathology and pathogenesis. *Am. J. Trop. Med. Hyg. 23:*1053, 1974.
5. Fergusson, A. R. Associated bilharziasis and primary malignant diseases of the urinary bladder, with observation on a series of 40 cases. *J. Pathol. Bacteriol. 16:*76–94, 1911.
6. Makar, N. *Urological Aspects of Bilharziasis in Egypt.* p. 51. S.O.P. Press, Cairo, 1955.
7. El-Sebai, I., El Bolkainy, M. N., Hussein, M. H. Cancer Institute registry. Medical Journal, Cairo University, *41:*175–181, 1973.
8. Chapman, D. The surgical importance of bilharziasis in South Africa. *Br. J. Surg. 53:*544–557, 1966.
9. Husain, I. Urinary bilharziasis. *Textbook of Tropical Urology*, Chapt. 13, edited by I. Husain. Churchill & Livingstone, London, 1984.
10. Zahran, M. M., Kamel, M., Mooro, H., Issa, A. Bilharziasis of urinary bladder and ureter. Comparative histopathological study. *Urology 8:*73–79, 1976.
11. Lehman, J. S., Jr., Farid, Z., Smith, J. H., Bassily, S., El-Masry, N. A. Urinary schistosomiasis in Egypt: clinical, radiological, bacteriological and parasitological correlations. *Trans. R. Soc. Trop. Med. Hyg. 67:*384–399, 1973.
12. Young, S. W., Farid, Z., Bassily, S., El-Masry, N. A. Urinary schistosomiasis in Egypt: further radiological correlations. *Trans. R. Soc. Trop. Med. Hyg. 67:*417, 1973.
13. Forsyth, D. M., MacDonald, G. Urological complications of endemic schistosomiasis in school children. *Trans. R. Soc. Trop. Med. Hyg. 59:*171, 1965.

14. Khafagy, M. M., El-Bolkainy, M. N., Mansour, M. A. Carcinoma of the bilharzial urinary bladder: a study of the associated lesions in 86 cases. *Cancer 30:*150–159, 1972.
15. Ghoneim, M. A. Urinary bilharziasis. *Textbook of Tropical Urology*, Chapt. 16, edited by I. Husain. Churchill & Livingstone, London, 1984
16. El-Bolkainy, M. N., Ghoneim, M. A., Mansour, M. A. Carcinoma of the bilharzial bladder in Egypt: clinical and pathological features. *Br. J. Urol. 44:*561–570, 1972.
17. Wallace, D. M. Urinary schistosomiasis in Saudi Arabia. *Ann. R. Coll. Surg. 61:*265–270, 1979.
18. El-Bolkainy, M. N., Ghoneim, M. A., El-Morsey, B. A., Nasr, S. M. Carcinoma of bilharzial bladder: diagnostic value of urine cytology. *Urology 3:*319–323, 1974.
19. Mauclarie, P. Quoted by 1895 Cordonnia, J. J. Urinary diversion. *Arch. Surg. 71:*818–827, 1955.
20. Ghoneim, M. A., Safwat, M. Necessity and indications of urinary diversion. *J. Egypt. Med. Assoc. 51:*1053–1070, 1968.
21. Awwad, H., Abdel-Baki, H., El-Bolkainy, M., Burgers, M., El-Badawy, S., et al. Preoperative irradiation of T_3 carcinomas in bilharzial bladder. *Int. J. Radiat. Oncol. Biol. Phys. 5:*787–794, 1979.
22. Gad El-Mawla, N., Muggia, E., Hamza, M. R., El-Marsi, B., Sherif, M., et al. 1978. Chemotherapeutic management of carcinoma of bilharzial bladder. A phase II trial with Hexamethylamine and VM-26. *Cancer Treat. Rep. 62:*993–997, 1978.
23. El Sebai, I. Bilharziasis and bladder cancer. *J Clin. 27:*100–105, 1977.
24. Ghoneim M. A., Ashamallah, A. G. Hammady, S., Gaballah M. A., Soliman H. S. Cystectomy for carcinoma of the bilharzial bladder: 138 cases 5 years later. *Br. J. Urol 51:*541–544, 1979.

16

Experimental and Clinical Investigations in Bladder Cancer

Nasser Javadpour, M.D., F.A.C.S.

The ultimate objectives of laboratory and clinical studies are elimination of bladder cancer and, therefore, the eradication of morbidity and mortality from this disease. During the last decade or so it has been increasingly apparent that bladder cancer is an environmental disease, related very closely to the diet, life style and a number of other factors, including exposure to carcinogens. A better understanding of the natural history, etiology, epidemiology and carcinogenesis has been achieved over the past decade. However, a number of problems still remain unsolved.

CELLULAR AND MOLECULAR MARKERS

The need for newer biologic markers for early diagnosis and monitoring bladder cancer needs no elaboration. Currently a number of tumor markers including ABO(H) blood antigens, T antigen, tumor-associated antigens and chromosome analysis are under study in a number of laboratories[5] (see Chapter 5 on tumor markers). The need for distinction between high risk and low risk superficial bladder tumors is essential in assessing, managing and determining the prognosis of these tumors in terms of recurrence, invasion, and potential for metastases. It has been reported that the value of detecting ABO(H) and T-antigen is additive.[5,9]

Also, the value of chromosome analysis and ABO(H) is complementary.[5] The clinical use of other markers such as plasminogen, hepatoglobulin, carcinoembryonic antigen and other oncofetal proteins have not been rewarding due to the lack of specificity and low frequency in bladder cancer. A number of other markers such as urinary polyamines, aminoisobutyrate, β-glucuronidase and urinary tryptophan metabolic products are under study at the present time.

LABORATORY MODELS

A number of bladder cancers have been induced in laboratory animals utilizing potent carcinogens. These carcinogens include N-(4-(5-nitro-2-furyl)-2-thiazolyl-foramide (FANFT), N-butyl-N-(4-hydroxybutyl)nitrosamine (BBN), N-methyl-N-nitrosurea (MNU), and a number of nitrosamines.

Currently, utilization of FANFT in mice, rats, hamsters, and dogs produces a reproducible, transplantable urothelial bladder tumor. This tumor appears to be analogous to the human transitional carcinoma in terms of histopathology and natural history. FANFT-fed rats initially develop hyperplasia of the bladder mucosa with progression to sessile or papillary carcinoma. This hyperplasia is reversible up to 6 weeks, but after 8 weeks the changes are irreversible and result in production of carcinoma in all rats or mice fed FANFT for 84 weeks. This tumor model has been utilized in screening of chemotherapeutic agents. A FANFT-induced tumor that is well characterized has been utilized in investigating the chemotherapy, immunology and immunotherapy of the bladder cancer.

Other carcinogens have been used in experimental animals. The mechanism of carcinogenesis appears to be multistage and require initiator and promotor (see Chapter 3, Carcinogenesis).

DIAGNOSIS AND STAGING

The role of cytology, various tumor markers, adequate biopsy and bimanual examinations are essential in the diagnosis and management of bladder cancer. Furthermore, the introduction of computed tomography has been helpful in the preoperative staging of the bladder tumor. It appears that the role of carcinoma *in situ* is important in deciding the appropriate therapy. Therefore, every attempt should be made to detect the presence of carcinoma *in situ* in pathologic specimens.

RADIATION THERAPY

The role of radiotherapy is controversial in bladder cancer. Over the past several decades radiotherapy has been utilized in conjunction with surgery in bladder cancer.[2, 12] It appears that the major role of radiotherapy, if any, is mostly in high grade and invasive tumors. There is no convincing control study to document the role of radiation therapy and critics of this modality have indicated that improvements reported after radiotherapy are simply reflecting a better patient selection and are partly because of the natural history of this disease. The proponents of radiotherapy in bladder cancer have indicated that bladder cancer cells are sensitive to radiation. Furthermore, radiotherapy before or after surgery will arrest the locally disseminated cancer cells (see Chapter 12 on radiotherapy). The role of radiosensitizers is also controversial and needs further study.

CHEMOTHERAPY

The utilization of intravesical and systemic chemotherapeutic agents has attracted the attention of a number of urologists and oncologists. It appears that intravesical instillation of thiotepa, doxorubicin (Adriamycin), mitomycin and a number of other agents has found its way in the armamentarium of contemporary urology.[7, 8, 12] A number of studies with appropriate controls have proven the efficacy of this approach in terms of decreasing recurrence of tumor. This approach has been used both as therapeutic and prophylactic measures. Systemic chemotherapy has also been reported in treatment of superficial bladder cancer.

However, the most trials have been in deep infiltrative and metastatic bladder cancer. The use of platinum, doxorubicin, cyclophosphamide and 5-fluorouracil (5FU) has been encouraging in this disease (see Chapter 14 on chemotherapy). However, the appropriate single agent or a chemotherapeutic regimen with maximal efficacy and minimal toxicity have not been recognized at the present time.

CLONOGENIC ASSAY

The direct cloning of tumor developed by Salmon and Hamburger is an *in vitro* chemosensitivity test for finding the most effective agent for a given tumor. The clonogenic assay and chemosensitivity is similar to culture and sensitivity of bacteria in certain aspects.

Method

The technique used for the growth of human cancer cells in agar is similar to that initially described by Hamburger and Salmon with certain modifications[8] (Fig. 16.1). A single cell suspension of cells is made by mechanical dissociation of the solid specimen by mincing, passing through needles and filtration through a 20-μm gauge nylon mesh. Malignant effusions were centrifuged, and the cells washed as previously described. The total number of nucleated cells is determined with a hemocytometer without any attempt to determine a differential

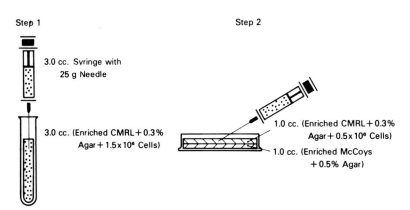

Step 1

3.0 cc. Syringe with 25 g Needle

3.0 cc. (Enriched CMRL + 0.3% Agar + 1.5 x 10⁶ Cells)

Step 2

1.0 cc. (Enriched CMRL + 0.3% Agar + 0.5 x 10⁶ Cells)
1.0 cc. (Enriched McCoys + 0.5% Agar)

Figure 16.1.   Plating of tumor cells in soft agar.

count of malignant or nonmalignant cells such as macrophages and polymorphonuclear cells.

The cells are cultured in 35-mm Petri dishes using two layers of selective media. The underlayer consists of 1.0 ml of McCoy's medium with 10% heat-inactivated fetal calf serum, various nutrients and 0.5% agar. Conditioned media may be used. The cells are resuspended in enriched CMRL media and 0.3% agar at a final concentration of 500,000 cells/plate. The cells are incubated at 37 °C in 6% carbon dioxide. The plates are examined using an inverted microscope after 7, 14, and 21 days of incubation.

For determination of drug sensitivities, the cells are incubated with chemotherapeutic agents for 1 hour at 37 °C. The cells are washed with McCoy's media and plated in triplicate as described above. The percentage survival of tumor colony-forming units is then compared to untreated controls. The current technical limitations need improvement (Table 16.1) before any meaningful clinical utilization. One can conclude that although the use of clonogenic assay and chemosensitivity remains an interesting and potentially useful technique, its routine use is premature at the present time.[11,12] Moreover, even if the current technical problems are solved, the effectiveness of this technique in any cancer, including bladder cancer, should be shown in randomized studies.[11]

CURRENT PROBLEMS AND FUTURE DIRECTIONS

Presently it appears that carcinogenesis plays an important role in carcinomas of the bladder. Therefore, the role of prevention in eradicating the environmental factors are essential. The need for developing further cell and serum markers that are clinically practical and reliable does not need any elaboration. This may identify the individual at risk. The role of more reliable techniques in diagnosis and staging is also essential. Controlled studies are needed to assess the exact role, dose and timing of radiotherapy of the bladder cancer. Intensive search for effective chemotherapeutic agents with maximal efficacy and minimal toxicity is also essential. Improvements in technique of clonogenic assay may be helpful in selecting the proper chemotherapeutic agents in this cancer. However, with the current limitations of clonogenic assay, caution should be exercised in interpretation of *in vitro* tests and

Table 16.1
Limitations and Problems with Clonogenic Assay

Low plating efficiency
Colony size
Tumor heterogeneity and lack of sufficient colonies for drug testing
Discrepancy between *in vitro* and *in vivo* sensitivity
Lack of prospective randomized clinical trials
Technical problems
    Questionable relevance of direct exposure of tumor cells *in vitro*
    Authenticity of tumor cells
    Preparation of single cell suspensions

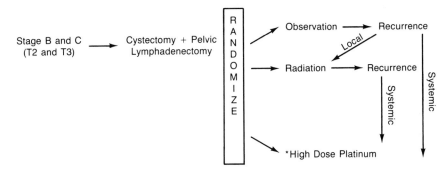

Stage B and C
(T2 and T3) → Cystectomy + Pelvic Lymphadenectomy

R A N D O M I Z E

Observation → Recurrence

Local

Radiation → Recurrence

*High Dose Platinum

Systemic

Systemic

*200 mg/m^2 in 250 ml of 3% saline.

Figure 16.2. Randomized clinical trial with surgery, radiation and high dose platinum in invasive bladder cancer.

applying it to the patient. Routine clinical and commercial utilization of this assay is premature at best.

The discovery of the bladder oncogene involving a multistep carcinogenesis is of interest and intense research should be in the future.[10, 11] The findings of glycosaminoglycans that normally protect the bladder cells from the introduction of carcinogenesis are significant. Recent studies have shown that the urinary levels of these glycosaminoglycans decrease in patients with bladder cancer as opposed to the controls.[7]

Finally we have embarked on a phase 2 and 3 in locally invasive bladder cancer with high dose platinum (Fig. 16.2).

REFERENCES

1. Brosman, S. A. Experience with BCG in patients with superficial bladder cancer. *J. Urol. 128:*27, 1982.
2. Droller, J. Controversial role of radiation therapy as adjunctive treatment of bladder cancer. *J. Urol. 129:*897, 1983.
3. Gonick, P., Kalathoor, R., and Fuscaldo, K. Chromosomal analysis as prognostic tool in transitional cell carcinoma. *Urology 16:*527, 1980.
4. Herr, H. W. Carcinoma *in situ* of the bladder. *Semin. Urol. 1:*15, 1983.
5. Javadpour, N., Roy, J., and Bottomly, Combined cell surface antigens and chromosomal studies in bladder cancer. *Urology 19:*29, 1982.
6. Pavone-Maculusa, M., and Ingagiola, G. B. Local chemotherapy in bladder cancer treatment. *Oncology 37:*71, 1980.
7. Parsons, L. C., and Dillard, J. The diminished excretion of urinary glycosaminoglycans in patients with bladder carcinoma. *Proceedings of American Urology Association*, Las Vegas, Nevada, 1983.
8. Soloway, M. S., and Murphy, W. M. Experimental chemotherapy of bladder cancer—systemic and intravesical. *Semin. Oncol. 6:*166, 1979.
9. Summers, J. L., Coon, J. S., Ward, R. M., Falor, W. H., Miller, A. W., and Weinstein, R. S. Prognosis in carcinoma of the urinary bladder based upon tissue blood group ABH and Thomsen-Friedenreich antigen status and karyotype of initial tumor. *Cancer Res. 42:*939, 1983.
10. Tabin, C. J., Bradley, Bargmann, C. L., *et al.* Mechanism of activation of a human oncogene. *Nature 300:*143, 1983.
11. Whitmore, W. F. Integrated irradiation and cystectomy for bladder cancer. *Br. J. Urol. 52:*1, 1981.
12. Weinberg, R. A. Alteration of genomes of tumor cell. *Cancer 52:*1971, 1983.
13. Yagoda, A. Advances in chemotherapy. In *Recent Advances in Urologic Cancer*, pp. 211–289, edited by N. Javadpour. Williams & Wilkins, Baltimore, 1982.

Index

Page numbers in italics denote figures; those followed by "*t*" or "*f*" denote tables or footnotes respectively.

Bleomycin, 161, 193*t*, 197*t*
Blood group(s), etiologic factor, 17
Blood group antigen(s) (*see* ABO(H) antigens)
BMH/UTCHS classification of urothelial carcinoma, 102*t*
Bone necrosis, post-radiotherapy, 175
Bracken fern(s), 20*t*, 21
7-Bromomethyl-benz(*a*)anthracene, 44
N-butyl-*N*-(4-hydroxybutyl)nitrosamine (*see* BBN)

Caffeine (*see* Coffee drinking)
Calculus(i), urinary, 40, 110, *111*
Canada, bladder cancer statistics, 8*t*, 13*t*
CAP, 192, 193*t*
Carcinoembryonic antigen, 221
Carcinogenesis
  growth patterns, histologic type and, 88
  hypothesis, 204
  multistage
    process of, 37
    rodent bladder, 43–45
    theoretical and practical importance, 46, 47
Carcinogen(s) (*see also* Promotors; specific carcinogens)
  chemical, 19, 20*t*, 37
  dosage effects, 38, *39*
  listing, 2*t*
Carcinoma *in situ*
  BCG immunotherapy, 132
  bilharzia and, 216
  clinicopathologic characteristics, 94–*96*
  cytology, 111–*113*
  evolution, *52*
  grading, 3
  growth patterns and, 88
  histopathology, 50–52
  multicentricity, 94
  natural history prediction, 80
  role in therapy determination, 222
  SCRA findings, 78*t*
  squamous cell carcinoma and, 96, 97
  transitional cell carcinoma and, 61*t*, 96
  WHO designation, 102
Case-control study(ies), defined, 6
Case-fatality, 7, 25, 26
Catheterization, urinary, 110
Cell division, promotion and, 42
Cell marker(s) (*see* Marker(s), tumor)
Cell surface antigens (*see also* ABO(H) antigens; T antigen)
  chromosomal analysis, determination with, 83
  perspective and limitations, 64, 65
  role in superficial bladder cancer prognosis, 84, 85
  stage and grade, correlation with, 63–65*t*
Cell type(s) (*see also* specific carcinomas)
  prognosis and, 163, 164
  topographical distribution and, 54*f*
Cercariae, 206
Chemical(s), carcinogenic, 19, 20*t*
Chemoradioimmunotherapy, 72, 73
Chemosensitivity determination, 224
Chemotherapy (*see also* specific therapies)
  adjuvant, 195, 196, 200
  advanced bladder cancer, 191–195*t*
  bilharzial bladder carcinoma, 218
  intra-arterial, 139–142, 196, 197*t*
  intravesical, 3
  loco-regional, 197–200*t*
  modification of radiation response, 161, 612

oral, 142
present role of, 194, 915, 223
systemic, 200
topical, 200
Chlornaphazine, 24, 38
Chromosome abnormalities
  analysis for
    correlation with stage and grade, 66–68*t*, 221
    with cell surface antigen testing, 83
  bladder cancer etiology and, 17
  superficial tumors and, 82, 144
Cigarette smoking (*see* Smoking, cigarette)
CISCA, 192, 193*t*
Cisplatin
  adjuvant therapy, 195, 196
  advanced cancer therapy, 191–195*t*
  anaphylaxis, 197*t*
  DDP radiation modification, 161, 162
  high dose clinical trial, *4, 225*
  intravesical, 142, 197*t*, 199, 200
  remission rate, 191, 192*t*
  tolerance, 196
Classification system(s)
  transitional cell tumors, 60–62*t*
  urothelial cancer, 101–130*t*
Clinical features, bladder cancer, 58, 61, 72, 136
Clonogenic assay
  limitations and problems, 224*t*
  method, *223*, 224
  role of, 4
Coffee drinking
  attributable fraction, 27*t*
  bladder cancer risk and, 23, 24, 29
  carcinogenic mechanism, 139
Cohort study(ies), defined, 6
Colon, complications following radiotherapy, 175
Computed tomography (CT)
  bilharzial bladder carcinoma, 213
  diagnosis, role in, 62, 63
  staging, value in, 72
  tumor extent and, 167
Concanavalin A-agglutinability, 45
Country(ies), incidence and mortality patterns, 7, 8*t*, 14*t*
CPE, 83
Cryotherapy, 145
Cyclamate (*see* Artificial sweetner(s))
Cyclophosphamide (Cytoxan)
  biological modifier, 161
  bladder cancer etiology and, 24
  in combination, 191–193*t*
  disseminated cancer, treatment of, 4
  multistage carcinogenesis and, 40
  papillary tumor treatment, 197*t*
  urothelium cytology, effect on, 115–*118*
Cystectomy
  bilharzial bladder carcinoma and, 217–219*t*
  cell surface antigens and, 82
  clinical trial, randomized, *4*
  indications, 148–150
  partial, 156, 157
  paramedian incision, left, 151, *152*
  patient positioning, 150, *151*
  plan of operation, 150–157
  preoperative period, 150
  radical
    compared with radiotherapy and salvage cystectomy, 186

reaction, 64
Squamous cell carcinoma
  bilharzial parasite and, 60
  cytologic distinctions, 106, *107*
  growth patterns, 87
  histologic patterns, 60, 61, *216*
  incidence, 15, *54*, 60
  prognosis, 163, 164
  relationship to carcinoma *in situ*, 96, 97
  SCRA testing, 81
Stage(ing), tumor
  bilharzial bladder carcinoma, 214, 216
  prognosis related to, 162, 163*t*
  superficial tumors, 136
  systems, comparison of, 70, 71*t*
  techniques used, 3
  transurethral ultrasonography, 62
  tumor markers and
    ABO(H) antigen loss and, 63, 77, 78*t*
    cell surface antigens and, 63, 65*t*66
    SCRA, chromosomes and, 68*t*
Stilbestrol, 212
Sublethal damage, radiotherapy, 179, 180
Superficial bladder tumor(s)
  BCG immunotherapy, 130, 132
  cystoscopic characteristics, 136, 137
  distinction between high and low risk, 221
  etiology, 138, 139
  immunological intervention, 128
  low-risk parameters, 3*t*
  natural history, 59
  prediction of invasiveness, 67–69
  prognosis, 82
  treatment, 139–146
Suprapubic pain, radiotherapy for, 173, 174
Suprapubic radium implantation, 144, 145
Surgery (*see* Cystectomy)
Survival
  radiation and, 184–186
  rates, 190

T antigen
  demonstration
    technique, 68, *69*, 79, 80
    with ABO(H) antigens, 70, 80
  loss, 144
  superficial tumor prognosis and, 82
  value of, 221
T1 lesions, radiotherapy, 168, 169*t*, 174*t*
T2 lesions, radiotherapy, 169*t*, 174*t*
T3 lesions, radiotherapy, 169–171*t*, 174*t*
T4 lesions, radiotherapy, 172, 174*t*
TAA (*see* Tumor-associated antigen)
Taxonomic Intracellular Analytic System (TICAS), 118
Teniposide (VM-26)
  in combination, 191–193*t*
  papillary tumor treatment, 197*t*, 198, 200
Testosterone, 40
12-*O*-Tetradecanoylphorbol-13-acetate (TPA), 42, 45
Thiotepa (triethylenethiophosphoramide)
  myelotoxicity, 197*t*
  papillary tumor treatment, 197–200*t*
  superficial tumor treatment, 139, 140
  urothelium cytology, effect on, 115–117
Thomsen-Friedenreich phenomenon, 79
TICAS (*see* Taxonomic Intracellular Analytic System)
TNM (Tumor, Node, Metastases) staging system, 70, 71*t*, 136

Tobacco, 19, 20*t* (*see also* Smoking, cigarette)
TPA (*see* 12-*O*-Tetradecanoylphorbol-13-acetate)
Transitional cell carcinoma(s)
  carcinoma *in situ* and, 96
  classification, 61*t*
  correlation with growth patterns, 87
  cytogenic studies, 144
  cytologic features, 102, 103, 102, 103
  cytotoxicity, 123–*125*
  endoscopic examination, 70
  etiologic factors, 139
  high grade neoplasm, 103, *104*
  histologic patterns, 60, 61
  incidence, 28, 60
  invasive, survival rate following cystectomy, 148
  low grade neoplasm, 103, *105*, 106
  multicentricity, 91*t*, 92*t*
  prognosis, 163
  radiosensitivity, 182, 183
  superficial, incidence of, 136
  T antigen and ABO(H) antigen determinations, 70
  tumor-associated antigens, 83
  WHO classification, 102*t*
Transuretheral resection (TUR)
  BCG immunotherapy, effect of, 130–*132*
  EORTC chemoprophylaxis trials, superficial tumors, 197–200*t*
  recurrence following, reduction by thiotepa, 140
Transurethral resection of bladder tumors (TURB)
  evaluations with radiotherapy treatments, 185
  prognosis, 164, 165
Triethylenethiophosphoramide (*see* Thiotepa)
Trigone
  involvement, incidence of, 50, 51, *54*
  tumor site, 137
Trihalomethane(s), 20, 21
Tryptophan
  carcinogenic metabolites, 18, 59, 139
    pyridoxine and, 199
    use as markers, 221
  multistage carcinogenesis, 40
Tryptophan metabolite(s), 18
Tryptophan metabolism, 59
Tumor-associated antigen(s) (TAA), demonstration of, 123-125
Tumor-specific transplantation antigens (TSTA), 123
Tween 80, potentiation of doxorubicin, 141

UICC (*see* Union Internationale Contre le Cancer)
Ulex europaeus extract, 76
Ultrasonography, 61
Umbrella cell(s), 106, *110*
Undifferented cell carcinoma(s), 61, 88
Union Internationale Contre le Cancer (UICC) system, 70, 71*t*
Uremia, post-radiotherapy, 174, 175
Ureter, bilharzial changes, 207*210*
Urethra
  reflux, 92, 97
  transection, *156*
Urinary diversion, 217
Urinary tract infection(s), 18
Urinary tract tumor(s), multicentricity, 88–*90*
Urine screening (*see* Cytology, urinary)
Urine specimen(s), for cytology, 100, 101
Urothelial cancer(s) (*see also* Adenocarcinoma(s))
  carcinoma in situ, *50–52*
  cytologic classification, 101, 102*t*